God Image Handbook
for Spiritual Counseling
and Psychotherapy:
Research, Theory, and Practice

God Image Handbook for Spiritual Counseling and Psychotherapy: Research, Theory, and Practice has been co-published simultaneously as *Journal of Spirituality in Mental Health*, Volume 9, Numbers 3/4 2007.

Monographic Separates from the *Journal of Spirituality in Mental Health*™

For additional information on these and other Haworth Press titles, including descriptions, tables of contents, reviews, and prices, use the QuickSearch catalog at http://www.HaworthPress.com.

The *American Journal of Pastoral Counseling*™ is the successor title to *Journal of Pastoral Psychotherapy* which changed title after Vol. 2, No. 1, 1989. The *American Journal of Pastoral Counseling*™, under its new title, begins with Vol. 1, No. 1, 1997.

God Image Handbook for Spiritual Counseling and Psychotherapy: Research, Theory, and Practice, edited by Glendon L. Moriarity, PsyD, and Louis Hoffman, PhD (Volume 9, No. 3/4, 2007). *Understand better the relationship between the emotional experience of God, mental health difficulties, and psychotherapy.*

The Formation of Pastoral Counselors: Challenges and Opportunities, edited by Duane R. Bidwell, PhD, and Joretta L. Marshall, PhD (Volume 8, No. 3/4, 2006). *Two dozen of the most prominent clinicians and scholars in the field reflect on "The Formation of Pastoral Counselors" from clinical, theological, and theoretical perspectives. This unique book explores the challenges to the personal and professional formation of pastoral counselors in a cultural and historic context that's radically different from the era when the profession first emerged as a specialized ministry. Contributors examine formation from a variety of contexts and perspectives, including spirituality and gender, address theological education and intercultural issues, and present emerging models for pastoral counselors.*

The Image of God and the Psychology of Religion, edited by Richard Dayringer, ThD, and David Oler, PhD (Vol. 7, No. 2, 2004). *"It is my hope that this anthology will open the door to further research on God-images, particularly investigating the implications of God-images for issues of race, culture, ethnicity, and racial oppression. It makes new inroads into empirical research about God-images, mental health, and clinical psychotherapy. Multiple religious traditions and perspectives, and the impact of both personified and non-anthropomorphic divine images, are sensitively presented in clients' own words." (Pamela Cooper-White, PhD, Professor of Pastoral Theology, Lutheran Theological Seminary of Philadelphia)*

International Perspectives on Pastoral Counseling, edited by James Reaves Farris, PhD (Vol. 5, No. 1/2, 3/4, 2002). *Explores pastoral care as practiced in Africa, India, Korea, Hong Kong, the Philippines, Central America, South America, Germany, and the United Kingdom.*

Pastoral Care and Counseling in Sexual Diversity, edited by H. Newton Malony, MDiv, PhD (Vol. 3, No. 3/4, 2001). *"A balanced and reasoned presentation of viewpoints." (Orlo Christopher Strunk, Jr., PhD, Professor Emeritus, Boston University; Managing Editor,* The Journal of Pastoral Care)

God Image Handbook
for Spiritual Counseling
and Psychotherapy:
Research, Theory, and Practice

Glendon L. Moriarty, PsyD
Louis Hoffman, PhD
Editors

God Image Handbook for Spiritual Counseling and Psychotherapy: Research, Theory, and Practice has been co-published simultaneously as *Journal of Spirituality in Mental Health*, Volume 9, Numbers 3/4 2007.

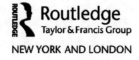

Routledge
Taylor & Francis Group

NEW YORK AND LONDON

First Published by

The Haworth Pastoral Press, 10 Alice Street, Binghamton, NY 13904-1580 USA

The Haworth Pastoral Press is an imprint of The Haworth Press, 10 Alice Street, Binghamton, NY 13904-1580 USA.

Transferred to Digital Printing 2010 by Routledge
270 Madison Ave, New York NY 10016
2 Park Square, Milton Park, Abingdon, Oxon, OX14 4RN

God Image Handbook for Spiritual Counseling and Psychotherapy: Research, Theory, and Practice has been co-published simultaneously as *Journal of Spirituality in Mental Health,* Volume 9, Numbers 3/4 2007.

The development, preparation, and publication of this work has been undertaken with great care. However, the publisher, employees, editors, and agents of The Haworth Press and all imprints of The Haworth Press, including The Haworth Medical Press® and The Pharmaceutical Products Press®, are not responsible for any errors contained herein or for consequences that may ensue from use of materials or information contained in this work.

The Haworth Press is committed to the dissemination of ideas and information according to the highest standards of intellectual freedom and the free exchange of ideas. Ststements made and opinions expressed in this publication do not necessarily reflect the views of the Publisher, Directors, management, or staff of The Haworth Press, or an endorsement by them.

Library of Congress Cataloging-in-Publication Data

God Image Handbook for Spiritual Counseling and Psychotherapy: Research, Theory, and Practice/Glendon L. Moriarity, Louis Hoffman, editors.
   p. cm
      "Co-published simultaneously as Journal of Spirituality in Mental Health, Volume 9, Numbers (3/4) 2007."
      Includes bibliographical references and index.
      ISBN 13: 978-0-7890-3439-7 (hard cover : alk. paper)
      ISBN 13: 978-0-7890-3440-3 (soft cover : alk. paper
   1. God (Christianity) 2. Image of God. 3. Pastoral counseling. 4. Pastoral psychology. 5. Psychotherapy–Religious aspects–Christianity. I. Moriarity, Glendon. II. Hoffman, Louis. III. Journal of spirituality in mental health.
BT103.G6182 2008
253.5–dc22

2007031307

This section provides you with a list of major indexing & abstracting services and other tools for bibliographic access. That is to say, each service began covering this periodical during the year noted in the right column. Most Websites which are listed below have indicated that they will either post, disseminate, compile, archive, cite or alert their own Website users with research-based content from this work. (This list is as current as the copyright date of this publication.)

Abstracting, Website/Indexing Coverage . . . . Year When Coverage Began

- *Academic Search Premier (EBSCO)*
  <http://search.ebscohost.com> 2007

- *Academic Source Premier (EBSCO)*
  <http://search.ebscohost.com> 2007

- *British Library Inside (The British Library)*
  <http://www.bl.uk/services/current/inside.html> 2007

- *Child Development Abstracts (Taylor & Francis)*
  <http://www.tandf.co.uk/> 2007

- *Contents Pages in Education (Taylor & Francis)*
  <http://www.tandf.co.uk> 2007

- *Current Abstracts (EBSCO) <http://search.ebscohost.com>* 2007

- *Current Citations Express (EBSCO) <http://search.ebscohost.com>* . . 2007

- *Educational Management Abstracts (Taylor & Francis)*
  <http://www.tandf.co.uk> 2007

- *Educational Research Abstracts (ERA) (Taylor & Francis)*
  <http://www.tandf.co.uk/era> 2007

- *Educational Technology Abstracts (Taylor & Francis)*
  <http://www.tandf.co.uk> 2007

- *Electronic Collections Online (OCLC)*
  <http://www.oclc.org/electroniccollections/> 2007

(continued)

Bibliographic Access

- *Cabell's Directory of Publishing Opportunities in Psychology <http://www.cabells.com>*

- *MedBioWorld <http://www.medbioworld.com>*

- *MediaFinder <http://www.mediafinder.com>*

- *Ulrich's Periodicals Directory: International Periodicals Information Since 1932 <http://www.Bowkerlink.com>*

Special Bibliographic Notes related to special journal issues (separates) and indexing/abstracting:

- indexing/abstracting services in this list will also cover material in any "separate" that is co-published simultaneously with Haworth's special thematic journal issue or DocuSerial. Indexing/abstracting usually covers material at the article/chapter level.
- monographic co-editions are intended for either non-subscribers or libraries which intend to purchase a second copy for their circulating collections.
- monographic co-editions are reported to all jobbers/wholesalers/approval plans. The source journal is listed as the "series" to assist the prevention of duplicate purchasing in the same manner utilized for books-in-series.
- to facilitate user/access services all indexing/abstracting services are encouraged to utilize the co-indexing entry note indicated at the bottom of the first page of each article/chapter/contribution.
- this is intended to assist a library user of any reference tool (whether print, electronic, online, or CD-ROM) to locate the monographic version if the library has purchased this version but not a subscription to the source journal.
- individual articles/chapters in any Haworth publication are also available through the Haworth Document Delivery Service (HDDS).

AS PART OF OUR CONTINUING COMMITMENT TO BETTER SERVE OUR LIBRARY PATRONS, WE ARE PROUD TO BE WORKING WITH THE FOLLOWING ELECTRONIC SERVICES:

AGGREGATOR SERVICES

- EBSCOhost • Ingenta • J-Gate • Minerva
- OCLC FirstSearch • Oxmill • SwetsWise

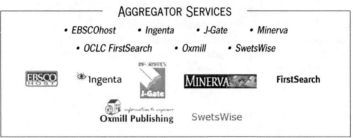

LINK RESOLVER SERVICES

- 1Cate (Openly Informatics) • ChemPort (American Chemical Society)
- CrossRef • Gold Rush (Coalliance) • LinkOut (PubMed)
- LINKplus (Atypon) LinkSolver (Ovid) • LinkSource with A-to-Z (EBSCO)
- Resource Linker (Ulrich's) • SerialsSolutions (ProQuest) • SFX (Ex Libris)
- Sirsi Resolver (SirsiDynix) • Tour (TDnet) • Vlink (Extensity)
- WebBridge (Innovative Interfaces)

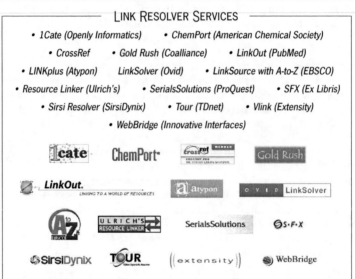

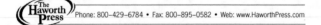
The Haworth Press
Phone: 800-429-6784 • Fax: 800-895-0582 • Web: www.HaworthPress.com

To Colin and Madeleine Moriarty,
I love you both with all of my heart (GLM)

In Memory of Robert J. Murney–Mentor, guide, and friend.
In Memory of Carl Davidson–Inspirational leader and friend (LH)

ABOUT THE EDITORS

Glendon L. Moriarty, PsyD, is a licensed psychologist and Associate Professor in the School of Psychology and Counseling at Regent University, where he supervises doctoral level trainees, teaches, and conducts research on psychodynamic psychotherapy and the psychology of religion. Dr. Moriarty is the author of *Pastoral Care of Depression: Helping Clients Heal Their Emotional Experience of God*. He has published articles, chapters, and presented on the integration of psychology and spirituality, the psychology of religion, and psychology and technology. In addition, he is the founder of the God Image Institute (www.godimage.com) the first agency in the country dedicated to helping people change their emotional experience of God. He was awarded multiple times for his contributions, receiving the Leadership Award, Fellowship Award, and being named among the Who's Who of Universities and Colleges. He is a member of the American Psychological Association, the Society for the Scientific Study of Religion, and the Christian Association for Psychological Studies.

Louis Hoffman, PhD, is Core Faculty member at the Colorado School of Professional Psychology, the Editor-in-Chief of the Colorado School of Professional Psychology Press, and Adjunct Faculty at the Graduate School of Psychology at Fuller Theological Seminary. He is also co-director of the God Image Institute, co-director of the Depth Psychotherapy Institute, and on the editorial board of *PsycCRITIQUES: APA Review of Books*. Dr. Hoffman is co-editor of the book *Spirituality and Psychological Health*. He has also authored and co-authored chapters for a number of books and journal articles on religious and spiritual issues in psychotherapy, existential-humanistic psychology, philosophical and historical issues in psychology, and LGBT issues in mental health.

God Image Handbook for Spiritual Counseling and Psychotherapy: Research, Theory, and Practice

CONTENTS

Foreword

The *God Image Handbook: Research, Theory, and Practice* addresses the professional needs of pastoral counselors, pastors, and clinicians specializing in religious and spiritual issues. The book intends to open a postmodern dialogue between the religious and scientific disciplines that converge in serving people who need religious and psychical help.

The editors have selected to focus their work on the impact that the internally elaborated God image has on the psychical and religious behaviors of each individual. They define the expression *God image* as 'the way a person emotionally or relationally experiences God.' Theoretically, they present the God image "as a psychological construct" which "exists across religious, cultural, academic, and theoretical boundaries." In other words, in our contemporary world reality, dominated by religious ideologies and conflicts, even those who have been minimally exposed to formal religious education form a conception of God that impact their view of themselves and of reality.

Form my point of view, the expression *God image,* useful as it is, needs some clarification. Conceived as a "construct" it risks being seen as an internal reality in its own right. It is useful to understand this construct as living and modifiable mental processes. The *God image* names an extraordinarily complex set of neurological and psychodynamic memory processes organized around the perceptual and fantasized conception of experiential realities and human relationships which have become linked to the individual's mode of connecting with or of avoiding the divinity. This becomes evident in the unavoidable interconnection that all authors in this volume describe so well between the sense of being oneself and the modality of experiencing God. It is also important to remember that fantasy and psychic defenses inflect modifications to the

[Haworth co-indexing entry note]: "Foreword." Co-published simultaneously in *Journal of Spirituality in Mental Health* (The Haworth Pastoral Press, an imprint of The Haworth Press) Vol. 9, No. 3/4, 2007, pp. xix-xx; and: *God Image Handbook for Spiritual Counseling and Psychotherapy: Research, Theory, and Practice* (ed: Glendon L. Moriarty, and Louis Hoffman) The Haworth Pastoral Press, an imprint of The Haworth Press, 2007, pp. xv-xvi. Single or multiple copies of this article are available for a fee from The Haworth Document Delivery Service [1-800-HAWORTH, 9:00 a.m. - 5:00 p.m. (EST). E-mail address: docdelivery@haworthpress.com].

Available online at http://jsmh.haworthpress.com
xv

memorial registration of human and religious experiences as a way of modulating the pain they may inflict. As several authors in the volume present it, we are not talking only about retrievable memories but also about memory processes embedded in modes of relating and of perceiving oneself and the realities of everyday life.

The editors, Glendon Moriarty and Louis Hoffman have organized the book as a comprehensive manual on the subject. The first part offers a review of the psychodynamic foundation and research that contribute to the understanding of the God image. The second part presents the contributions of seven skilled clinicians using different theoretical and technical approaches to help those who come to them with their personal and religious problem. The case presentations make this section very rich and enlightening. The variety of approaches indicates that they are many ways of helping people and that the integrity, respect, commitment, and technical competence of the therapist is not only the common denominator they all share but also a significant factor in their therapeutic efficacy. It is important to remember that when people appear in the therapist's office they obtain help at a particular cross sections of their lives. At another junction of their existence they may have different needs and conflicts and may require another approach. The reader will benefit from sharing in the struggles of the people presented and by witnessing how their therapists help them. It is worth noticing that all the therapists invited and insisted that each person assumed psychic responsibility for his or her life and moved from feeling an impotent victim of destiny to an active agent in the world. Having enjoyed watching them change, I only regret, as a psychoanalyst, that the editors did not include and example of psychoanalytic psychotherapy.

The final section addresses future developments and explores the implications of race, culture, gender orientation, and economic conditions of the psychic organization of the God image. Today, we should also consider the impact of religious and ethnic wars on children's elaboration of the God image.

This book is a contribution to the field. It gathers in one volume most of what is know today about the God image and offers much to reflect about short term and longer therapeutic interventions to help people wrestle with their God image and their suffering and dysfunctional lives. The handbook should become a referential resource for pastors, pastoral counselors, and clinicians specializing in religious and spiritual issues.

Ana-María Rizzuto, MD
March 20, 2007

Acknowledgments

Glen and Louis would like to thank . . .

First, we would like to thank the contributors to this volume. We were very deliberate in who we invited to participate in this volume. It has been a great pleasure to work with a group of professionals who have contributed so many great things to the field. We believe the strength of *The God Image Handbook* is in the dialogue; we thank you for sharing your voice, perspective, and time.

Second, we would also like to thank the faculty at the God Image Institute who contributed in many unseen ways to the current volume: Rodney Hesson, Michael Mitchell, Nicholas Gibson, Jay Gattis, Clarence Leung, Steve Simpson, and Peter Kalve.

Third, we would like to offer special thanks to William Schmidt. He has been a tremendously supportive editor. He has offered encouragement, helped us learn to trust our own judgment, and been remarkably available throughout this entire process. We would also like to thank the many others at Haworth who have helped us with this project, but have not played as visible a role.

Glen Moriarty would like to thank . . .

I want to begin by thanking my wife, Nicole. She is a wonderful spouse and mother of our beautiful twins, Colin and Madeleine. I am also grateful for her continual confidence in me and in all my projects.

I also want to thank my colleagues at Regent University. Dean Hughes and Bill Hathaway have been supportive of this project. I am thankful for their proactive leadership and for providing an atmosphere that encourages growth for young professionals. Thanks also to my fellow faculty members. The community they have created is invaluable to me.

[Haworth co-indexing entry note]: "Acknowledgments." Co-published simultaneously in *Journal of Spirituality in Mental Health* (The Haworth Pastoral Press, an imprint of The Haworth Press) Vol. 9, No. 3/4, 2007, pp. xxi-xxii; and: *God Image Handbook for Spiritual Counseling and Psychotherapy: Research, Theory, and Practice* (ed: Glendon L. Moriarty, and Louis Hoffman) The Haworth Pastoral Press, an imprint of The Haworth Press, 2007, pp. xvii-xviii. Single or multiple copies of this article are available for a fee from The Haworth Document Delivery Service [1-800-HAWORTH, 9:00 a.m. - 5:00 p.m. (EST). E-mail address: docdelivery@haworthpress.com].

Available online at http://jsmh.haworthpress.com
xvii

I also owe big thanks to Louis Hoffman. He has been a tremendous friend to me, godparent of my son Colin, and a true brother. Louis has a ton of integrity and honor. It is a real privilege to work with him and have him as a close friend.

Louis Hoffman would like to thank . . .

First, I would like to thank the greatest blessing in my life: my wife, my partner, and my friend. Thank you for you patience, support, and for being a part of my life. For all the words I've written, I can never seem to find the ones to express what you mean to me. Thank you, too, for not throwing my laptop out the window when it was getting the attention that you deserved.

I would also like thank Brittany Garrett-Bowser and Robert Murney, who helped me find the courage to make writing part of my career and my life; my brother, John Hoffman, who continually pushes me to become a stronger writer and thinker; H. Newt Malony, who provided early encouragement to pursue writing and academia; Sandra Knight, whose collaboration on many projects, including one chapter in this book, has been greatly valued and helped further my thinking about diversity issues; and Sue Cooper, who always understood, valued, supported, and encouraged my decisions to focus more on the writing portion of my career.

Special thanks are also due to the administration, faculty, staff, and students at the Colorado School of Professional Psychology (COSPP). Many of these people have helped me to develop my thinking about the issues I write about in this book. COSPP has provided wonderful encouragement and flexibility to pursue writing and has created an exemplary academic environment to grow as a person and a professional. I feel blessed to be a part of this community.

Members of the GLBT Religious Research team, including Sandra Knight, Margie Arms, John Hoffman, Scott Boscoe-Huffman, Debye Galaska, Beth Peterson, and Tracy Mahlock, deserve special thanks. Each of the individuals is making important contributions to understanding the impact of diversity on religious experience. I look forward to future collaborations and to reading your future contributions to the field.

Last, I wish to thank my colleague and good friend, Glen Moriarty. It has been a great honor to share this project with Glen, who is one of the great talents among the young professionals in our field. I know we will be reading the contributions of Glen for many, many years to come. But mostly, I wish to thank Glen for his friendship.

About the Contributors

John Allmond, MA, is a doctoral trainee in the School of Psychology and Counseling at Regent University. He graduated from Lee University with a Bachelor's in Psychology. He is currently working on a dissertation related to assessing God image interventions across professional and spiritual disciplines. He has worked as a clinician for several years, primarily focusing on case management with adults diagnosed with severe psychological disorders and in-home counseling with at-risk youth.

Scott Boscoe-Huffman, MA, is a graduate student in clinical psychology, working on his PsyD, at the Colorado School of Professional Psychology (COSPP). His Bachelor of Arts from Florida Atlantic University was received in 1990. He received his Masters of Arts in Psychology from COSPP in August of 2006. His areas of research interest include religion, race, gender and sexual orientation. He has spent the last fifteen years in program development, supervision, training, fund development and management in non-profit organizations as a counselor, program director and executive director. In these roles, he was responsible for either direct creation or oversight of non-profit agency programs. In addition, he served as a counselor for many of these disenfranchised clients. The populations he served included the acutely mentally ill, persons infected with HIV/AIDS, and foster children. Although his concentration is clinical, he plans to continue his research practice throughout his professional career.

Carrie Doehring, PhD, is Associate Professor of pastoral care and counseling at Iliff School of Theology. She has taught in masters and doctoral programs at Boston University's School of Theology, as well as in the Counseling Psychology and Religion PhD Program in the Graduate School of Arts and Sciences. In addition, she is ordained in the Presbyterian Church. Her three book publications are *Internal Traumatization,* an empirical study of women's images of God and their history of childhood abuse, and *Taking Care: Monitoring Power Dynamics and Relational Boundaries in Pastoral Care and Counseling*, a book about clergy sexual misconduct, and *The Practice of Pastoral Care: A Postmodern Approach*, a book about pastoral care that is oriented to premodern, modern, and postmodern approaches to religious knowledge.

Fernando Garzon, PsyD, is Associate Professor in the Center for Counseling and Family Studies at Liberty University. He has a PsyD in Clinical Psychology from Fuller Theological Seminary and a BA in Biology from

Wake Forest. His interest areas include spirituality in psychotherapy and counselor education. Correspondence regarding this chapter may be sent to the author at Liberty University, 1971 University Blvd., Lynchburg, VA 24502 or fgarzon@liberty.edu.

Nicholas J. S. Gibson, PhD, (Psychology of Religion, University of Cambridge, 2006) is Assistant Research Coordinator of the Psychology and Religion Research Group at the University of Cambridge. His research interests include religious and social cognition, psychology of religion, and the integration of psychology and theology.

Christopher Grimes, PsyD, is a graduate of the Forest Institute of Professional Psychology. He earned a Doctor of Psychology in Clinical Psychology from Forest and is a Licensed Psychologist in private practice in Independence, Missouri, a suburb of Kansas City. He specializes in working with individuals wishing to integrate their faith and spirituality into the therapy process.

Todd W. Hall, PhD, Dr. Hall's writing and research focuses on relational approaches to spiritual development that are informed by multiple areas and disciplines including attachment theory, relational psychoanalytic theories, neurobiology of attachment, and emotion research. Dr. Hall developed the Spiritual Transformation Inventory (STI), a web-based measure of Christian spirituality that is being used in a national assessment project conducted by the Coalition of Christian Colleges and Universities, and also by churches and seminaries. He has served as a consultant to numerous organizations on spiritual assessment, including the National Institute of Mental Health. Dr. Hall has participated in several grant-funded studies of spiritual development across the college years. He was most recently a co-investigator on a Templeton funded longitudinal study of spiritual transformation conducted at Biola. Dr. Hall has co-edited a book on spiritual formation, and published numerous journal articles in journals such as the *Journal of Psychology and Christianity, Journal of Psychology and Theology, Journal for the Scientific Study of Religion, International Journal for the Psychology of Religion, Mental Health, Culture and Religion, and the Journal of Family Psychology.* He has presented over 40 papers at national conferences on the topic of relational spiritual development. Dr. Hall is currently working on several books on spiritual formation. His forthcoming book with Biola colleague Dr. John Coe (*Christianity and Psychology: Reclaiming the Self for the Spiritual Formation of the Church*) will be part of IVP's forthcoming worldview series. Dr. Hall recently wrote a workbook for the STI titled: *Furnishing the Soul: How Relational Connections Prepare Us for Spiritual Transformation,* and he is completing a book with the same name. Dr. Hall also conducts *Furnishing the Soul* seminars for churches and Christian universities.

Louis Hoffman, PhD, is a core faculty member at the Colorado School of Professional Psychology and also maintains a private practice in Colorado Springs, Colorado. He is co-director of the God Image Institute and the Depth Psychotherapy Institute. His interests include religious and spiritual issues in psychotherapy, existential and depth psychotherapy, diversity issues, and philosophical issues in clinical psychology. Co-author of *Spirituality and Psychological Health*, Dr. Hoffman has also authored numerous book chapters, journal articles, and conference papers as well as being a published poet.

Brad Johnson, PhD, is Associate Professor of psychology in the Department of Leadership, Ethics and Law at the United States Naval Academy, and a Faculty Associate in the Graduate School of Business and Education at Johns Hopkins University. He is a clinical psychologist and fellow/supervisor of the Institute for Rational Emotive Behavior Therapy in New York. Prior to joining the Naval Academy faculty, Dr. Johnson spent four years as a faculty member and director of research for the APA-approved clinical doctoral program at George Fox University. He has been a member of Oregon's Board of Bar Examiners and an oral examiner for Oregon's Board of Psychologist Examiners. Dr. Johnson has authored numerous articles and book chapters, as well as three books in the areas of ethical behavior, mentor relationships, psychotherapy outcomes, and the integration of psychology and spirituality.

James W. Jones, PhD, is Professor of Religion and Adjunct Professor of Clinical Psychology at Rutgers University. He has published nine books on psychoanalysis and spirituality, including: *Contemporary Psychoanalysis and Religion*; *Religion and Psychology in Transition*; *Terror and Transformation: the Ambiguity of Religion in Psychoanalytic Perspective*; *and In the Middle of This Road We Call Our Life*. His books have been translated and published in Japan, China, Latin America, and Europe and he lectures regularly in Europe and America. The Division of Psychology of Religion awarded him the William Bier Award at the annual meeting of the American Psychological Association; and in 2002, he was nominated for the Oskar Pfister Award.

Sandra Knight, PhD, is a licensed psychologist in private practice for over 30 years and retired Dean of Clinical Training and faculty member at the Colorado School of Professional Psychology. She is the Past President of Mental Health Association of El Paso County, Director of the City and County Mental Health Responders to Critical Incidents (MHRCI), and

Chair of the Client Care Advisory Board of Nurse Family Partnership. Her interests include spiritual issues in psychotherapy, diversity issues, and treatment of complex trauma disorders.

Glendon L. Moriarty, PsyD, is a licensed psychologist and Assistant Professor in the School of Psychology and Counseling at Regent University. Dr. Moriarty is the author of *Pastoral Care of Depression: Helping Clients Heal Their Relationship with God.* He is also the founder of the God Image Institute (www.godimage.com), the first agency in the country dedicated to helping people change their emotional experience of God.

Jacqueline L. Noffke, PsyD, earned her degree from Rosemead School of Psychology in La Mirada, California. She is currently earning her post-doctoral hours for licensure at the Center for Discovery and Adolescent Change, a residential facility for the treatment of eating disorders in southern California. Her specialties include psychoanalytically-informed psychotherapy, attachment theory, and working with spiritually-committed clientele and those with eating disorders.

Kari O'Grady received a BS degree in psychology from Brigham Young University. She is currently a doctoral candidate in the APA accredited PhD program in Counseling Psychology at Brigham Young University. She is the co-author of several publications and presentations on the topics of spirituality, psychotherapy, and multiculturalism, including: Out of obscurity: The faith factor in physical and mental health (*Contemporary Psychology: APA Review of Books, 2003*), Treating the religiously committed client (*Psychologists' Desk Reference* (2nd ed., 2004), New York: Oxford University Press), Spirituality and therapeutic process case study (*Spirituality and the Therapeutic Process: A Guide for Mental Health Professionals*, APA, under contract). Her doctoral dissertation examined scientists' and health professionals' beliefs and experiences regarding inspiration in research and practice.

P. Scott Richards, PhD, is co-creator of the ecumenical and eclectic Theistic approach (along with Allan Bergin) and is well-known for his book, *A Spiritual Strategy for Counseling and Psychotherapy.* He has co-authored two additional books that were published by the American Psychological Association: *Casebook for a Spirituality Strategy for Counseling and Psychotherapy* and the *Handbook of Psychotherapy and Religious Diversity.* Dr. Richards is a licensed psychologist and an associate professor of educational psychology at Brigham Young University where he is the Coordinator of the PhD program in Counseling Psychology.

Sharon Stewart is a native of Texas. She received her Master's degree in psychology in 2001. Sharon is now a PsyD candidate at the Colorado

School of Professional Psychology. Currently, she lives in Europe where she is also fulfilling her internship requirements. The treatment of trauma is an area of particular interest to Sharon.

Michael Thomas, MA, is currently in his fourth year of the Doctor of Psychology program at Regent University. He graduated with a Bachelor of Science degree in Biblical Studies from Philadelphia Biblical University and with a Master of Arts in Clinical Psychology from Regent University. His current research focuses on helping hurting Christians grow in experiencing God's love and grace in their lives. He served as a pastor for three years prior to beginning his graduate training. He has also worked with at-risk youth, and adults in the Christian community.

PART I
FOUNDATIONS

Chapter 1

Introduction and Overview

Glendon L. Moriarty, PsyD
Louis Hoffman, PhD

Psychological difficulties are pervasive and influence multiple domains of life, including the religious and spiritual domains. People who identify with theistic perspectives and are encountering emotional difficulties often experience conflict in their personal experience of God. They intellectually understand the theological components of their faith, but have difficulty emotionally grasping them.

This common experience occurs because people have multiple ideas of God, the two most common being the God concept and the God image. The God concept is an abstract, intellectual, mental definition of the word "God" (Lawrence, 1997; Rizzuto, 1979). It represents what people think about God rather than what they feel about God. Most indi-

[Haworth co-indexing entry note]: "Introduction and Overview." Moriarty, Glendon L., and Louis Hoffman. Co-published simultaneously in *Journal of Spirituality in Mental Health* (The Haworth Pastoral Press, an imprint of The Haworth Press) Vol. 9, No. 3/4, 2007, pp. 1-9; and: *God Image Handbook for Spiritual Counseling and Psychotherapy: Research, Theory, and Practice* (ed: Glendon L. Moriarty, and Louis Hoffman) The Haworth Pastoral Press, an imprint of The Haworth Press, 2007, pp. 1-9. Single or multiple copies of this article are available for a fee from The Haworth Document Delivery Service [1-800-HAWORTH, 9:00 a.m. - 5:00 p.m. (EST). E-mail address: docdelivery@haworthpress.com].

viduals profess a God concept characterized by love, strength, and wisdom. The God image, on the other hand, is the complex, subjective emotional experience of God. It is shaped by a person's family history and causes their experience of God to resemble their relationship with their parents. Familiarity is comfortable so people pattern future relationships after what they learned with their caregivers. People who struggle with mental health issues often have a God image that is distant, critical, and judgmental because they had parents that were distant, critical, and judgmental.

Clients suffering with a negative experience of God often want to explore and resolve these issues through the psychotherapy process. Therapists are usually willing to discuss these issues, but feel limited in their ability to conceptualize and treat God image difficulties. Despite the recent interest in spirituality and mental health, clinicians have few resources that directly address the God image. The main integration texts briefly mention the God image, but do not detail how therapists can assess and change it through the therapy process.

The *God Image Handbook: Research, Theory, and Practice* fills this gap by providing a comprehensive, multi-perspective volume built upon strong philosophical and research foundations to provide 7 clinical approaches to working with the God image in psychotherapy. Each approach or theoretical orientation views the God image through a template that emphasizes: Background and Philosophical Assumptions, God Image Development, God Image Difficulties, God Image Change, and Strengths and Weaknesses. In addition, contributing authors further illustrate each orientation through case examples with the following headings: Client History, Presenting Problem, Case Conceptualization, Treatment Plan, Interventions, Duration of Treatment, Termination, and Therapeutic Outcomes.

HISTORICAL AND CONTEMPORARY RELEVANCE

The idea of the God image has been ruminating in unconscious and conscious realms of Western thought since at least the 1800s in the writings of Feuerbach (1841/1989), Nietzsche (1892/1954), and Freud (1913/1950, 1927/1961), among others. However, it wasn't until Rizzuto (1979) wrote *The Birth of the Living God* that a language and research agenda began to emerge to formally explore the experience of God.

Truly, it is hard to underestimate the value of Rizzuto's work. It is as relevant today as it was when she first began writing about the God image. As we began to formulate the concept of The *God Image Handbook*, we knew that we owed a great debt to Rizzuto's work that could not be encapsulated in words. Many of Rizzuto's predecessors assumed that if the experience of God could be explained by psychological and cultural forces, then this means God does not exist. For them, God became a product of wish fulfillment, the psychological need for security, and personal and cultural history. Rizzuto knew well that these factors influenced how people experience God, but also demonstrated that this does not mean that God does not exist.

The next important phase in the development of the God image research could best be termed the assessment phase. Many luminaries in the psychology of religion attempted to capture and quantify the emotional experience of God (Benson & Spilka, 1973; Gorsuch, 1968; Lawrence, 1997). Although many authors in this volume strongly critique quantitative, self-report, God image measures (see Gibson, Chapter 12), they represent an important new development that played an important role in the increased consideration of the God image in the psychological and research literature. Contemporary researchers of the God image still debate how to best measure the experience of God and whether it is possible to adequately distinguish the emotional or relational experience of God from religious cognitions or beliefs. This book does not answer these important questions; however, it does further the dialogue.

Many other important research developments could also be noted. Kirkpatrick (1997, 2004; Kirkpatrick & Shaver, 1990) made significant contributions to the research literature from an attachment perspective although not utilizing the language of the God image or God concept. Kirkpatrick's research was influential in distinguishing between the two primary models: the *correspondence model* and the *compensation model*, which are discussed in Chapter 1. Hall (Hall, Halcrow, Hill, Delaney, & Teal, 2005; Hall & Porter, 2004) has been influential in developing theories to reconcile these seemingly opposite models.

Thus far, most of the God image literature has been set in the context of a modernist paradigm. Modernism's tendency was to use science and research to explain away metaphysics. If science offered a concrete answer, it was assumed to be more valid and truthful than what religion had to offer. In this context, it was easy for Freud and others to explain God away. Postmodernism, however, responded by critiquing the absolute authority of religion (premodernism) and science (modernism), opening a door for dialogue.

This book reflects such a postmodern dialogue. For many of the readers of this volume, religion holds the trump card when conflict arises.

For others, science trumps religion. However, for many, science and religion are continuously engaged in a dialogue as each sharpens the other in the pursuit of greater understanding. Part of the process of achieving greater understanding occurs through being aware of the limitations of the God image literature while remaining in dialogue with differing perspectives.

LIMITATIONS OF THE CURRENT LITERATURE

The God image, or the way a person emotionally or relationally experiences God, has exploded in the psychological literature in last 10 years. The number of journal articles, conferences papers, and books on this topic dramatically increased over this time. However, the dialogue has encountered a number of significant challenges.

A primary limitation in the development of the God image literature is the challenge in locating this information. Many important contributions have been made through conference presentations, dissertations, and articles in journals which are often difficult to track down. One goal of this volume is to bring many of the notable contributors together so that key and different viewpoints can be found in one work. Second, some of the contributors to the God image literature have not adequately addressed the different perspectives. This can cause readers to form an incomplete understanding of a complex and multifaceted construct–the emotional experience of God. This work attempts to overcome this limitation by giving voice to many different perspectives. The goal is to view the God image through a variety of lenses, so that the reader has a nuanced perspective.

A third limitation is the lack of consistent use of language. Different words have been used to describe the emotional experience of God. Some of the monikers include: the God representation, the God concept, the God schema, and, of course, the God image. We, somewhat ambivalently, have decided to use the term "God Image." It isn't necessarily the best term, but it is the term that is most frequently cited in research, theory, and assessment. Other semantic issues involve confusing the God image with *images of God* or *the image of God*, which reflect distinct, but related constructs. Whereas the God image refers to *the way a person emotionally or relationally experiences God*, images of God refer to *pictures or images in which God is illustrated either graphically or mentally*. Although images of God are related and often represent aspects of the God image, it is still a distinct construct. The image of God, or imago dei, on the other hand, is a theological concept referring to human beings as created in the *image of God.*

A fourth limitation involves the lack of practical information on how to conceptualize and work with the God image in therapy. Clinicians regularly encounter the Sacred in their work, but often struggle with theoretical frames, or language, to help them understand the perceived experience of God. If they do have a frame, then they often lack interventions to help the individual who is facing spiritual struggles. A primary goal of this work is to outline how to practically understand and address the God image through a variety of theoretical orientations.

In this volume, the God image literature is advanced through addressing these limitations while furthering the dialogue. The authors in this book offer a number of very different perspectives, and techniques, on how to work with the God image. Additionally, the work brings together many of the important and influential thinkers in the God image literature and the literature on religious and spiritual issues in therapy.

RELIGIOUS AND THEORETICAL DIVERSITY

In approaching this book, we felt it was important to integrate, but also reach beyond our own personal beliefs about faith and the God image. The God image, as a psychological construct, exists across religious, cultural, academic, and theoretical boundaries. As we identified the important leaders in the field who would contribute to this book, we were intentional about seeking out scholars from different religious perspectives, different theoretical backgrounds, and different academic backgrounds. One limitation of this is that most of the authors are rooted in the Christian tradition. Future dialogues should be more inclusive of divergent religious viewpoints beyond Christianity.

The diversity this book represents serves two important intentions. First, it is our hope that this book represents a dialogue as well as a scholarly contribution. The astute reader will quickly notice that although the authors of this book differ on important theoretical and religious beliefs, they share a respect for these differences and openness to different perspectives. Through dialogue, we hope to advance theory and research developments.

Second, the diversity serves a pedagogical purpose. Most clinicians utilizing the God image in therapy work with clients from various religious perspectives and worldviews. It is our belief that to work more effectively with a diverse clientele it is essential that clinicians are exposed to a variety of different religious, cultural, and theoretical perspectives. Therapists with a myopic vision or understanding often unintentionally impose their beliefs and values upon their clients. Hopefully the diverse perspectives in this book will help clinicians avoid this dangerous ethical pitfall.

ETHICAL ISSUES

Over the many years that we have written, presented, and taught about the God image, one of the common questions which surfaces is, "What gives you the right to tell someone what their image of God ought to be?" This is an important and valid question; however, it misses the intention of most clinicians who utilize the concept of the God image in therapy. Yet, this is one of the great dangers of this work.

The authors of this book do not intend to suggest that there is a correct way that all people should see God; rather, we are concerned that many people distort their experience of God in a manner that causes unnecessary psychological and spiritual suffering. Any time a therapist ventures into religious and spiritual issues in psychotherapy, they begin wading into dangerous ethical grounds. It is common for a therapist to believe that because they are personally religious and also a therapist or counselor that they are adequately prepared to deal with religious and spiritual issues in therapy. This is a dangerous and naïve assumption, particularly when helping people explore and attempt to change the way they think about God and experience God.

We propose a couple of important ethical guidelines to help therapists and counselors avoid this trap. First, it is important to carefully consider the context of the therapy. For pastors and pastoral counselors, there is much greater latitude in intentionally and directly addressing religious beliefs; however, for therapists and counselors practicing in private practice or non-religious contexts, to do so would be unethical. In these settings, therapists can assist clients in understanding, exploring, and changing beliefs and values; however, therapists should help empower clients to make these changes instead of suggesting specific directions.

Second, therapists need to be aware of their own beliefs, biases, and values, especially when they may contradict client values. Additionally, they should be aware of their own God image or experience of God. One of the most common instances is when therapists impose their values or beliefs on clients is when they make false assumptions of agreement or when they are not aware of their own beliefs and values (Hoffman, Grimes, & Mitchell, 2004). The ethical therapist is a self-aware therapist.

Awareness should also include a broader awareness of religious and spiritual diversity. Without understanding different perspectives, it is often difficult to understand our own. As awareness of cultural diversity can assist therapists in working effectively with clients from different cultural backgrounds, awareness of religious diversity can help therapists understand clients from different religious backgrounds. However, it is also important not to use knowledge about cultural or religious differences to make assumptions about people. There is often as much within group difference as between group difference. In other words, agreement should not be assumed just because you share the same religious, sectarian, or denominational affiliation.

Third, therapists should recognize the difference between exploring religious and spiritual issues and making religious or spiritual interventions. In exploration, the therapist and client seek to better understand the client's beliefs and where they come from; conversely, religious interventions entail the therapist using techniques that are more directive and may incur particular values. Therapists desiring to use more active religious interventions should have specialized training and supervision before implementing these approaches.

Fourth, therapists should be informed about the ethical issues involved in working with religious and spiritual issues in therapy, such as using an informed consent. Although this section provides an introduction to some of the ethical issues we believe to be most pertinent to God image work, Richards and Bergin's (2005) *A Spiritual Strategy for Psychotherapy and Counseling* is recommended for a more thorough overview of ethical issues when working with spiritual issues in psychotherapy. Tan's (1994, 1996) work also offers helpful guidelines and is highly recommended.

ORGANIZATION AND OVERVIEW OF THE GOD IMAGE HANDBOOK

The *God Image Handbook* consists of three main sections. The first section of the book explores the research and psychodynamic foundations that support the God image. In Chapter 1, Christopher Grimes provides a comprehensive review of God image research. Distinguished scholar James Jones illustrates the psychodynamic evolution of the God image in Chapter 2.

The second part of the book will be of particular interest to therapists and clinicians. The authors of the different chapters are considered some of the foremost clinicians and researchers in their respective areas. The section provides seven different approaches to working with the God image. These approaches include: attachment therapy, time-limited dynamic psychotherapy, existential integrative, a neuroscientific approach, rational emotive behavioral therapy, theistic, and a liberal protestant pastoral approach.

The final section of the book addresses future directions of God image research and clinical work. Nicholas Gibson provides an important and innovative look at measuring the God image. He offers critiques of the current measures and offers practical solutions to overcoming some of our most difficult challenges when faced with assessing the God image. Glen Moriarty next compares and contrasts the different therapy approaches outlined in Part 2. Finally, Hoffman, Knight, Boscoe-Huffman, and Stewart discuss the future directions of God image research and theory with emphases on racial, cultural, gender, and economic considerations.

CONCLUSION

God image work is an exciting and growing field. Much has been written on this subject and much more will be written in the years to come. In this introduction, we have attempted to paint with broad strokes what we see as some of the foundations of God image work.

The contributors to this volume have built on this foundation through literature reviews and practical chapters on how to work with the God image in the consulting room. In addition, they have pointed out that we still have a ways to go, particularly in regards to measuring the God image and better understanding the relationship between the God image and diversity issues.

We hope The *God Image Handbook* is the beginning of a dialogue that will continue to grow and expand over time. Although we have intentionally included diverse perspectives and viewpoints, the constraints of the volume prevented us from including other, equally important voices. We are committed to an open and collaborative dialog and would welcome your thoughts and feedback. Please visit us on the Web at www.godimage.com. We look forward to working with you to further advance God image clinical work and research.

REFERENCES

Benson, P.& Spilka, B. (1973). God image as a function of self-esteem and locus of control. *Journal of Scientific Study of Religion.* 12(3): 297-310.

Feuerbach, L. (1989). *The essence of Christianity* (G. Eliot, Trans.). Amherst, NY: Prometheus. (Original work published in 1841)

Freud, S. (1950). *Totem and taboo* (J. Stratchey, Trans.). New York: Norton & Company. (Original work published in 1913)

Freud, S. (1961). The future of an illusion (J. Stratchey, Trans.). New York: Norton & Company. (Original work published in 1927)

Gorsuch, R. (1968). The conceptualization of God as seen in adjective ratings. *Journal for the Scientific Study of Religion,* 7, 56-64.

Hall, T. W., Halcrow, S., Hill, P., Delaney, H., & Teal, J. (2005, April). *Attachment and spirituality.* Paper presented at the Christian Association for Psychological Studies International Conference, Dallas, TX.

Hall, T. W. & Porter, S. L. (2004). Referential Integration: An emotional information processing perspective on the Process of Integration. *Journal of Psychology and Theology, 32,* 167-180.

Hoffman, L, Grimes, C. S. M., & Mitchell, M. (2004, July). *Transcendence, suffering, and psychotherapy.* Paper presented at the Bi-annual Conference of the International Network for Personal Meaning, Vancouver, British Columbia, Canada.

Kirkpatrick, L. A. (1997). A longitudinal study of changes in religious beliefs and behavior as a function of individual differences in adult attachment style. *Journal for the Scientific Study of Religion, 36,* 207-217.

Kirkpatrick, L. A. (1998). God as a substitute attachment figure: A longitudinal study of adult attachment style and religious change in college students. *Personality and Social Psychology Bulletin, 24,* 961-973.

Kirkpatrick, L. A. (2004). *Attachment, evolution, and the psychology of religion.* New York: Guilford Press.

Kirkpatrick, L. A. & Shaver, P. R. (1990). Attachment theory and religion: Childhood attachments, religious beliefs, and conversion. *Journal for the Scientific Study of Religion, 29,* 315-334.

Lawrence, R. T. (1997). Measuring the image of God: The God image inventory and the God image scales. *Journal of Psychology and Theology, 25,* 214-226.

Nietzsche, F. (1954). *Thus spoke Zarathustra: A book for none and all* (W. Kaufmann, Trans.). New York: Penguin. (Original work published in 1892)

Richards, P. S. & Bergin, A. E. (2005) *A spiritual strategy for counseling and psychotherapy* (2nd ed.). Washington, DC: American Psychological Association.

Rizzuto, A. M. (1979). *The birth of the living God: A psychoanalytic study.* Chicago: University of Chicago Press.

Tan, S.Y. (1994). Ethical considerations in religious psychotherapy: potential pitfalls and unique resources. *Journal of Psychology and Theology, 22,* 389-394.

Tan, S.Y. (1996). Religion in clinical practice: implicit and explicit integration. In E.P. Shafranske (Ed.), *Religion and Clinical Practice of Psychology* (pp. 365-386). Washington, DC: American Psychological Association

doi:10.1300/J515v09n03_01

Chapter 2

God Image Research:
A Literature Review

Christopher Grimes, PsyD

SUMMARY. The purpose of this article is to provide a summary of the empirical research on the God image construct. Contemporary research is placed against the backdrop of older studies in order to provide a comprehensive review of the literature. The God image is discussed as a multi-dimensional construct and the relationship of the God image to other variables including family dynamics and attachment processes are discussed. The relationship between the God image and psychopathology and treatment is also reviewed. Finally, consideration is given to areas needing further investigation. doi:10.1300/J515v09n03_02 *[Article copies available for a fee from The Haworth Document Delivery Service: 1-800-HAWORTH. E-mail address: <docdelivery@haworthpress.com> Website: <http://www.HaworthPress.com> © 2007 by The Haworth Press. All rights reserved.]*

GOD IMAGE RESEARCH: A LITERATURE REVIEW

The development of research methods to assess an individual's experience of God is wrought with difficulties (Bassinger, 1990). These diffi-

[Haworth co-indexing entry note]: "God Image Research: A Literature Review." Grimes, Christopher. Co-published simultaneously in *Journal of Spirituality in Mental Health* (The Haworth Pastoral Press, an imprint of The Haworth Press) Vol. 9, No. 3/4, 2007, pp. 11-32; and: *God Image Handbook for Spiritual Counseling and Psychotherapy: Research, Theory, and Practice* (ed: Glendon L. Moriarty, and Louis Hoffman) The Haworth Pastoral Press, an imprint of The Haworth Press, 2007, pp. 11-32. Single or multiple copies of this article are available for a fee from The Haworth Document Delivery Service [1-800-HAWORTH, 9:00 a.m. - 5:00 p.m. (EST). E-mail address: docdelivery@haworthpress.com].

Available online at http://jsmh.haworthpress.com
© 2007 by The Haworth Press. All rights reserved.
doi:10.1300/J515v09n03_02

culties arise, in part, from attempts to quantify a transcendent experience. Despite the ambiguities of such work, the study of individual's cognitive and emotional experience of God is a worthy pursuit because of the impact these experiences have upon the person. Researchers continue to find evidence of a relationship between spiritual belief, religious practice, and psychological well-being (Ervin-Cox, Hoffman, and Grimes, 2005; Koenig, 1998), and knowledge gained from research of the God image can guide therapeutic interventions in order to move individuals toward psychological wellness and spiritual wholeness.

The emphasis in this chapter is on reporting the findings of researchers who have investigated the God image as a psychological construct and have themselves reported their findings in scholarly writings. The literature review presented here is selective with special attention paid to recent research articles recorded in peer reviewed journals, while older studies have been incorporated as needed to help set a backdrop to understand recent findings.

Definition of Terms

The construct of the God image emerged from the work of Rizzuto (1979), who built upon the psychoanalytic theories of Freud and objects relations theory to develop a means of conceptualizing individual's experiences of God. The God image as a psychological construct is concerned with how an individual feels toward God, and how they feel God feels about them. The God image is primarily an unconscious phenomenon, as compared to the God concept. The God concept, as a distinct construct, referrers to an individual's cognitive understanding of God. Hoffman (2005) summarizes the God concept as being largely conscious and rational, based upon what a person is taught about God, and influenced by such things as religious teachings of parents, spiritual leaders, and religious texts. Comparatively, Hoffman notes that the God image is more complex and is emotional, experiential, and unconscious in nature.

Unfortunately, researchers investigating the God image have not always distinguished between the constructs God image and God concept, tending to lump to two constructs together and sometimes using the terms "God image" and "God concept" interchangeably in their writings. While some have argued that the God image and God concept may be redundant constructs (Piedmont & Muller, 2006), others have suggested that the majority of research carried out on the God image has in fact been measuring the God concept while neglecting the more unconscious and experiential components of religious experience (Hill & Hall 2002; Hoffman, Grimes, & Acoba, 2005). This author stands in agreement with Hill and Hall, and Hoffman et al. that there is a valid theoretical distinction to be made between the God image and God concept. However, that the two constructs have not been well delineated in the professional literature complicates the task of compiling a literature review solely on the God image. Therefore, the God image, as defined for the purpose of this review, is consistent with the broader definition historically given in the literature and may often overlap with the God concept. More will be said about this limitation of the research later.

DIMENSIONS OF THE GOD IMAGE

Early investigations of the God image focused on studying the words individuals used to describe their God image. Gorsuch (1968), for example, developed an adjective checklist to assess an individual's God image. Certainly, the words individuals associate with God and use to describe God's attributes can give indications of their God image, and other researches have built upon Gorsuch's work Research investigating the nouns ascribed to God and the adjectives used to describe God's attributes suggest an individual's God image is multi-dimensional. Roof and Roof (1984) reported on data collected in the General Social Survey wherein respondents were asked when they thought about God how likely the image of Judge, King, Lover, Master, Father, Redeemer, Friend, Healer, Mother, Liberator, Spouse, and Creator were to come to their mind. Their results indicated that Creator was the most dominant God image, while the image of God as a Spouse was the least popular. Not surprisingly, Roof and Roof found that those nouns which corresponded to traditional images of God from religious teaching were more popular than the more familiar-personalist images. Following this trend, the paternal image of Father was considered extremely likely to come to mind for 61% of the respondents while the image of Mother was considered extremely likely to come to mind for only 25% of the respondents. Roof and Roof interpreted this finding to suggest that Americans tend to hold a more traditional paternal image of God.

Nelsen, Cheek, and Au (1985) used factor analysis to further analyze the data from the General Social Survey of 1983 and came to a different conclusion than Roof and Roof (1984). Nelsen et al.'s analysis distinguished two primary factors, one maternal (God as Healer) and the other paternal (God as King). The most frequently reported concepts from the General Social Survey data (Creator, Healer, Friend, Redeemer, and Father) all fell in the maternal factor set. Although the respondents were far more likely to choose Father than Mother as a descriptor of God, the meaning of the Father descriptor fell within the more maternal, God as Healer, factor. Whereas traditionally the God as Father image referred to a punitive and powerful figure, Nelson et al.'s results suggest that God as Father imagery may sometimes suggest a more supportive, nurturing figure.

In another study investigating the language used to describe God, Janssen, De Hart, and Gerardts (1994) used open ended questions to elicit adolescents' God images. Content analysis was performed on the adolescents' responses and a hierarchical model was developed to distinguish the attributes of God and the acts of God. Regarding the specific words used to described God, Jansen et al. found there seemed to be no common words to described God. They state,

> There is neither a common stock of words nor a common stock of significants . . . Different individuals use different terms; the same individuals use different terms at different moments. The image of God is shrouded in mist: There is no vocabulary or formulas or common poetry to lift that shroud. (p. 110)

This quote encapsulates the challenges of God image research illustrating the extreme subjectively of the language used to describe the experience of God.

While the specific words used to describe the experience of God varied significantly, there was commonality among the concepts used to describe God. The adolescents in Jansen et al.'s (1994) study most often described God as a form of activity, while only less that one third described God as a being having certain qualities. The most commonly mentioned act of God was the wielding of power to correct or to help and support people.

Kunkel, Cook, Meshel, Daughtry, and Hauenstein (1999) focused their study of God image dimensions on an approach which emphasized individual's internal constructions. Previous qualitative research on the dimensions of individual's God image limited the range of possible responses to those options specified by the researches and their instruments. To avoid these limitations Kunkel et al. employed multi-dimensional scaling analysis hoping to capture individuals' meaning while acknowledging and accommodating for the ambiguity and variability of responses.

The results of Kunkel et al. (1999) study suggest that God images are organized along two dimensions of anthropomorphic verses mystical and punitive versus nurturant. Each of these dimensions overlap, and several distinct regions were suggested by the research, as represented in Figure 1. For example, human images tended to be grouped by role (i.e. Man, Woman, Brother) and regulating functions (i.e. Teacher, Ruler, Judge, and Lawmaker). There were clusters representing both powerful and benevolent images, as well as distant and mysterious images. There was one cluster composed of vengeful images as well. In examining the structure of the map and comparing adjacent clusters the researchers found that images of God as regulating or controlling may bridge human roles with powerful roles when it comes to a reflection of God's perceived influence on human life. Likewise, inspirational God images may bridge benevolence and mystery. Overall, congruent with earlier research (Dickie, Eshleman, Merasco, Shepard, Vander Wilt, Johnson, 1997; Nelson et al., 1985), participants tended to view God as masculine, powerful, and nuturant.

The breadth and diversity in participants God images was consistent with previous findings suggesting the varied and multidimensional aspects of the God image. A strength of Kunkel et al.'s (1999) study is the freedom allowed participants through the open ended response format employed. Interestingly, the God image list produced by respondents overlapped considerably with items used by previous investigators, including many of the items of the General Social Survey analyzed by Roof and Roof (1984) and Nelsen et al. (1985).

GENDER DIFFERENCES IN DIMENSIONS

Previous authors have speculated that given Christianity's tradition of using masculine language to describe God, men and women would respond differently to a male-imaged God leading to the development of distinguishable God images between the genders (Johnson, 1988). Jansen et al. (1994) found some support for this hypothesis in their research of the words adolescents use to describe God, finding that girls preferred words that indicated support and help while boys' text evidenced a preference for words indicating creation and power. Krejci (1998) compares the God images of men and women using multidimensional scaling analysis. Krejci's study differed from most previous studies in that it used multi-dimensional scaling analysis to uncover schemas that serve as a foundation for images of God and operate at an implicit

FIGURE 1. Kunkel et al.'s (1999) findings suggest that God images are organized along the dimensions of anthropomorphic versus mystical and punitive versus nurturant with distinct regions within and between the dimensions. (This figure is provided for the purpose of illustration only, the reader is referred to Kunkel et al.'s original article for a more detailed figure.)

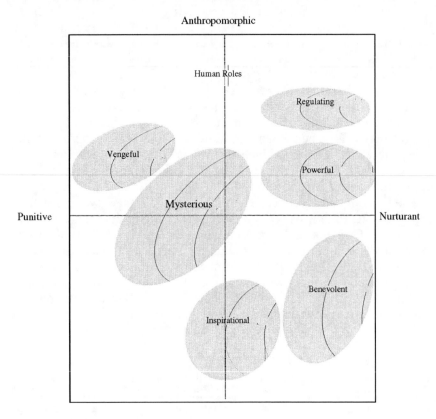

level, whereas most studies to date had relied on measuring individual's explicit rating of God images. His analysis suggested females and males utilize the same God image dimensions. Both genders organized their God schemas along three opposing images. While the expectation that men and women would develop different God images was not confirmed, the salience of the three dimensions did vary between genders. The three dimensions resulting from this research were: judging-nurturing, controlling-saving, and concrete-abstract. The judging-nurturing dimension was the overall most salient dimension. Controlling-saving was more salient for women than men, and it appears that women are more likely to image God along the saving end of this continuum while men are more likely to image God as controlling. The abstract-concrete dimension was the least utilized.

GOD IMAGE AND OTHER VARIABLES

In understanding the God image, it is useful to know how the God image is related to other variables. Researches exploring the relationship between the God image and other variables provide insight into how the God image relates to variables such as self-esteem, level of education, and belief system. There has also been much work done exploring the relationship of the God image to variables from participants' family of origin.

SELF-ESTEEM AND SELF-IMAGE

Theories of self-concept and self-esteem note that self-evaluation is at least partially related to how an individual perceives he or she is evaluated by others. One can hypothesize, as did Francis, Gibson, and Robbins (2001), that if one believes God views them as unworthy and miserable sinners their self-concept will tend to be more negative. In the same vein, individuals who view themselves in a depreciating and unworthy manner would tend to have similar views of others and God. On the other hand, if one perceives that God views them as unconditionally acceptable and accepted it would be anticipated that their self-concept would tend to be more positive in nature.

In previous research, Benson and Spilka (1973) explore this relationship between God images and scores on a self esteem inventory. They found, consistent with above notion, that self esteem scores were positively correlated with loving God images, but negatively correlated with rejecting, impersonal, vindictive, and controlling God images. Spilka, Addison, and Rosensohn (1975) supported these finding with further research suggesting that among male adolescents a positive self-image was negatively related to a wrathful God image, and among female students a positive self image was negatively related to a deistic God image and positively related to a loving, traditional, and kind God image.

Francis et al. (2001) selected a large sample of participants from secondary schools in Scotland and assessed the self worth and God images of each participant using brief measures. Their findings confirmed the basic findings of the Benson and Siplka (1973) and Spilka et al. (1975), again suggesting a positive relationship between self-worth and images of God as loving and forgiving, and a negative relationship between self-worth and images of God as cruel and punishing.

Belief System

Noting that parental images contribute to an individuals God image, Tamayo and Desjardins (1976), investigated whether on not an individual's belief system, defined as "a set of predispositions to perceive, feel toward, and respond to ego-involving stimuli and events in a consistent way" (p. 133) was related to their God image being more maternal or paternal. Tamayo and Desjardins' hypothesis was that the God image of concrete individuals would be more similar to the father image than the mother image, and that concrete individuals would show a preference for paternal values (authority, law, order, rules) which meet their need for structure and order. Because abstract individuals are more able to live with uncertainty and ambiguities and are able to integrate complex phenomena, the researchers predicted the individuals with an abstract belief system would have a God image consisting of a mixture of both parental images.

Tamayo and Desjardins's (1976) results support their hypothesis that individual with an abstract belief system have a parentally blended God image; one that consist of both paternal as well as maternal characteristics. Also, the paternal characteristic of the God image were significantly more emphasized by concrete individuals when compared to the emphasis on paternal characteristics of the abstract group. However, when considered alone, the concrete group emphasized both paternal and maternal characteristics equally. The researchers offer tentative explanations for this finding suggesting that the demand characteristics of the experimental situation and the measures used may have contaminated the responses received from the concrete individuals. More research is needed in this area.

Level of Education

In a study designed to investigate the influence of field of study, level of education, and gender on the conceptual images of mother, father, and God, Tamayo and Dugas (1977) found individual's field of study and level of education both affected their God image. Participants for this research were French Canadian undergraduate and graduate students. The research compared arts students to science students, undergraduate to graduate students, and males to females with regard to representation of mother, father, and God based on results of a semantic differential measure. Differences were found in the God images of art and science students; the God image of arts students was more maternal than paternal, while for the science and graduate students God was equally modeled on maternal and paternal images. Differences were also observed between the undergraduate and graduate students; undergraduate students modeled their image of God more on their parental images than did graduate students, perhaps suggesting that as individuals obtain higher intellectual development and professional training the similarity between their God image and parental images decrease. Interestingly, for the entire sample, the mother image, not the father, was the found to be the most accurate symbol for the representation of God, contradicting earlier theories (Freud, 1951, 1960) and research findings (Roof & Roof, 1984; Tamayo & Desjardins, 1976; Vergote, Tamayo, Pasquali, Bonami, Pattyn, & Custers, 1969) where the God image was shown to be either more paternal than maternal, or equally related to both images. These results taken together seem to indicate that either the father or the mother image can become the most accurate symbol of the God image, and the reader will note below how later researches have explained this complex relationship.

PARENTAL DYNAMICS IN FAMILY OF ORIGIN

Individuals may not be consciously aware of how their relationships with parents influence their experience of God. For example when asked directly whether they could see any correspondence among their God image and their parental image most respondents (56%) saw no resemblance to either father or mother figures, research has consistently reported a relationship between parental dynamics of one's family of origin and their God image. When a conscious resemblance is mentioned the mother is hardly ever referred to, instead, keeping with the classical picture of God as masculine and fatherly, the father is the most often mentioned by those who indicate a resemblance between their parental image and God image (Jansen et al., 1994). In fact the most widely researched variables with regard to the God image are those relating to family of origin and the influence of relationships with parents on participants' God image. Early researchers have demonstrated the possibility that the God image is sometimes significantly correlated with the mother image only (Nelson & Jones, 1957) or both the mother and father images (Strunk, 1959). Others provided support for a relationship between the God image and the preferred parent (Nelson, 1971).

Although most previous investigators considered the influences of maternal and/or paternal relationships, few examined the parental relationship as a composite. Noting this shortcoming, Birky and Ball (1987) investigated the relationship between an individual's "composite" parental image and their image of God. Some previous investigations (Nelsen et al. 1985; Roof & Roof, 1984; Tamayo & Desjardins, 1976; Vergote et al., 1969) comparing either one's mother or father image with their God image had led to discrepant conclusions regarding which image, the father or mother, had the most correspondence to one's God image. Birky and Ball asked subjects to rate traits descriptive of God, their father, their mother, and also to make ratings of their parents as a composite unit. The results did not indicate a singular importance of either the father or the mother in regard to correspondence to the subjects God image. The main contribution of Birky and Birky's research is their inclusion of the parental composite rating, which was found to be the closest to the God image rating, suggesting that for a God representation to be most fully understood, the influences of both parents must be examined as a composite and not only as singular representations themselves.

Recently, an increasing amount of research has considered attachment theory as an explanatory model for understanding the nature of individual's God image. Kirkpatrick (1992; Kirkpatrick & Shaver, 1990) was among the first to suggest attachment theory as a theoretical framework for understanding the nature of individuals' God images. While historically psychoanalytic theories have dominated as the main theories for conceptualizing individual religious experiences, these constructs have proven difficult to research. Classical psychoanalytic and object relations constructs lend themselves to case studies and qualitative methods of inquiry (i.e., Rizzuto, 1979), but contemporary research psychology has tended to value empirical quantitative research methods. The constructs of attachment theory are more conducive to this sort of research and, as Kirkpatrick notes, the God of most Christian traditions corresponds very closely to the idea of a secure attachment figure. Research into attachment styles and the God image focus on the idea of God serving as a secure base and on God's perceived availability/responsiveness, which provides comfort and security for the individual.

The God image may serve as an attachment figure, either in addition to or in lieu of relationships with parents, spouses, or lovers.

Much of the research conducted on individual differences in God images fit well within the attachment framework. The adjectives that individuals use to describe their experience of God correspond closely with the notion of secure attachment. For example, participants report they experience God as "loving" "protective," and "not distant," "not inaccessible" (Gorsuch, 1968; Spilka, Armatas & Nussbaum, 1964). Additionally, research findings on the link between parent-child relationships and the God image have been consistent with attachment theory (Nelson, 1971; Strunk, 1959). Also, the reported positive association between God images and self-concept or self-esteem (Benson & Spilka, 1973) is consistent with attachment theory's understanding of the relationship between models of self and models of attachment figures. Individuals who experience their attachment figures as loving and caring tend to view their self as lovable and worthy of being cared for, and visa versa.

From the research of Kirkpatrick and others, two hypothesis have arisen to explain the function of the God image within the context of attachment behavior. The first of these hypotheses, the compensation model, is supported by the research of Kirkpatrick and Shaver (1990). This model suggests that God can become a substitute attachment figure and the individual's God image compensates for needs of security and availability not fulfilled in the childhood parental relationships.

Kirkpatrick and Shaver (1990) used a modification of Benson and Spilka's (1973) Loving and Controlling God-image scales modified to include a Distant God-image scale. Perceptions of participants' parental religiosity was measured through items asking each respondent to rate their parents in terms of church attendance, commitment to religion and frequency with which religious issues were discussed in the home. Participants were also provided with a description of the secure, avoidant, and anxious/ambivalent patterns of attachment and rated their mother and father separately with regard to their recollection of their childhood relationship with each parent. Among the results of this study, was the finding that adults that had been reared by relatively non-religious mothers tended to report a God image that was characterized as loving, benevolent, and protective. With regard to maternal attachment, those reporting avoidant attachments scored highest in religiosity and had the highest mean scores on the loving God scale.

The above results lend support for the compensation hypothesis, suggesting that an individual's God image may serve as a substitute attachment figure and may develop in part out of needs to compensate for a lack of secure attachment with parents. However, other research suggests the correspondence hypothesis. The correspondence model states an individual's God image corresponds to their other interpersonal relationships. For example, an individual with a secure attachment style would be likely to have a God image that is characterized as loving and available. A study by Kirkpatrick and Shaver (1992) demonstrated this to be accurate for their participants. Adult attachment styles were compared cross-sectionally to a variety of religious variables, including one's God image. Individuals with a secure attachment style had a more loving and less distant God image compared to individuals with insecure attachment styles, suggesting a correspondence between interpersonal relationships and religious beliefs.

The findings which support the compensation hypothesis in one study and the correspondence hypothesis in a later study may seem paradoxical. However, Kirkpatrick (1997) notes that both are consistent with different aspects of attachment theory when consideration is given to the dynamics of attachment and the possibility of change over time as previously insecure attached individuals find substitute attachment figures. In order to understand the potential longitudinal change in adult attachment and religious variables, Kirkpatrick (1997) followed-up earlier research (Kirkpatrick & Hazen, 1994) to test the hypothesis that insecure respondents would report more positive perceptions about their relationship with God. The results of this longitudinal study provided further support for the compensation hypothesis. In an all women sample, females evidencing an insecure attachment style were more likely to have experienced a new relationship with God and were more likely to have reported having a religious experience or conversion between the initial study and the follow-up research. Kirkpatrick interprets these results to suggest that a relationship with God may serve as a compensatory function for individuals with insecure attachment styles. The anxious attached individuals were more likely than avoidant attached individuals to report an intensely emotional religious experience. It is supposed that avoidant attached individuals may experience their relationship with God in a less dramatic, more private manner.

While Kirkpatrick (1990) had used retrospective accounts of childhood relationships with parents, Dickie, Eshleman, Merasco, Shepard, Vander Wilt, and Johnson (1997) attempted to eliminate retrospective bias through directly exploring the relationships between children's images of God and their image of the parents. Building on the theoretical perspective of Kirkpatrick's compensation hypothesis, Dickie and colleagues expected that as children mature and become less dependent on parents the child's God image would shift to include more powerful and nurturing qualities to compensate for the expanding relational distance between the child and their parents who had been serving as the attachment figure.

As expected, Dickie et al. (1997) found evidence that children's perceptions of mother and father are related to their perceptions of God; children perceived God as similar to their parents in qualities of nurturance and power. As predicted by attachment theory, children's God images increase in these qualities with maturity; as children become more independent of parents, God becomes the substitute attachment figure. Dickie and colleagues did not differentiate between the participants attachment style, making it difficult to determine if God as a substitute attachment figure serves as a compensatory or corresponding attachment figure. The results of this study do not indicate, for example, whether or not insecure children experience God as more nurturing and powerful than secure children, as predicted from Kirkpatrick's (1990) work.

Dickie et al.'s (1997) results provide support for both the correspondence and compensation hypotheses. Younger children may fit the correspondence model, while through maturity and increasing separation from parents older children may developed a God image which compensates, in part, for maturational challenges. Other researches have suggested alternative explanations to resolve the correspondence-compensation hypothesis discrepancies. Granqvist and Hagekull (1999) proposed a revised correspondence hypothesis suggesting that securely attached children acquire religious beliefs and behavior through socialization. That is, children who have developed a secure attachment to their caregivers are more likely to be successfully socialized into their attachment figure's system of religious attitudes and behavior, and this would account for the strong correspondence in God image. Granqvist and Hagekull found support for this revised compensation hypotheses through research into adult's religiousness. Religiousness is a broad construct, but it would be expected to be related to individual's God image.

Preliminary empirical support for Granqvist and Hagekull's (1999) revised correspondence hypothesis with regard to the God image is found in the research of Herthel and Donahue (2001) who tested the hypothesis that parents' God images would influence their parenting style which in turn would influence their children's God images. They suggest parents socialize children to hold views of God similar to their own, in part through parenting styles. The results of Herthel and Donahue's study indicated youth's images of parents were predictive of the youth's God image, and parents' God images were predictive of the youth's God images. Additionally, parents' image of God as loving was a strong predictor of their children's image of parents as loving, suggesting that parents who experience God as loving parent their children in a loving manner thus conveying this loving God image to the child. Finally, congruent with most theories of attachment, the mothers' God image, more than the fathers', influenced the children's God image suggesting that mothers continue to serve as the primary attachment figure and dominate socializer in families.

Broader Family Context

Harking back to the work of Roof and Roof (1984) and the questions of the General Social Survey, Lee and Early (2000) utilized four God-image items (Mother vs. Father, Master vs. Spouse, Judge vs. Lover, and Friend vs. King) from the survey to assess an individual's God image in order to study the relationship between God images and family values. Their hypothesis was that more maternal and gracious images of God (Mother, Spouse, Lover, Friend) would be positively associated with progressivism and negatively associated with traditionalism within families. Families were given a list of 14 family arrangements and asked to answer whether or not each arrangement was a "family" to assess their alignment with progressive family values. Traditional family values were measured by a separate scale. Indeed, the more maternal and gracious images of God were positively correlated with progressive family attitudes, and negatively correlated with the measure of traditional values, suggesting that God-images are predictive of family attitudes in the sense that God-image are assumed to develop prior to social attitudes about families.

THE GOD-IMAGE IN PATHOLOGY AND TREATMENT

Relatively few empirical studies have been conducted to investigate the relationship between pathology and the God image. Two studies reported here address more severe pathology including dissociative disorders and character disorders, and another reported study examines depression. Bowman, Coons, Jones, and Oldstrom (1987) studied the God images in a small sample of seven women with multiple personality disorder (now referred to a Dissociative Identity Disorder or DID).

The diagnosis of Dissociatve Identity Disorder is controversial, and the generalization of Bowman et al.'s findings is risky due to the extremely small sample size and absence of statistical analysis with regard to the significance of the reported results. Yet their observations regarding the relationship between the God image and personality development are interesting.

Bowman et al. (1987) theoretical perspective is that personalities are developed through partial identification with parents or other important figures from early life. With the correlation between God image and images of self and parents being known, Bowman and colleagues hypothesized each DID patient would have multiple God images corresponding to their multiple personality, and also that patient's God images would show splits similar to the splits in their parental images. Each participant who had previously been diagnosed with DID was interviewed using a religious ideation interview which included questions relative to their God image. In order to assess differences between participants' multiple personalities, each participant was interviewed twice with a primary and a secondary personality being assessed.

No one patient's two personalities espoused the same God image; instead each personality held conflicting parts of the total God image. While all the primary personalities reported a confident belief in God's existence, two of the secondary personalities interviewed denied any belief in God. The primary personalities, while reportedly certain of God's existence, were as a group largely ambivalent in their God images. Bowman and her colleagues were not surprised by the primary personalities observed ambivalence about God, suggesting it makes sense when put in context of the conflicting parental behaviors these primary personalities experienced leading to the eventual personality split. The conflicted God images correspond to the conflicting images of parents and of themselves (Benson & Spilka, 1973).

The secondary personalities in Bowman et al.'s (1987) study were reportedly clear cut and succinct in their God images. This observation corresponds to the object relations theory of multiple personalities which holds that the secondary personalities are formed as a defensive maneuver to resolve the ambivalent feelings caused by conflicting object representations of the parents. Additionally, while the primary personalities reported strong interactions with God and frequent attendance of religions services, the secondary personalities rejected interactions with God and reported rare involvement in religious services. Again, generalization of these observations are dangerous, but they do point to the complexity of the God image, and suggest severe trauma experiences may impact its development.

A growing area of research is the relationship between religiosity and psychological distress. In a study of the relationship between religious strain and psychological distress, with a clinical sample of 54 individuals seeking treatment at an anxiety and depression clinic, Exline, Yali, and Sanderson (2000) found depression to be associated with an alienating God image. Exline and colleagues assessed participants with regard to their religiosity and the comfort and/or strain associated with their religiosity. As expected, the experience of religious strain was associated with both depression and suicidality. Interestingly, of all the potential religious strains assessed, feeling alienated from God was the major predictor of depression. These results suggest that the pessimistic appraisal of self, other, and world associated with the experience of depression may also affect the person's God image. However, as noted by the researchers, the reverse may also be true. A negative God image may color the individual's perceptions of self, other, and world leading to depression and other forms of psychological distress.

Psychological problems are often observed to be related to the religious experience of the patient. Schaap-Jonker, Eureling-Bontekow, Verhagen, and Zock (2002) provide evidence that the God image can be influenced by pathological personality traits. Individuals with personality traits consistent with borderline, avoidant, schizotypal, schizoid, dependent, and paranoid personality disorders evidence more negative feelings toward God. More specifically, individuals with personality traits consistent with the schizotypal, avoidant, obsessive-compulsive, and paranoid disorders often view God's actions as negative. The greater the level of pathology, the more negative are the implications for the God image. Schapp-Jonker et al. (2002) were able to characterize God images according to personality disorder clusters. Participants scoring high on cluster A (paranoid, schizoid, and schizotypal) personality traits have a God image of a passive, aloof, distant, and unsupportive God, paralleling the way individuals with these personality traits relate to others. Similarly, individuals scoring high on cluster C traits (avoidant, dependent, and obsessive-compulsive) experience God as being dominate and punishing, in accordance with how individuals with obsessive-compulsive personality disorder relate to others with their controlling, rigid adherence to rules and regulations. Participants with cluster B traits (antisocial, borderline, and histrionic) tended to be less predicable in their God images.

Only a few empirical studies have explored the effect that psychotherapy may have on the God image. However, from these few studies there is evidence that psychotherapy does have a positive effect on individuals' God images. In an investigation of the relationship of inpatient treatment of depression and patients' God image, Tisdale, Key, Edwards, Brokaw, Kemperman, and Cloud (1997) found inpatient treatment had a significant positive effect on patients' personal adjustment and God image. The inpatient treatment program was grounded in object relations theory and included an integration of religious teachings and practices. Measures at discharge of patients' personal adjustment and God image indicated a significantly more positive views of themselves as well as a significant shift in their God image toward closeness, lovingness, being present and being accepting. Follow-up assessments suggested these changes were maintained up to a year after treatment.

Further evidence that individuals' God image can change as they achieve personal growth is found in Cheston, Piedmont, Earnes, and Lavin (2003) research. These researchers found a significant positive relationship between personal growth and positive change in the God image for individuals who participated in outpatient therapy compared to a no-treatment control group. Therapy patients ratings of God's perceived neuroticism (tendency to experience negative affect such as anxiety, depression, and hostility) declined significantly at the end of the study while their ratings of God's perceived agreeableness (tendency to show compassion rather than be antagonistic) had significantly increased compared the control group's God image ratings . Additionally, the God image of individuals evidencing a high degree of emotional change became more emotionally stable, less assertive, and more compassionate and loving through the course of therapy. More research is needed to explore this relationship between the growth that occurs through the therapy process and changes in individual's God image.

CONCLUSION AND AREAS FOR FUTURE INVESTIGATION

Within all the research domains noted above there is opportunity for further investigation in order to help behavioral scientists and clinicians more fully understand the depth and breadth of the dynamics of the God image construct. It is evident the God image is a multidimensional construct (Kunkel et al., 1990), but further investigation is needed to differentiate those variables which influence the various dimensions including developmental tasks and the environmental context. The compensation-correspondence hypotheses model (Kirkpatrick and Shaver, 1990; Kirkpatrick, 1997; Dickie et al., 1997; Granqvist and Hagekull, 1999; Herthel and Donahue, 2001) has added greatly to our understanding of the varying ways family dynamics and attachment may influence the development of the God image within the individual. Yet, there still are lingering questions regarding how these apparent contradictory explanations coincide. There is much clinical usefulness to be found in the knowledge researchers have provided on the God image construct and its relationship to the interpersonal and intrapsychic dynamics of the person. However, more research is needed in clinical treatment settings to address the relationship between the God image and mental illness including how psychological treatments influence individual's experience of God. With all the areas that been investigated, there are some that have yet to be explored. Very little research has investigated issues of diversity related to the God image construct, and more about this is mentioned below. Additionally, with the increasing sophistication of research methodologies and means of statistical analysis it is important to revisit the issues of epistemological concerns of previous God image research in order to encourage further development of means to assess the complexities of the God image construct.

Diversity

Few attempts have been made at differentiating the God image of individuals of different social-cultural backgrounds including racial background and sexual orientation. Hoffman et al. and Hoffman, Knight, Boscoe-Huffman, and Stewart (2006) are among the few researchers who have addressed issues of diversity in relation to the God image. Hoffman et al.'s (2005) research examined the influence of various expressions of diversity on the God image through comparison of a broad set of demographic variables to individual's God image. In their assessment of racial identity, the researches used a measure of "Whiteness" to differentiate how strongly each participant identified themselves as White. Their findings suggest that individual's identifying themselves as multiracial and partially Whites were less likely to report a God image typified by egocentrism (focusing on the self in relation to God) or benevolence, while those who identified themselves as non-White were more likely to report a God image typified by egocentrism or benevolence. Although this initial research of Hoffman et al. (2005) begins to answer questions regarding racial identity and the God image, much more work is needed in order to provide an understanding of how the dimensions of the God image may vary among individuals of different racial-ethnic backgrounds.

Although research on racial-ethnic diversity is sparse, research on sexual orientation and the God image is nearly non-existent. Hoffman et al. (2006) discuss the theoretical considerations related to the homosexual's experience of God. Included among these are issues related to whether or not the individual views a homosexual lifestyle as sinful or immoral. The individual's understanding of their sexual behavior would be expected to have an impact upon the individual's experience of God, and visa-versa, the individual's God image would be expected to influences feelings of guilt, shame, or pride associated with their lifestyle. Hoffman (2004) notes, religious experiences can be filled with paradoxes for gay and lesbian individuals. They may hold an image of God characterized by love, acceptance, and nurturance, but consistently experience rejection and judgment from other religious believers. Research into the impact of the paradoxical and confusing experiences on the individual's God image is an area that remains largely unexplored.

Epistemological Concerns

This chapter began with a statement pointing out the inevitable difficulties created for social scientists in researching religious experience. In many ways the process of measuring the God image is still in development and researchers have had expected difficulty devising a reliable and thorough measure of the God image do largely to the subjectivity with which individuals experience God. In the majority of the research reported in this chapter, investigators have used quantitative surveys, checklists, or questionnaires to elucidate individual's God image. Unfortunately, few investigators have given attention to qualitative and/or experiential methods for assessing the God image in order to adequately assess the dynamic relational factors of the construct.

The God image may be more flexible and shifting than previous research would lead one to believe (Hill & Hall, 2002). Hoffman, Grimes, and Acoba (2005) have noted the limitation of most quantitative measurement of the God image, which is the inability to move beyond the conscious conceptions of God to asses the unconscious processes related to the God image. They suggest, based on the work of Hall and Porter (2004), that not only may God images change over the person's lifespan, but also different experiences of God may occur concurrently at different levels of processing. Additionally, the God image may change, at least partially, due to the environment and contextual cues.

Future research will need to evaluate these assumptions through the development of research methods able to assess the fluidity and unconscious processes which contribute to the God image. Although challenging, research into the God image construct is a worthy endeavor and future research findings will no doubt shed more light on this sometimes mysterious construct.

REFERENCES

Bassinger, D. (1990). The measurement of religiousness: Some "philosophical" concerns. *Journal of Psychology and Christianity, 9,* 5-13.

Benson, P., & Spilka, B. (1973). God image as a function of self-esteem and locus of control. *Journal for the Scientific Study of Religion, 12,* 297-310.

Birky, I. T., & Ball, S., (1987). Parental trait influence on God as an object representation. *Journal of Psychology, 122,* 133-137.

Bowman, E. S., Coons, P. M., Jones, R. S., & Oldstrom, M. (1987). Religious psychodynamics in multiple personalities: Suggestions for treatment. *American Journal of Psychotherapy, 41,* 542-554.

Cheston, S. E., Piedmont, R. L., Eanes, B., & Patrice, L. (2003). Changes in client's images of God over the course of outpatient therapy. *Counseling and Values, 47,* 96-108.

Cox, R., Ervin-Cox, B., & Hoffman, L. (Eds.). (2005). *Spirituality and psychological health.* Colorado Springs: Colorado School of Professional Psychology Press.

Dickie, J. R., Eshleman, A. K., Merasco, D. M., Shepard, A., Vander Wilt, M., & Johnson M. (1997). Parent-child relationships and children's images of God. *Journal for the Scientific Study of Religion, 36,* 24-43.

Ervin-Cox, B., Hoffman, L., & Grimes, C. S. M. (2005). Selected literature review on spirituality and health/mental health. In R. Cox, B. Ervin-Cox, & L. Hoffman (Eds.), *Spirituality and psychological health.* Colorado Springs: Colorado School of Professional Psychology Press.

Exline, J. J., Yali, A. M., & Sanderson, W. C. (2000). Guilt, discord, and alienation: The role of religious strain in depression and suicidality. *Journal of Clinical Psychology, 56,* 1481-1496.

Francis, L. J., Gibson, H. M., & Robbins, M. (2001). God images and self-worth among adolescents in Scotland. *Mental Health, Religion & Culture, 4,* 103-108.

Freud, S. (1950). *Totem and taboo* (J. Strachey trans.) New York; Norton & Company. (Original work published in 1938).

Freud, S. (1961). *The future of an illusion* (J. Strachey trans.). New York: Norton & Company. (Original work published in 1927).

Granqvist, P., & Hagekull, B. (1999). Religiousness and perceived childhood attachment: Profiling socialized correspondence and emotional compensation. *Journal for the Scientific Study of Religion, 38,* 254-273.

Grosuch, R. L. (1968). The conceptualization of God as seen in adjective ratings. *Journal for the Scientific Study of Religion, 7,* 56-64

Hall, T. W., & Porter, S. L. (2004). Referential integration: An emotional information process perspective on the process of integration. *Journal of Psychology and Theology, 32,* 167-180.

Hertel, B., & Donahue, M. (1995). Parental influences on God images among children: Testing Durkheim's metaphoric parallelism. *Journal for the Scientific Study of Religion, 34,* 186-199.

Hill, P. C., & Hall, T. W. (2002). Relational schemas in processing one's image of God and self. *Journal of Psychology and Christianity, 31,* 365-375.

Hoffman, L. (2004, October). *Cultural constructions of the god image and God concept: Implications for culture, psychology, and religion.* Paper presented at the joint meeting of the Society for the Scientific Study of Religion and Religious Research Association, Kansas City, MO.

Hoffman, L. (2005). *A developmental perspective on the God image.* In R. H. Cox, B. Cox, & L. Hoffman (Eds.), *Spirituality and Psychological Health.* Colorado School of Professional Psychology Press, Colorado Springs, CO.

Hoffman, L., Grimes, C. S. M., & Acoba, R. (2005, November). Research on the experience of God: Rethinking epistemological assumptions. Paper presented at 2005 Annual Meeting of The Society for the Scientific Study of Religion, Rochester, NY.

Hoffman, L., Hoffman, J., Dillard, K., Clark, J., Acoba, R., Williams, F., Jones, T. (2005, April). Cultural diversity and the God image: Examining cultural difference in the experience of God. Paper presented at the Christian Association for Psychological Studies International Conference, Dallas, TX.

Hoffman, L. Knight, S., Boscoe-Huffman, S., & Stewart, S. (2006, August). *Religious experience, gender, and sexual orientation.* Paper presented at the American Psychological Association Annual Convention, New Orleans, LA.

Jansen, J., De Hart, J., & Gerardts, M. (1994). Images of God in adolescence. *The International Journal for the Psychology of Religion, 4,* 105-121.

Johnson, R. (1988). The theology of gender. *Journal of Psychology and Christianity, 7,* 39-49.

Kirkpatrick, L. A. (1992). An attachment-theoretical approach to the psychology of religion. *International Journal for the Psychology of Religion, 2,* 3-38.

Kirkpatrick, L. A. (1997). A longitudinal study of changes in religions belief and behavior as a function of individual differences in adult attachment style. *Journal for the Scientific Study of Religion, 36,* 207-217.

Kirkpatrick, L. A., & Hazan, C. (1994). Attachment style, gender, and relationship stability: A longitudinal analysis. *Personal Relationships 1,* 123-42.

Kirkpatrick, L. A., & Shaver, P. R. (1990). Attachment theory and religion: Childhood attachment, religious beliefs and conversion. *Journal for the Scientific Study of Religion, 29,* 315-334.

Koenig, H. G. (1998). *Handbook of religion and mental health.* San Diego: Academic Press.

Krejci, M. J. (1998). Gender comparison of God schemas; A multidimensional scaling analysis. *The International Journal for the Psychology of Religion, 8,* 57-56.

Kunkel, M. A., Cook, S., Meshel, D. S., Daughtry, D., & Hauenstein, A. (1999). God images: A concept map. *Journal for the Scientific Study of Religion, 38,* 193-202.

Lee, C., & Early, A. (2000). Religiosity and family values: Correlates of God-image in a protestant sample. *Journal of Psychology and Theology, 28,* 229-239.

Nelson, M. O. (1971). The concept of God and feeling toward parents. *Journal of Individual Psychology 27*, 46-49.

Nelson, M. O., & Jones, E. M. (1957). An application of the Q technique to the study of religious concepts. *Psychological Reports, 3*, 293-297

Nelsen, H., Cheek, Jr., N. H., & Au, P. (1985). Gender differences in images of God. *Journal for the Scientific Study of Religion, 24*, 396-402.

Piedmont, R. L., & Muller, J. (2006, August). Are God image and God concept redundant constructs? Poster presented at the 2006 Annual Convention of the American Psychological Association, New Orleans, LA.

Rizzuto, A. M. (1979). *The birth of the living God: A psychoanalytic study.* Chicago: University of Chicago Press.

Roof, W. C., & Roof, J. (1984). Review of the polls: Images of God among Americans. *Journal for the Scientific Study of Religion, 23*, 201-205.

Schaap-Jonker, H., Eurelings-Bontekoe, E., Verhagen, P., & Zock, H. (2002). Image of God and personality pathology: An exploratory study among psychiatric patients. *Mental health, religion & culture, 5*, 55-71.

Spilka, B., Addison, J., & Rosensohn, M.. (1975). Parents, self, and God: A test of competing theories of individual-religion relationships. *Review of Religions Research, 16*, 154-165.

Spilka, B., Armatas, P., & Nussbaum, J., (1964). The concept of God: A factor analytic study. *Review of Religious Research, 16*, 154-165

Strunk, O. L., Jr.. (1959). Perceived relationships between parental and deity concepts. *Psychology Newsletter, 10*, 222-226

Tamayo, A., & Dugas, A. (1977). Conceptual representations of mother, father, and God according to sex and field of study. *The Journal of Psychology, 97*, 79-84.

Tamayo, A., & Desjardins, L., (1976). Belief systems and conceptual images of parents and God. *Journal of Psychology 92*, 131-140.

Tisdale, T. C., Key, T. L., Edwards, K., J., Brokaw, B. F., Kemperman, S. R., & Cloud, H. (1997). Impact of God image and personal adjustment, and correlations of the God image to personal adjustment and object relations development. *Journal of Psychology and Theology, 25*, 227-239.

Vergote, A., Tamayo, A., Pasquali, L., Bonami, M., Pattyn., M. R., & Custers, A. (1969). Concept of God and parental images. *Journal for the Scientific Study of Religion, 8*, 79-87.

doi:10.1300/J515v09n03_02

Chapter 3

Psychodynamic Theories
of the Evolution of the God Image

James W. Jones, PsyD, PhD, ThD

SUMMARY. This paper discusses the clinical, psychodynamic approach to understanding the internal God-image. Such an approach reveals the ways in which these internal images are rooted in and linked to the person's developmental history and their character and personality style. The works of Freud, Rizzuto (and its grounding in the theories of Fairbairn and Winnicott), Spero, and their utilization by other writers are discussed and evaluated in some detail. Theological and pastoral implications of this work are also alluded to here. doi:10.1300/J515v09n03_03 *[Article copies available for a fee from The Haworth Document Delivery Service: 1-800-HAWORTH. E-mail address: <docdelivery@haworthpress.com> Website: <http://www.HaworthPress.com> © 2007 by The Haworth Press. All rights reserved.]*

INTRODUCTION

For decades researchers have investigated people's images of God. For example, an early study by Spilka and colleagues found that images of God

[Haworth co-indexing entry note]: "Psychodynamic Theories of the Evolution of the God Image." Jones, James W. Co-published simultaneously in *Journal of Spirituality in Mental Health* (The Haworth Pastoral Press, an imprint of The Haworth Press) Vol. 9, No. 3/4, 2007, pp. 33-55; and: *God Image Handbook for Spiritual Counseling and Psychotherapy: Research, Theory, and Practice* (ed: Glendon L. Moriarty, and Louis Hoffman) The Haworth Pastoral Press, an imprint of The Haworth Press, 2007, pp. 33-55. Single or multiple copies of this article are available for a fee from The Haworth Document Delivery Service [1-800-HAWORTH, 9:00 a.m. - 5:00 p.m. (EST). E-mail address: docdelivery@haworthpress.com].

Available online at http://jsmh.haworthpress.com
© 2007 by The Haworth Press. All rights reserved.
doi:10.1300/J515v09n03_03

as loving were associated with higher levels of self-esteem while images of God as wrathful, controlling, or uninvolved were associated with less self-esteem (Spilka et al., 1964; Benson & Spilka, 1973). In a study that creates problems for Freudian theory, Vergote and his colleagues found that people's images of God consistently resembled their maternal relationship rather than their image of their father (Vergote & Tamayo, 1981). Later studies have found that children tend to model God on whichever parent is more salient in the child's life (Dickie, Eshleman, Merasco, Shepard, VanderWilt, & Johnson, 1997) and that for young adults their own self-concept and level of self-esteem are more significant influences on their concept of God than are their parental characteristics (Buri & Mueller, 1993). Recent studies have also underscored the importance of self-esteem in the development the individual's personal image of God (Dickie, Ajega, Kobylak, & Nixon, 2006).

These studies involve people's conscious beliefs about God's existence (or non-existence) and nature. Most are carried out by personality psychologists using empirical methods to ascertain the correlations between beliefs about God and other variables (personality traits, religious involvement, gender, various behaviors, etc.). At the same time, researchers who are primarily clinicians working with patients, mainly from a psychodynamic perspective, have also been studying and reflecting on the psychological nature of religious belief and practice. Their studies suggest that conscious beliefs about God rest upon and carry more elaborate and complex unconscious dynamics.

These two approaches are more complementary than contradictory. The correlational approach uncovers possible connections between beliefs about God and aspects of a person's personality and behavior. The clinical, psychodynamic approach suggests ways in which these beliefs are rooted in and linked to the person's developmental history, their character, and personality style. Such a clinical, psychodynamic approach is the topic of this chapter.

In addition, since this book is primarily directed at pastoral counselors, pastors, and clinicians specializing in religious and spiritual issues, I will be indicating a few of the theological implications of this material. There is not space to develop these in any depth but it is important for the theologically sensitive reader to keep in mind that these psychological models, like all psychological models, have theological implications–that is implications for understanding human nature, religious experience, claims about the possibility of religious knowledge, and (as we shall see in the next few pages) even about the nature of God.

Sigmund Freud

Like most clinical, psychodynamic theorizing, psychoanalytic discussions of an internalized God image begin with Sigmund Freud. According to Freud, children (remember he's speaking here primarily about male children) internalize a representation of the father as they resolve the Oedipal Complex. This internalization forms the nucleus around which the internal God image is built. For Freud, God is a father figure, pure and simple. For Freud, the origin of the internalized God image is in the Oedipal period. The result is an internalized image of a patriarchal deity of law, guilt, and subjugation. Freud's treatise *Totem and Taboo* (1913/1950) casts this oedipal drama backward in time so that the origin of the individual's religion becomes the model for the origin of culture. Freud begins his history of culture and religion with, "there is a violent and jealous father who keeps all the females for himself and drives away his sons as they grow up" (p. 41). Once the Oedipal situation was set up, the result was inescapable. Eventually the sons murdered the primordial father (1913/1950, pp. 141-142). Thus, the history of culture parallels individual development; instinct-driven ambivalence for the father is the key to both. After the sons acted out their jealousy and hatred, the other side of their ambivalence emerged: love replaced hate. At first the sons hated their father who stood in the way of their boundless desire for power and sex. But they loved and admired him too. After murdering him, their affection for him, which they had had to deny in order to kill him, reappeared as guilt and remorse. This is how guilt, on which all religion depends according to Freud, originated (1913/1950). He stated, "We cannot get away from the assumption that man's sense-of-guilt springs from the Oedipus complex" (1931/1962, p. 78).

The murderous sons of the primal father, the harbingers of all religion and civilization, had to find a way to make peace with their returning repressed guilt. The solution was to identify with the father and internalize his image. Thus patriarchal theism was born. Freud remains convinced that the root of all images of God is a "longing for the father" (Freud, 1913/1950, p. 148). An ambivalent relationship to one's father is the core of all religion: "Religion, morals, society and art converge in the Oedipus complex. . . . The problems of social psychology, too, prove soluble on the basis of one single concrete point - man's relation to his father" (1913/1950, p. 157). Superego masochism is the foundation of morality, religion, and civilization. This oedipal legacy of patriarchal theism becomes the lens through which all religious history is to be seen. "The god of each of them is formed in the likeness of the father, his personal relation to God depends on his relation to his father . . . at bottom God is nothing other than an exalted father." (1913/1950, p. 147). Freud is convinced that the murder of the father and its continual replay in fantasy and culture is the unconscious center of all images of the divine.

In dissolving the Oedipus complex, the males of the species, the creators of culture, simultaneously renounce their attachment to their mother and internalize an image of their father. For it is the internalized image of the father, as ego-ideal, that is foundation of culture and religion. In the resolution of the male Oedipus complex the connection to the mother is displaced by an identification with the father. The same displacement of the feminine by the masculine takes place in psychoanalytic theorizing, as the pre-oedipal, mother-dominated period is downplayed in favor of the developmental centrality of the oedipal, father-dominated stage. And, keeping to the parallel between individual and cultural development, Freud confesses he can find no place "for the great mother goddesses, who may perhaps in general have preceded the father gods" (1913/1950, p. 149). This oversight surely parallels the fact that he can find no place in his theory for the pre-oedipal, maternal period in human development except its displacement by a normative patriarchy. With the coming of the oedipal period individually and prehistorically, the normative ethos of patriarchy returned. "With the introduction of father deities a fatherless society gradually changed into one organized on a patriarchal basis . . . it gave back to fathers a large portion of their former rights" (1913/1950, p. 149).

Freud's analysis of religion depends on this very specific idea about the believer's internal image of God. The patriarchal God of law and guilt is the only image of God Freud will consider. If he were to give up that paternal representation of God as normative, his argument would lose much of its force. Freud reproduces the exclusive, patriarchal monotheism of Western religion in his theory of the exclusively oedipal and paternal origins of culture, religion, and morality. Freud must insist that religion is essentially patriarchal, for that is the only religion that fits within the frame of the oedipal drama and that can easily be derived from the instinct theory. "Without prejudice to any other sources or meanings of the concept of God, upon which psychoanalysis can throw no light, the paternal element in that concept must be a most important one" (1913/1950, p. 147).

Freud's analysis points to the deep psychodynamic connections between patriarchal cultures, paternalistic images of the deity, and guilt-engendering religions. Such connections, common in the history of religion, are not coincidental but can be explained by the Oedipus complex understood not as biological necessity but as cultural expression. Exploring oedipal dynamics reveals the ways males in a patriarchal culture identify with the father and internalize the motifs of dominance and submission, detached and impersonal experiences of power, and the need for distance. The divine, when encountered in the context of these masculine identifications, is experienced in terms of dominance and submission and transcendental power and control. And when morality is worked out in the same context, the result is an ethics of law backed up by sacred power and dominance. The result is patriarchal divine image of law and power in which submission to the law of the father is the primary moral imperative and guilt the main religious emotion. Such a psychodynamic conclusion has an important theological implication: any attempt to rethink the gender categories of Western religion will involve more than just substituting *she* for *he* in reference to God in theological and liturgical texts. Any such theological reformation means transforming traditional models of divine authority and power and rethinking the nature of ethics.

In one or two places Freud speaks of the "father of personal pre-history"–a shadowy, psychoanalytic postulation of a pre-Oedipal relationship with the father. It is not really an internalization or an identification, rather this phrase appears to refer to a more primitive, pre-verbal relationship with the father. According to Freud, this pre-Oedipal relationship with the father is totally wiped out, repressed beyond recall, by the sexually charged Oedipal/Electra dynamics. For Freud this "father of personal pre-history" is not connected with the internalized God image. God is wholly and completely a recapitulation of the patriarchal, Oedipal father of guilt and authority. The internal image of God does not arise from the pre-Oedipal period for Freud, but only as a result of Oedipal dynamics.

Ana-María Rizzuto

For Freud, the father was the major object internalized by the developing (male) child. While remaining loyal to the centrality of instinctual drives in shaping the personality, Melanie Klein broadened Freud's account to include the mother and any other significant figures in the child's early life. W. R. D. Fairbairn extended this model even further (see Jones, 1996). For Fairbairn one's entire personality is structured by the internalization of interpersonal experiences. Fairbairn's is a consistently relational model of personality development, leaving little role of the instinctual drives that were the centerpieces of Freud's and Klein's theories. For Fairbairn, personality and behavior are organized around and motivated by a primary drive to establish and maintain connections with others.

Fairbairn (1943) maintained all aspects of the personality are connected to experiences with others that have been internalized. Internalization is not a mechanical recording of impressions. It is not a kind of psychological photography, although Fairbairn's term *internal image* suggests that misunderstanding. Rather, internalization is an active, constructive processes by which relational experiences structure and transform the personality.

Among the psychoanalytic investigators who have approached religion in terms of the process of object relations is Ana-María Rizzuto. As a clinical practitioner, she conducts her research in a patient centered way that produces a very experience-near account of the origin of the internalized God image that differs significantly from Freud's account (McDargh, 1997).In her pioneering study entitled *The Birth of the Living God* (1973), she investigated "the possible origins of the individual's private representation of God" (Rizzuto, 1979, p. 3). Rizzuto collected information on the family, developmental history, and religious convictions of several psychiatric patients and then had them draw pictures of their families and their gods. From this project she proposed several theses that draw upon object-relations models of personality like that of Fairbairn:

1. The child internalizes his interactions with the world in terms of a variety of "object representations." These are complex phenomena that may include, among other things, somatic sensations, affects, and concepts.
2. These discrete memories are consolidated into ever more complex sets of representations. For example, an internal representation of the child's mother may be an amalgamation of sensations of being held and rocked, the sound of her voice, all the feelings it generated, and the need to idealize her.
3. An internal representation of God is the apex of this process of consolidating object representations into a coherent inner object world; it is compounded out of the bits and pieces of object representations the child has at her disposal. The internal God image, Rizzuto says "is created from representational materials whose

sources are the representations of primary objects" (Rizzuto, 1979, p. 178).

Rizzuto uses Kohut's concept of mirroring to explain the early creation of the God representation out of the experience of the mother (Rizzuto, 1979). Our earliest sense of self, she suggests, grows from seeing our self mirrored in our mother's reactions. For Rizzuto, this early experience of mirroring, which forms the basis of a cohesive sense of self, lies at the core of our God representation. All other images that are joined to it in the elaboration of our private God representation are colored by that core mirroring experience (or lack of it) with the mother.

The child's development of a cohesive sense of self makes use of a representation of God to mirror and focus the self's integrative processes. This internalized God image serves to consolidate the bits and pieces of a person's inner representational world. The term *religion* comes from the Latin word *religio* which means, among other things, "to bind together." Psychodynamically religion binds self-experiences together. Rizzuto writes that "the sense of self is in fact in dialectical interaction with a God representation that has become essential to the maintenance of the sense of being oneself" (Rizzuto,1979, p. 5).

In addition, she says that every child is an implicit philosopher, wondering about the origin of the world, and each needs the idea of God to answer the question "why?" The idea of God is, also, developmentally necessary to ground our earliest awareness of the existence of things.[1] One significant and controversial implication of Rizzuto's work is that everyone, of necessity, forms some internal God representation in order to end the infinite regress of questions about the origin of the world and to consolidate the representational fragments born of his or her early life (McDargh, 1997). This representation is there whether or not the person, as Rizzuto says, "uses it for belief" (Rizzuto, 1979, p. 200). Often when students have spoken at great length with me about how they do not believe in God, I ask them to tell me about the God they do not believe in. *And they always answer.* They have a very clear idea of who or what God is, even though they don't believe in "him." And I must observe in passing that their images are often of a God that I wouldn't believe in either. However cognitively compelling it may be, total atheism for Rizzuto is a psychodynamic impossibility. Everyone has some image of God, even if the person rejects it as an object of faith.

Rizzuto (1979) suggests that the God representation is reworked, added to, and transformed as the individual goes through life and brings new experiences to his or her inner representational world. Whether one becomes an atheist or a devotee is determined by whether or not one's image of God fits or can be reworked to fit one's needs at any given developmental stage. In Rizzuto's words,

> Belief in God or its absence depends upon whether or not a conscious identity of experience can be established between the God representation of a given developmental moment and the object and self-representations needed to maintain a sense of self. (p. 202)

For example, one of her subjects' image of God was so tinctured with masochistic anger and destructive rage (from the subject's experience with his father) that he was unable to make use of it as he grew up; he rejected any idea of God because the pain associated with it was intolerable. This raises an important point for the psychology of religion. Freud considered atheism as normative; atheism required no further analysis, only religious belief did. Rizzuto's work makes clear that the lack of belief in God is just as much a product of the individual's personal history and psychodynamic development as is belief in God. Atheism too should be subject to analysis (Jones, 1996, 1991).

Every developmental stage is also a crisis of belief since it demands that the God image be reworked to fit a new conception of self. If the God image is too brittle or rigid, it cannot be reworked and must be rejected in order for development to continue. As Rizzuto writes, her "central thesis is that God as a transitional representation needs to be recreated in each developmental crisis if it is to be found relevant for lasting belief" (Rizzuto, 1979, p. 208). Given the plasticity of the idea of God, it can be continually refashioned and so need not be discarded as the person encounters new experiences requiring incorporation into his or her ever-developing sense of self. However fixed it may appear from the outside, internally the life of faith is an ongoing series of major and minor transformations and adjustments in the central image of God. Creedal formulations and ritual actions may remain unchanged from childhood to old age, but their inner meaning to the believer is continually being updated on the basis of new experiences.

In treating the internal God image in terms of object relations, Rizzuto's language often contains the same ambiguity found in Fairbairn. Rizzuto frequently speaks of internalizations, including those relating to God, as "images," "object-representations," "objects," and "perceptual memories"–terms conveying an image of a tiny snapshot of the object within our heads. In keeping with this model of internalizations, much of her study is taken up with drawing connections between a patient's parental representations and the origins and transformations of his or her God representation. Although it is clear that the internalization of objects cannot be separated from our relationship with them, Rizzuto tends to focus more on the internalized objects themselves and less on the internalized relationships (Jones, 1991).

For Rizzuto, the root of the internalized God image is the interpersonal experience of being mirrored. The heart of the internal God image is the experience of presence, of standing in relationship to another. This is strikingly different from Freud's model. For him the experience at the core of the internalized image of God is of feeling guilty, of being judged, of dependency on a superior power. Hers is a model of religion built on a sense of presence; his is a model of religion built around law and guilt. This is an important theological point. Rizzuto and Freud represent not only two different models of personality–a relational model and a drive model in textbook language–but implicitly they also represent two different theologies. Hers is a pre-Oedipal religion of presence and relationship; his is an Oedipal religion of law and authority.

How might these two different implicit theologies be related psychologically? Perhaps they represent two different religious trajectories built around two different psychodynamic core experiences. Or perhaps they are related developmentally. Does the pre-Oedipal religion of presence develop first with an Oedipal religion of law and authority layered on top of it? Does the paternal, Oedipal religion obliterate the earlier maternal religion? Or transform it? Or does the earlier one remain as a necessary foundation?

In any case, there is an important point here on the boundary of theology and psychoanalytic psychology. Conscious beliefs about God, whether devout or atheistic, rest on unconscious processes and come with a long and complicated developmental history. Rizzuto's research implies that attempts to inculcate or transform a person's conscious beliefs about God by purely conscious means (preaching, theological lecturing, reading, or debating) are slightly naïve. Such beliefs are not purely cognitive but rather involve potent affects, strongly held sensibilities about self and world, and deeply felt wishes and fears. They are also carriers of profound, early interpersonal experiences and developmental processes. Beliefs about God's existence or non-existence, and God's nature are objects of incredible emotional investment and to more fully understand them involves understanding more than their cognitive content.

We should note that this much of Rizzuto's theorizing is entirely based on Fairbairn's model. Winnicott's (1971) notion of transitional objects plays no role in her understanding of the origin and development of the internal internalized God image. It is only after having worked out what is basically a Fairbairnian model of internalized object-relations (a model Winnicott rarely uses), that she picks up Winnicott's idea that religion (and all of culture) is located in the "transitional sphere."

For Winnicott (1971), healthy development requires not the imposition of Freud's "reality principle" and the renouncing of illusion but just the reverse. The "facilitating environment" is so finely attuned to the infant's desires that the child learns to actualize, not suppress, his or her spontaneous wishes. If the reality principle is introduced too quickly, rather than mature rationality, the result is a compliant "false self'" and loss of access to the spontaneous and creative "true self" within. For Winnicott, the child must first consolidate a coherent sense of self made up of spontaneous desires and actions before confronting the harsh and unresponsive external world.

Gradually the child learns to accommodate external reality, facilitated by "transitional objects," which cushion the move from subjectivity to acknowledging the independence of the external world. These transitional objects (the proverbial blanket or teddy bear) both exist in the external world and are given their meaning and special status by the child's imagination. Thus they stand midway between the narcissistic world of the infant's experience and the reality-based world of adults.

Whereas Freud's demarcation of health and sickness is driven by a hard and fast distinction between reality and illusion, in *Playing and Reality* Winnicott (1971) moves beyond this dichotomy by proposing a "third area of human living, one neither inside the individual nor outside in the world of shared reality" (Winnicott, 1971, p. 110). Between inner and outer lies *interaction.* Neither the objective environment nor the isolated individual but, rather, the interaction between them defines this third domain, for it "is a product of the *experiences of the individual . . .* in the environment" (Winnicott, 1971, p. 107). This intermediate reality is interpersonal from its inception. Beginning in the interactional space between the mother and infant, it remains an interpersonal experience as it gradually spreads out from the relation to the mother to the "whole cultural field," for the "place where cultural experience is located is in the *potential space* between the individual and the environment" (Winnicott, 1971, p. 100). Key to the infant's move into the outside world is the use of the "transitional object," which "is not *inside . . . n*or is it *outside"* (Winnicott, 1971, p. 41). Rather, it occupies that intermediate space that is interactional and thus carries for the infant the security of that first interpersonal experience (Winnicott, 1971, p. 4). Even when the baby plays alone, he or she is still operating interpersonally; the experience of play carries echoes of those first a interactions, for the "playground is a potential space between the mother and the baby or joining mother and baby" (Winnicott, 1971, p. 47). Winnicott's theory is not primarily about certain kinds of objects–teddy bears and blankets–but about certain kinds of relational experiences.

Encompassing inner and outer reality, the transitional experience transcends the dichotomy of objectivity and subjectivity, for it is an "intermediate area of *experiencing,* to which inner reality and external life both contribute" (Winnicott, 1971, p. 2). In Freud's positivistic epistemology, which rigidly dichotomized objectivity and subjectivity, there was no place for a way of knowing that was neither subjective nor objective but contained elements of both. Winnicott (1965) calls this transitional realm paradoxical:

> In health the infant creates what is in fact lying around waiting to be found. . . .Yet the object must be found in order to be created. This has to be accepted as a paradox and not solved by a restatement that by its cleverness seems to eliminate the paradox. (p. 181)

The world of the infant's experience (and our own adult world) is both created and found, constructed and discovered. We are neither the passive recipients of brute facts imposed on us from outside nor (in health) do we make our own realities out of nothing. Human knowing is an active, creative process (Jones 1997b) in which reality is simultaneously discovered and constructed. According to Winnicott (1971),

> This area of playing is not inner psychic reality. It is outside the individual, but it is not the external world . . . Into this play area the child gathers objects or phenomena from external reality and uses these in the service of some sample derived from inner or personal reality. In playing, the child manipulates external phenomena in the service of the dream and invests chosen external phenomena with dream meaning and feeling. (p. 51)

Heuristically we can separate subject and object, but, for Winnicott, they are, in actual experience, two sides of the same process.

Rizzuto's theory of the internal God image blends Fairbairn's idea of an internalized object with Winnicott's idea of a "transitional object."

Rizzuto follows Winnicott (1971) in explicitly locating the reality of God in this "transitional space," half way between hallucination and physical reality. Rizzuto (1979) notices and remarks on a significant difference between God and all other transitional objects. The others are eventually outgrown and put away. As every parent knows, in the course of childhood, the closet overflows with discarded transitional objects–teddy bears, toys, bits of blankets, favored outfits. But, notes Rizzuto, God is not among them. In the normal course of things, the psychic history of God is the reverse of that of other transitional objects, "instead of losing meaning, God's meaning becomes heightened" (p. 179). Because God is a "nonexistent" object and the God representation, unlike teddy bears and security blankets, is infinitely plastic, the person can throughout life "create a God according to his needs" (Rizzuto, 1979, p. 179).

It is worth questioning whether that is a sufficient explanation for this difference between God and the rest of the inhabitants of the transitional world. Winnicott, to whom Rizzuto is indebted for this argument, takes it in a slightly different direction. When speaking about transitional objects, Winnicott (1971) is really calling attention to a certain capacity for *experience,* writing that transitional phenomena point to "an intermediate area of *experiencing* to which inner reality and external reality both contribute" (p. 2). Teddy bears and security blankets are left behind, but the capacity to transcend the dichotomies of inner and outer, subjective and objective, continues to grow and becomes the basis for human creativity in the arts and sciences. Winnicott writes that the transitional object,

> is not forgotten and it is not mourned. It loses meaning, and this is because the transitional phenomena have become diffused, have become spread out over the whole intermediate territory between inner psychic reality and the external world . . . that is to say, over the whole cultural field. (p. 14)

Imaginative play represents more than world of ghosts, goblins, and fairy tales; it is the source of the plays of Shakespeare and the formulae of Einstein. Watching a child play with a teddy bear, Winnicott saw a child developing the capacity to write a novel or invent a machine or propose a theory.

Rizzuto focuses too much on the transitional *object* and not enough on the transitional *experience.* Thus she often makes God sound like a supernatural version of the teddy bear and then speculates on why the deity is not discarded like other such "objects." But what is important here is not an object but a capacity for experience and perhaps one's God is not discarded because it is the carrier of that capacity par excellence. Winnicott's analysis of transitional processes goes beyond describing the functions of blankets and teddy bears to evoking a transitional domain of experience, intermediate between shear objectivity and pure subjectivity, which is a domain of creativity and transformation. Winnicott's theory is not only about objects but also about a certain kind of experience. Religion certainly involves the use of various sacred physical objects (books, buildings, statues and paintings, groves of trees, etc.) and special objects of belief like divine beings and powers. These may profitably be described as transitional objects in the way that Rizzuto, Meissner, Pruyser, and others do (Jones, 1997a). But a living religion also consists in certain transforming experiences, including experiences of the divine, which escape the dichotomy of subjectivity and objectivity. Here, too, Winnicott's discussion of the transitional realm may be fruitfully applied (Jones, 1997a).

According to Winnicott (1971), the child's transitional objects carry the child's first relational experience with the mother, conveying her presence when she is absent. Likewise the internal God image begins with the mother's presence and mirroring and it too carries a sense of presence when no one else is present. The core of the internal God image is the mother-child relationship. This is the psychological foundation of the God who is always there. Like other transitional objects, the internal internalized God image carries that experience of maternal presence, even when the mother herself is absent. The major attributes of the deity in many traditions–that God sees us, knows our hearts and minds, is always there–these are transitional functions in Winnicott's sense.

Several criticisms have been raised about Rizzuto's schema. Beit-Hallami (1992) and others have suggested that this claim about the universality of the internal internalized God image is an implicit religious apologetic. For them, it is too short a distance from saying that the internal God image is a reality to saying that God is a reality. Clearly writers must take extreme caution here in order to make it clear that they are talking about an internal, unconscious and psychological process and *not* a theological object of devotion or belief. Rizzuto certainly is clear on this score. Whether such a dynamic process occurs in the developing minds of children is an empirical question that cannot be used to argue for (or against) a divine reality.

Almost the reverse objection is raised by Moshe Helevi-Spero (1992) and Stanley Leavy (1986). They claim that Rizzuto's reliance on Winnicott makes God into a teddy bear or security blanket, thereby diminishing the reality and majesty of God. Winnicott has a very robust model of developmental transformation. A child playing with blocks or finger painting is not the same as Einstein coming up with an equation or Picasso painting a canvass; but for Winnicott child's play is the precursor and psychological foundation for adult creativity. Saying that, however, does not diminish the power of scientific investigation or artistic invention. Likewise, saying that religious belief and practice have psychological and developmental precursors and foundations should not diminish their power and importance in adult lives.

I have a different concern about her use of Winnicott. Hers is really a theory of the origins of mental representations and internalized objects. She follows Fairbairn and other object-relations theorists closely in this regard. In contrast to Fairbairn, Klein and others, Winnicott does not write much about internalized objects or mental representations. Rizzuto tends to equate transitional objects with internal mental representations; but these constructs may not refer to the same thing. Transitional objects are, in the first place, physical objects, not mental representations. Part of Winnicott's point is that transitional objects are intermediate between inner and outer realities. Mental representations are totally internal, even if they are the internalization of one's experience of someone in the external world. Rizzuto's discussion of how the internal God image is a different type of transitional object really results in a discussion of how the internal internalized God image is not a transitional object at all.

> God is a special type of transitional object because unlike teddy bears, dolls, or blankets made out of plushy fabrics, he is created from representational materials whose sources are the representations of primary objects . . . God is also a special transitional object because he does not follow the usual course of other transitional objects. Generally, the transitional object is gradually allowed to be decathected . . . God, on the other hand, is increasingly cathected . . . Instead of losing meaning, God's meaning becomes heightened. . . . (Rizzuto, 1979, p. 178)

Rizzuto has synthesized three different theoretical constructs: (1) Freud's notion of God as an internally generated internal object, constellated by the resolution of the Oedipal complex, (2) the Klein/Fairbairn notion of internalized object representations which are experiences with external objects taken inside and transformed, and (3) Winnicott's notion of a transitional object. The result is a model that is creative and a picture that is a bit confusing. For example, internal objects a'la Freud or Fairbairn never disappear from the psychic economy. They may be repressed but they remain potent, exactly what Rizzuto does say about the internal internalized God image. Transitional objects (as every parent knows) do disappear, they are, as Winnicott (1971) says, eventually "put aside."

The aspect of transitional phenomena that Rizzuto refers to most often in her discussion of the internal God image is that they are "both created and found." The internalized God image is both created by the child's inner representational processes and found in the wider culture. Rizzuto's is a story of our finding and re-finding God. Like Winncott's transitional objects, our internalized God image and the God we use for belief or reject is both created and found. This is primarily an epistemological issue and reflects the place where Winnicott's influence on the psychology of religion has been strongest—in our understanding of religious knowledge (Jones 1996, 1992). Others besides Rizzuto, including William Meissner and Paul Pruyser, have found Winnicott's notion of transitional phenomena, which transcend the modern dichotomy between objectivity and subjectivity, a viable way of locating religious claims epistemologically. And I have argued at length myself that Winnicott's theorizing is epistemologically suggestive, not just in the domain of religion but in all domains of human understanding (Jones 1997b, 1996). Here, in terms of understanding human understanding and the place of religion in it, rather than in terms of the psychological origin of religious phenomena, is (I think) Winnicott's greatest contribution to the psychology of religion (Jones, 1997a).

Along the same lines, Rizzuto engages in a rather long discussion of the role of imagination in human understanding. She cites the common childhood experiences of imaginary playmates and the creation of fictional characters and scenarios that perpetuate the child's imaginative inner world. Part of Rizzuto's book is a deliberate attempt to validate the importance of fantasy and the imagination for mental health, as opposed to Freud's empirical austerity (see, for example, Rizzuto, 1979, pp. 46-53). God is, for Rizzuto, a creation of the imagination, but that is precisely the source of his power and reality. We cannot live without the creations of our imagination and Rizzuto stresses their psychological importance.

We have forgotten the powerful reality of nonexistent objects, objects of our creation . . . . The fictive creations of our minds . . . have as much regulatory potential in our psychic function as people around us in the flesh . . . . Human life is impoverished when these immaterial characters made out of innumerable experiences vanish under the repression of a psychic realism that does violence to the ceaseless creativity of the human mind. In this sense, at least, religion is not an illusion. It is an integral part of being human, truly human in our capacity to create nonvisible but meaningful realities . . . Without those fictive realities human life becomes a dull animal existence. (Rizzuto, 1979, p. 47)

By "real" Rizzuto clearly means powerful. Such "fictive" entities as "muses, guardian angels, heroes . . . the Devil, God himself . . . unseen atoms, imaginary chemical formulas" (p. 27) can have a powerful impact on human lives and their psychic power constitutes their reality. Imaginary playmates and abstract ideas perform an indispensable psychological function in the lives of individuals and cultures, and so the imaginative capacity demands respect rather than denigration. God is seen as different, she says, because parents and the wider culture sanction the existence of God in a way that they do not reinforce the child's imaginary playmates or fantasies of being a pirate or visitor from outer space. Parents engaging in God-talk themselves confers on it a realism and respect not given to talk of gremlins or imaginary siblings.

So Rizzuto is assimilating the internalized God image to two well-established childhood experiences: (1) Winicott's transitional objects which are external objects put in the service of inner processes, and (2) imaginary playmates which are almost entirely inner created realities projected outward. Such a claim can be read in either of two ways. It can be read as claiming that God is simply an imaginary playmate or transitional object. Such a claim goes beyond the disciplinary boundaries of psychology whose role cannot be to say what God is or is not; and, I think, goes beyond the claim Rizzuto herself is making. Or her argument can be read as claiming that the same psychological processes that go into the making of imaginary playmates and the use of transitional objects also go into the constellation of the internalized God image. This is an empirical claim to be answered by an in depth analysis of the psychological processes that go into an individual's inner God image. This, I think, is closer to Rizzuto's own claim here. Her position is, I think, only that the internalized God image shares some psychological characteristics and functions with both imaginary playmates and transitional objects. But one can still ask, while remaining within the disciplinary boundaries of psychology, whether or not this is a complete *psychological* account of the origin and function of beliefs about God.

Moshe Halevi Spero

A rather different analysis of the internalized God image is articulated by Moshe Halevi Spero (1992). His presentation has both clinical and epistemological components. Clinically, Spero insists that not accepting a religious patient's view that God is objectively real may constitute a profound failure of empathy, which can shipwreck the therapy. It is not sufficient that the therapist listen respectfully and interpret nonreductively. For Spero, establishing a working alliance with a religious patient requires empathizing with the patient's conviction that God exists (Spero, 1992; see also McDargh, 1993). Making such a stance psychologically coherent requires that Spero articulate a psychological framework in which God's existence makes sense. This he attempts in *Religious Objects as Psychological Structures*, where he seeks to "link the therapeutic process directly to an underlying religious structure with built-in potential for relationship with God" (Spero, 1992, p. 97). Spero asserts that, God "holding forth the possibility of being discovered or known may be further assumed to have created mechanisms or faculties through which discovery is indeed possible" (p. 140). According to Spero, God has implanted in the human psyche certain "deocentric intrapsychic endowments," (p. 139) which serve as precursors of the experience of God. Made directly by God, such structures are *a priori*, existing before psychological experiencing. Created in the image of God, the infant has some primordial, preverbal awareness of God's presence. Spero quotes Roy Shafer to the effect that "it is conceivable that some objects have existed as internal objects from their beginnings" (Spero likes this sentence so much he quotes it twice, see Spero 1992, pp. 89 & 191).

Such primordial awareness may constitute "deep preconceptions on the order of an 'archaic heritage' that *disposes* the psyche towards God's presence" (Spero, 1992, p. 142). The individual's personal God representation *is* not, however, a direct consequence of this primordial awareness of the deity. The personal God representation is internally generated, an "amalgamation of suitable material, some of which *is supplied* by family and social input, which is then projected and given quasi-objective form" (p. 138). Spero is therefore arguing for two lines of religious development. One involves the internalization of our experience of objects in our ordinary world and the constellation of a *private* God representation in much the same way as described by Rizzuto (1979), McDargh (1983), and others. The second, and this is the core of Spero's position, involves "an objective God object moving on its representational pathway toward internalization" (Spero,1992, p. 138). Such a deocentric process of internalization is possible because there is both an objectively real God and a literally God-given compatibility between the developmental structures of the human psyche and that objective God they are designed to grasp. Although the term "internalized God representation" is widely used in the literature (see Rizzuto, Mc-Dargh, Meissner, and others) to cover variations on the first, intrapsychic processes, Spero insists that only the second, deocentric process can *truly* be said to yield an internalized God representation.

> While the line of development for the objective, *human* object may, indeed, yield anthropocentrically based, internal or endopsychic gods, only the line of development from the objective object known as God can legitimately be said to yield an *internalized* God representation. For only in the later case has something *really* external and *objectively* of God been taken inward. (Spero, 1992, p. 138)

This then raises the obvious question, "To whom do we relate, to God or to the representation of God?" (Spero, 1992, p. 42). The answer is equally obvious: to both. That is, we relate to God through our representation of God just as we relate to our parents through our internalized representation of them.

Spero (1992) wants to preserve both what he takes to be the religiously essential claim that God is objectively real and the clinically essential claim that our representation of God is fashioned by the vicissitudes of our development. He preserves them both by articulating two separate lines of development: an intrapsychic one and a deocentric one. These lines interact, and at any given moment an individual's religious experience is a conjunction of his or her internalized experience of the real God and his or her private, intrapsychically generated God representation. Thus Spero does not naively identify our experience or representations of God with God. Such a literal identification would involve us in idolatry and would render clinical analysis of an individual's religious experience sacrilegious. Thus, Spero gives the clinician free reign to analyze and interpret the individual's religious expressions and beliefs while also preserving God's objective reality by locating our connection to the real God in a separate, semi-autonomous developmental realm.

Spero (1992) wants to make room within psychoanalysis for the existence of God by making God into another external object that we internalize and project back onto our intrapsychic representations in a way precisely analogous to our relationships with parents and other primary objects. So, in answering the question whether we relate to an objective God or to our God representation, Spero quotes Sandler's discussion of our relationship to our mother, in which he says, "The internal image of the mother *is* thus not a substitute for an object relationship, but is itself an indispensable part of the relationship" (Spero, 1992, p. 142). The same, for Spero, can be said of our relationship to God. Spero appears to disregard any disciplinary limits on psychology's capacity to discuss God and not just the human experience of God. Spero rejects Kant's insistence on the limitations of finite human cognitive and psychological structures to grasp the infinite. Rather, Spero believes that God fashioned the human mind in order to know God, and so our faculties are designed to correlate with the divine reality.

Within the context of particular religious faith, which begins from the premise of God's existence, such a position makes sense, although every religious person is not required to accept Spero's pre-Kantian epistemology. Spero (1992) asserts that "we have no idea what God, indeed, *is* like" (p. 29), so it is not clear what sort of knowing of God comes to us through our primordial experience and divinely created categories. From a perspective encompassing world religions, the pluralism of experiences and articulations may be too broad to fit within this framework. Spero acknowledges that "God is apparently known in different ways by different people during different eras" (p. 69); but it is not clear that the same set of cognitive and psychological structures can be correlated with, say, the divine lawgiver of Mount Sinai and the universal Brahma of classical Hinduism. Or is the sacred encountered through a different set of psychological processes in the different religious traditions?

As long as Spero stays strictly within the Orthodox Jewish context out of which he is writing, the particularities of his exposition are no problem. If, however, the student of religion or psychotherapist wants to use Spero's model to make sense of the plurality of world religions, some broadening of the categories will be necessary. More specifically, the primordial awareness might be understood as a generic drive for something sacred and transcendent to serve as the ground of value and the source of meaning and purpose to life. Such a primordial drive may be structured and expressed differently as it is refashioned by the interpersonal experiences, cognitive categories, and cultural formulations that mediate the experience of the sacred to each individual.

Such a primordial awareness bears some relationship to what Christopher Bollas (1987) calls the "unthought known." These are the bodily sensations, primitive smells, and sights associated with objects, and the experience of interacting with them, that the child incorporates before the dawning of mental representation and language, "all children store the quality of an experience that is beyond comprehension, and hold onto it in the form of a self-in-relation-to-object-state" (Bollas, 1987, p. 246). We "know" such primordial experiences but cannot think them or speak of them. We know them as a "felt sense" (the term is from Eugene Gendlin) of elation or dread, affirmation or negation. Such precursor experiences force themselves into awareness through fantasies, aesthetic experiences, the ways the subject relates to others, and transference. They may also be carried by the individual's religious longings and expressions.

The human root of religious experience would thus be in the preverbal domain. The immediate appeal (or lack thereof) of certain religious images and symbols may be in part because they evoke (or fail to evoke) that "primordial" (Spero, 1992) or "unthought" (Bollas, 1987) realm of experience. In more traditional terms, the "imago Dei" of western theology or the "remembering soul" of Platonic and Neo-Platonic philosophy or the Atman of Hinduism may well be found in the realm of preverbal experience. Part of the ineffable quality of religious experience may result from its tapping into the trace of a relationship that cannot simply be processed "through mental representation or language" (Bollas, 1987, p. 3).

CONCLUSION

McDargh (1993) makes a distinction, useful for organizing this material, between two relational approaches to the psychoanalysis of the individual's God image: the "God relational" approach and the "faith relational" approach. Spero is the paradigm of the God relational approach. This model,

concerns itself with the complex correspondence between such object representations of "God" and the individual's genuine, evolving relationship to what the client, and also the therapist, may

be able to ontologically affirm as–and here language limps badly–
the very God. (McDargh 1993, p. 183)

The God relational perspective is explicitly theological in that it in-
quires after the specific theological contents of a person's belief and
presupposes the patient and the therapist can speak directly about a normative concept of God.

Rizzuto (and Freud too), on the other hand, illustrate the "faith relational perspective." This approach focuses "not upon the *what,* i.e., specific religious contents, but rather upon *how* the representational world
functions, regardless of content" (McDargh,1993, pp. 183-184). Thus,
the "faith relational perspective" eschews normative discussions of
God's nature as a part of therapy and instead "attempts a more inclusive
formulation of what constitutes 'religious material' in order to accommodate the widest range of human spiritual experience" (McDargh,
1993, p. 183). This perspective is less confessionally theological and
more grounded in the disciplines of religious studies or the study of
comparative religions.

The strength of a God relational approach is that meets the believer on
his or her own terms and immediately accepts the fundamental premise of
faith regarding the objectivity of the divine, however distorted by psychopathology any given individual's rendition of the divine may be in the eyes
of the therapist. Such an approach makes sense for those therapists working in an explicitly denominational context. For them Spero's formulation of the divine object in terms of primordial consciousness and
pre-established psychological structures provides a coherent psychological
account of the place of the divine object in the human psyche.

The faith relational approach uses a more functional, rather than con-
tent-based, definition of religion and religious material. Thus it opens a
wider range of material to analysis. Secular ideologies, less traditional
spiritualities, even militant atheism can be analyzed with the tools
forged in the psychoanalytic study of religion (Jones, 1996). Such an
approach seems appropriate for therapists working in religiously pluralis-
tic or secular settings.

REFERENCES

Beit-Hallahmi, B. (1992). Between religious psychology and the psychology of religion. In M. Finn & J. Gartner (Eds.), *Object relations theory and religion* (pp.
119-128). Westport, CT.: Praeger.

Benson, P., & Spilka, B. (1973). God image as a function of self-esteem and locus on control. *Journal for the Scientific Study of Religion, 12*, 297-310.

Bollas, C. (1987). *The shadow of the object.* New York: Columbia University Press.

Buri, J. & Mueller, R. (1993). Psychoanalytic theory and loving God concepts. *Journal of Psychology, 127*, 17-27.

Dickie, J., Ajega, L., Kobylak, J., & Nixon, K, (2006). Mother, father, and self: Sources of young adults' God concepts. *Journal for the Scientific Study of Religion, 45(1),* 57-71.

Dickie, J., Eshleman, A,, Merasco, D., Shepard, A., VanderWilt, M., & Johnson, M. (1997). Parent-child relationships and children's images of God. *Journal for the Scientific Study of Religion, 36(1),* 25-43.

Evans, E. (2001). Cognitive and contextual factors in the emergence of diverse belief systems. *Cognitive Psychology, 42*, 217-266.

Freud, S. (1962). *Civilization and its discontents.* New York: Norton. (Original work published in 1930)

Freud, S. (1964). *The future of an illusion* (W. Robson-Scott, Trans.). Garden City, NY: Doubleday. (Original work published in 1927)

Freud, S. (1950). *Totem and taboo* (J. Strachey trans.). New York: Norton. (Original work published in 1913)

Jones, J. (1996). *Religion and psychology in transition: Psychoanalysis, feminism and theology,* New Haven, CT: Yale University Press.

Jones, J. (1991). *Contemporary psychoanalysis and religion: Transference and transcendence,* New Haven, CT: Yale University Press.

Jones, J. (1997a). Playing and believing: The uses of D. W. Winnicott in the psychology of religion. In J. Jacobs & D. Capps (Eds.), *Religion, society and psychoanalysis: Readings in contemporary theory* (pp. 106-126) Denver, CO: Westview Press.

Jones, J. (1997b). The real is the relational: Relational psychoanalysis as a model of human understanding. In J. A. Belzen (Ed.), *Hermeneutical approaches in psychology of religion* (pp. 51-64) Atlanta: Rodopi.

Jones, J. (1992). Knowledge in transition: Towards a Winnicottian epistemology. *The Psychoanalytic Review, 79(2),* 223-237.

Leavy, S. (1986). A Pascalian meditation on psychoanalysis and religious experience. *Cross Currents, 26*, 147-155.

McDargh. (1997). Creating a new research paradigm for the psychoanalytic study of religion: The pioneering work of Ana-Maria Rizzuto. In J. Jacobs & D. Capps (Eds.), *Religion, Society and Psychoanalysis* (pp. 181-199) Denver, CO: Westview Press.

McDargh, J. (1993). Concluding clinical postscript: On developing a psychotheological perspective. In M. L. Randor (Ed.), *Exploring sacred landscapes.* New York: Columbia University Press.

McDargh, J. (1983). *Psychoanalytic object relations theory and the study of religion.* Lanham, MD.: University Press of America.

Rizzuto, A. M. (1979). *The birth of the living God.* Chicago: University of Chicago Press.

Spero, M.H. (1992). *Religious objects as psychological structures: A critical integration of object relations theory, psychotherapy and Judaism.* Chicago: University of Chicago Press.

Spilka, B, Armatas, P, & Nussbaum, J (1964). The concept of God: A factor-analytic approach. *Review of Religious Research. 6,* 20-35.
Vergote, A. & Tamayo, A. (Eds). (1981) *The parental figures and the representation of God.* The Hague: Mouton.
Winnicott, D. (1971). *Playing and reality.* New York: Routledge.
Winnicott, D. (1965). *The maturational process and the facilitating environment.* London: Hogarth.

doi:10.1300/J515v09n03_03

PART II
CLINICAL THEORY AND APPLICATIONS

Chapter 4

Attachment Psychotherapy and God Image

Jacqueline L. Noffke, PsyD
Todd W. Hall, PhD

SUMMARY. This chapter integrates attachment theory, emotional information processing theory, and affective neuroscience in order to provide a theoretical framework for understanding the development and transformation of God image. Repeated relational experiences with primary caregivers are encoded subsymbolically as "implicit relational representations" or a visceral sense of what it is like to be a self with others. These implicit relational representations then function as templates for interpreting subsequent interpersonal interactions and organizing individuals' characteristic approaches of relating to others, including God. Thus, these implicit filters bias believers' experiences of God toward the content and quality of their experiences within human attachment relationships. We propose a model of transformation of the God image that

[Haworth co-indexing entry note]: "Attachment Psychotherapy and God Image." Noffke, Jacqueline L., and Todd W. Hall. Co-published simultaneously in *Journal of Spirituality in Mental Health* (The Haworth Pastoral Press, an imprint of The Haworth Press) Vol. 9, No. 3/4, 2007, pp. 57-78; and: *God Image Handbook for Spiritual Counseling and Psychotherapy: Research, Theory, and Practice* (ed: Glendon L. Moriarty, and Louis Hoffman) The Haworth Pastoral Press, an imprint of The Haworth Press, 2007, pp. 57-78. Single or multiple copies of this article are available for a fee from The Haworth Document Delivery Service [1-800-HAWORTH, 9:00 a.m. - 5:00 p.m. (EST). E-mail address: docdelivery@haworthpress.com].

involves both nonverbal relational information and an integration of this code with the verbal code within the therapeutic relationship. In therapy, adaptive relational experiences recruit new neural networks, establishing the neuronal basis for different ways of experiencing, representing, and being with God. We illustrate this model of transformation of the God image with a case study. doi:10.1300/J515v09n03_04 *[Article copies available for a fee from The Haworth Document Delivery Service: 1-800-HAWORTH. E-mail address: <docdelivery@haworthpress.com> Website: <http://www.HaworthPress.com> © 2007 by The Haworth Press. All rights reserved.]*

INTRODUCTION

There is now a substantial body of research suggesting that psychological and spiritual functioning are highly related in some very important ways (see Brokaw & Edwards, 1994; Hall, Halcrow, Hill & Delaney, 2004). Research within the fields of attachment, affective neurobiology, and emotional information processing indicate that patterns of infant-caregiver emotional communication are internalized by infants and serve as templates for interpreting subsequent interpersonal interactions and organizing their characteristic approaches of relating to others. To believers, God is both an external and internal figure with whom they relate. Thus, the psychological processes and mechanisms that automatically and nonconsciously mediate how individuals process emotional information with humans also influence the form and quality of their relationships with God. Benner (1998) refers to this relationship between psychological and spiritual functioning as the "psychospiritual unity of personality." Therefore, in order to begin to describe the formation, possible difficulties, and means of transforming believers' images of and relational patterns with God, we must examine these processes at a general level. This chapter integrates the complimentary theories from attachment, affective neurobiology, and emotional information processing specifically with regard to the development, pathologies, and methods of changing general relational schemas. This information and an extended clinical example are then used to illustrate these same processes with regard to believers' internal models of God.

BRIEF BACKGROUND ON ATTACHMENT THEORY

Current conceptualizations within attachment theory assert that the set goal of infants' attachments to caregivers is a sense of "felt security"

(Sroufe & Waters, 1977). In infancy and throughout the lifespan, the attachment bond and its corresponding strategies for achieving felt security are established through shared emotional communication (Siegel, 1999). Caregivers' sensitivity to infants' signals of distress provides an experience of a haven of safety and comfort, which soothes distress and enables infants to use their caregivers as a secure base from which to confidently explore the environment.

Caregivers, however, differ in their attunement to infants' cues, resulting in varying influences on infants' confidence in and desire for contact and exploration. As a result of repeated patterns of emotional communication, infants develop internal organizations of the emotions, sensations, behaviors, and "cognitions" involved in their efforts to maintain felt security with a particular attachment figure (Bowlby, 1969). For instance, the ability of secure infants to soothe themselves following separation is an indication of an internal model of a caregiver who is a consistent source of comfort, resulting in an expectation that "homeostatic disruptions will be set right" (Pipp & Harmon, 1987, p. 650). Insecure attachment models do not provide infants with an internalized sense of felt security, thus impairing their capacities for regulating their own emotions. As a result, insecurely-attached infants develop compensatory strategies that involve restricting certain emotions or behaviors and emitting only the social signals to which their internalized caregivers are capable of responding in order to achieve a moderated sense of felt security (Bowlby, 1969). Subsequently, these internal relational models serve as templates for interpreting and responding to future attachment figures, thereby, influencing believers' images of and relational patterns with God.

Development of Implicit Relational Representations of God

From the perspective of attachment theory, individuals' images of and relational patterns with God are considerably influenced by the internalization of early attachment experiences with emotionally-significant others. Current research in affective neuroscience helps explicate the process and content of this internalization. During the first three years of life, the "low road" brain circuit (LeDoux, 1996), particularly in the right hemisphere is dominant with respect to brain activity and development. The right, low road brain circuits process information in rapid, parallel, holistic fashion, producing nonverbal representations of sensations and images, as opposed to the sequentially-processed, semantic representations of objects that dominate the "high road" brain circuits, particularly in the left hemisphere (LeDoux, 1996).

In addition, the right cortical hemisphere contains extensive reciprocal connections with the limbic and subcortical regions and, so, is dominant for the processing and expression of emotional information. Specifically, the right hemisphere is primarily responsible for the reading of social and emotional cues and for representing and responding to the body's physiological reactions. These right limbic circuits account for the unique contribution of the right hemisphere in regulating homeostasis and integrating cortically-processed information concerning the external environment with subcortically-processed information regarding the internal visceral environment (Schore, 2003). In other words, in infancy and throughout the lifespan, the right hemisphere nonverbally depicts the "gist" or social meaning of events, rapidly producing a "gut-level" sense of the self in relation to others and initiating mechanisms for regulating affective homeostasis.

There is strong evidence that, from the time of birth, infants naturally and automatically seek others with whom to enter intersubjective states of shared affect attunement (Beebe & Lachmann, 2002; Stern, 1985). According to Schore (2003), the infant's right hemisphere is psychobiologically attuned to the output of the caregiver's right hemisphere as a means of organizing and regulating immature mental and bodily states. This linking of the infant's and caregiver's minds occurs through affective interactions, which are primarily communicated through nonverbal social signals. The infant's right hemisphere, which is dominant for the recognition of the caregiver's face, affective expressions, and the prosody of the caregiver's voice, synchronizes with and is, thereby, regulated by the output of the caregiver's right hemisphere, which is behaviorally manifested through such nonverbal signals. This affective synchrony enables the infant's mind to regulate itself in the moment and to use the output of the caregiver's right cortex as a template for the hard-wiring of its expanding cognitive-affective capacities for attending to, appraising, and responding to variations in both external and internal information. It is in this manner that the emotional state of the sender directly shapes that of the receiver, recruiting in the infant brain processes that are similar to those experienced by the caregiver.

Given the right hemisphere's nonverbal, imagistic mode of processing and the significant involvement of subcortical regions in the processes of emotional arousal and appraisal, the psychobiological impact of these affect-regulating interactions between infant and caregiver are encoded implicitly, or without conscious, verbal awareness (Schore,

2003). In other words, affect attunement and misattunement create a nonverbal, visceral sense of what it is like to be a self with a particular other. Bucci (1997) refers to this implicit relational information as a product of subsymbolic emotional processing. According to Bucci, there are three modes of emotional processing: (a) subsymbolic; (b) nonverbal symbolic; and (c) verbal symbolic. Subsymbolic processing is nonverbal or "analogic," involving the processing of variations within continuous dimensions such as the motoric, visceral, and sensory. The nature of subsymbolic processing is that an individual's knowledge does not exist in symbolic form and, thus, cannot be easily communicated in words and is not under direct control. Rather, subsymbolic knowledge is communicated and modified in the modality in which it exists. For instance, dancers teach and learn their craft in the format of feeling and movement. The primary medium of the nonverbal symbolic code is imagery. Images can be processed sequentially, as in the verbal symbolic code, or in a parallel, continuous manner, as in subsymbolic processes. Language is the quintessential example of the symbolic code. Words function clearly as symbols, referring to entities outside of themselves. In the symbolic mode, information is processed one message at a time and can be directly controlled by the processor.

At the neuronal level, the subsymbolic sense of what it is like to be a self with an attachment figure is represented in the circuits that are activated as a result of the specific patterns of emotional communication. Once established, these circuits reinforce their connections with each other (Schore, 2003). In other words, a pattern of neuronal activation recruits similar patterns in the future. Thus, this nonconscious knowledge of what it is like to be with a specific other becomes encoded in implicit memory as a relational expectation, what we are referring to as an "implicit relational representation" (see Hall, 2004). For instance, a caregiver's consistent amplification of positive emotion and alleviation of uncomfortable affect recruits and perpetuates brain processes in the infant corresponding to a visceral sense of an effective, lovable self in the presence of encouraging others. Formation of such mental models is a fundamental way in which implicit memory allows the mind to create generalizations of past experiences, so that rapid regulation, interpretation, and prediction of future attachment-related behaviors can occur.

Mental models of attachment, thus, enable infants to establish coherent strategies for regulating their emotions following internal and external stressors by providing a template for predicting caregivers' degrees of emotional availability and responsiveness to specific signals of distress. Based on these relational templates, infants begin to preferentially emit the social signals to which caregivers are capable of responding. In other words, implicit relational representations shape infants' characteristic approaches to affect-regulation and, consequently, interpersonal interaction (Bowlby, 1969). For instance, based on their mental model that their distress will be comforted, securely-attached infants develop the capacity for autoregulation of emotion, freeing them to seek intimacy as an end in itself.

Due to their inconsistent and/or rejecting implicit relational representations, insecure infants experience a chronic, implicit concern with achieving felt security and rely on alternative, maladaptive mechanisms to compensate for their deficits in autoregulation. Avoidant/dismissive individuals accommodate to their attachment figures' consistent rebuffs of their bids for nurturance by deactivating their attachment system activation as a strategy for modulating their distress and increasing their sense of felt security. Ambivalent/preoccupied individuals respond to their caregivers' inconsistent availability by hyperactivating their attachment system as a strategy aimed at ensuring receipt of comfort (Main, Kaplan, & Cassidy, 1985). In this way, implicit memory is the means by which past events affect future interpersonal perceptions and responses, creating stable patterns of relationship.

With regard to the development of believers' images of and relational patterns with God, it is asserted that the religious forms provided by caregivers, religious instruction, and culture strongly influence individuals' explicit religiosity, such as theological belief and religious practice. To a large degree, the transmission of religious belief and practice occurs at the symbolic level of information processing. Yet these externally-fashioned understandings and interactions with God are reshaped according to individuals' implicit relational representations. The perceptions of the self and others and the interactional patterns infants develop to maintain felt security are represented in self-perpetuating neural networks that are automatically and nonconsciously elicited by attachment-related stimuli with God. Thus, past emotional experiences impact the appraisal process of present interactions with God without the experience of something being remembered. In Bucci's (1997) terms, symbolic belief is, therefore, not necessarily reflective of and does not have direct impact on individuals' subsymbolic interpretations of and responses to emotional information. In other words, it is possible that believers' symbolic and subsymbolic systems may contain discrepant expectations of God.

DIFFICULTIES DUE TO INSECURE

Implicit Relational Representations of God

The implicit relational representations established as a result of internalized caregiver responses to infants' emotional cues influence individuals' perceptions of the availability and responsiveness of future attachment figures and their capacities for autoregulation. Given the "psychospiritual unity" of personality, individuals' relationships with God are impacted in these respects also. With regard to God image, attachment research indicates that individuals with histories of insecure attachment tend to perceive God as controlling, less accepting and nurturing, and/or distant (Granqvist & Hagekull, 2005; Kirkpatrick & Shaver, 1992).

Internalized forms of noncontingent emotional communication not only produce negative images of God but also result in an impaired sense of felt security, prompting the insecurely attached to rely on maladaptive, compensatory strategies to re-establish homeostasis. For instance, some insecurely attached believers remain unconscious of their negative God images or do not experience the painful affect associated with their conscious, negative beliefs. In other words, their painful, gut-level experiences of God are dissociated from awareness.

Bucci (2003) asserts that maladaptive mental models of the self and others inherently involve a level of dissociation, which is nonconsciously but deliberately maintained in order to avoid the disorganizing affect elicited when divergent images of the self and/or others are experienced simultaneously. According to Bucci (2003), individuals consolidate separate representations of the sensations, feelings, and cognitions elicited, for example, by caregivers' expressions of anger or love. In adaptive development, infants' distress is managed by caregivers' soothing actions, enabling infants to reconcile both the negative and positive forms of subsymbolic activation and the representation of the caregiver into an integrated schema. These infants consolidate an image of the caregiver as a source of both love and anger, neither of which is overwhelming in intensity.

Maladaptive functioning results from dissociation among components of emotional schemas. For example, a schema of the mother as rageful, with its corresponding terror or rage responses in the child, is disorganizing and incompatible with an image of the mother as the child's source of comfort. In response, the child may dissociate the terror or attack responses from recognition of the mother as the source of the sense of danger so that the child feels afraid or angry but is spared the recognition that these feelings are directed at the child's main attachment figure. On the other hand, due to the child's conflicting feelings toward the mother, the child may be unable to integrate a sense of soothing with the image of the mother as comforter. As a result, the child may dissociate the experience of being soothed from the image of the mother as comforter, producing an emotionally-flat representation of motherly comfort. In other words, the subsymbolic affective core is dissociated from symbolic beliefs about the object.

This "cutting of the subsymbolic cord" that occurs in dissociation results in implicit appraisal and response patterns that continue to organize interpersonal relationships along maladaptive lines despite maintenance of contrary, symbolic beliefs (Bucci, 2003). For instance, when one of the authors (T.H.) asked a client about her relationship with her mother early on in the therapy, the client reported that the relationship was supportive. However, she nonverbally expressed signs of anxiety. Despite her positive beliefs about the relationship, the client implicitly experienced her mother as communicating that the client was only acceptable when she presented herself as strong and competent. Outside of the client's awareness, this implicit relational representation influenced how she interacted with her mother and other significant attachment figures, leading the client to feel shame about and to hide her vulnerability. Thus, dissociation between believers' theological beliefs and their painful, subsymbolic activation leaves them without any means of bringing the meaning of their negative God images into relationship with themselves, others, or God in order to create opportunities for their transformation.

While all maladaptive mental models involve a level of dissociation, individuals' internalized patterns of emotional communication determine the emotional experiences that trigger a sense of danger and the particular coping strategies on which they rely. Affective neurobiology research suggests that those with avoidant/dismissive attachment rely on a generalized process of dissociating subsymbolic experience from symbolic awareness as their characteristic approach to affect regulation. Dismissive parents have been shown to provide minimal degrees of affective attunement to their infants and to use words that are disconnected from the nonverbal aspects of communication (Siegel, 1999). Over time, this emotionally-barren and noncooperative pattern of communication establishes an implicit representation of the attachment figure as nonresponsive in the infant's mind, rendering emotional closeness uncomfortable. In order to achieve a moderated sense of felt security, the avoidant infant learns to decrease awareness of socially-generated emotional states, resulting in isolation from others and the self.

Despite physiological activation in response to social interactions, the dissociation between affective experience and language and the dominance of logical, left-hemisphere representations that characterize the infant-caregiver relationship become reflected in the infant's mind (Siegel, 1999). Supporting this research, Byrd and Boe's (2001) investigation of prayer as a function of attachment revealed that, despite dismissive believers' presumed physiological activation to attachment-related interactions, they tend to use forms of prayer that minimize a sense of closeness with God, dissociating their attachment arousal from a more rational relationship with God. In other words, avoidant believers experience a more distant, intellectualized relationship with God and remain defensively self-sufficient from Him, replicating their early experiences of feeling completely responsible for their care and of interacting with a caregiver who is removed and unmoved by their needs.

The means preoccupied believers use to increase their sense of felt security with God are equally maladaptive. Unlike dismissive caregivers' consistent nonresponsiveness to their infants' cues, preoccupied caregivers are unreliably available and attuned. Preoccupied caregivers appear to experience frequent, implicitly-triggered anxiety about whether their internalized attachment figures will soothe them. As a result, these caregivers become flooded with anxiety, rendering them inconsistently sensitive to their infants' actual signals. This causes them to intrude on their infants' states with their own needs. Ambivalent infants appear to interpret their caregivers' inconsistency as reflecting their own unlovableness, resulting in intense preoccupation as to whether their distress will be soothed. In response, preoccupied individuals maximize their attention on the unpredictable attachment relationship and intensify their expressions of distress as a means of attempting to ensure comfort (Siegel, 1999).

For instance, research indicates that preoccupied believers primarily engage in help-seeking prayer, evincing their implicit mistrust of God's reliability and their attempts to maintain the perceived fragile bond by approaching Him in a clingy manner (Byrd & Boe, 2001). In addition, a number of attachment studies indicate that insecure attachment–particularly preoccupied attachment–is associated with sudden conversion and increases in religious belief and activity following attachment disruptions. Such precipitous increases in religious involvement are viewed as an example of the hyperactivating strategy and as serving the primary function of providing an external source of temporary felt security. In other words, relationship with God is not pursued as an end in itself but as a means to self-regulation (Noffke, 2006). In the end, the decrease in anxiety that preoccupied believers experience after seeking comfort from God in a clingy manner recapitulates their assumption that they are unlovable and that nurturance is not reliably available, rendering them overly-dependent on emotionally intense religious experiences to achieve a sense of security with God.

TRANSFORMING INSECURE IMPLICIT RELATIONAL REPRESENTATIONS OF GOD

Given the automatic, nonconscious nature of implicit memory, insecure believers' opportunities for experiencing interpersonal safety and responsiveness from God or the church are often blocked because these experiences are interpreted through the filter of negative attachment models. In order for individuals to develop more positive images of and relational patterns with God, it is necessary to create new neural networks that correspond to experiences of others as available and responsive and of the self as loved. Bucci (2003) provides an understanding of the therapeutic action that brings about such change. As previously described, Bucci (2003) asserts that maladaptive functioning results from the dissociation of the subsymbolic, affective core of an experience from symbolic processing. As a result, individuals respond to their senses of danger according to their attachment-specific affect-regulation strategies but are unaware of their arousal and/or toward whom the emotion is directed. Thus, structural change of the maladaptive schema occurs through referential activity or the process of linking subsymbolic experience to images and words.

For this process to occur, the client must communicate the contents of the schema, and the therapist must understand and generate an intervention that connects words or imagery back to the client's emotional core. Given its dissociated nature, the affective core is primarily communicated through the nonverbal aspects of the client's communication. Through the process of right-brain-to-right-brain synchrony, the therapist begins to experience the somatic and motoric components of the client's subsymbolic state and to connect this activation within herself to symbolic forms. The therapist then articulates some understanding of the state elicited within her to activate the referential activity that is missing within the client.

Incorporating Bucci's (1997, 2003) theory with the attachment and neuroaffective research previously summarized, the authors present a conceptualization of the process of transforming implicit relational representations. It is asserted that an attachment bond must be facilitated between the therapist and client so that the relationship is ascribed sufficient significance to elicit the negative implicit relational representations and to be internalized as an attachment object. However, elicitation of an implicit relational model automatically leads to arousal and evaluation processes that tend to perpetuate the experience of the therapeutic relationship according to the negative self and/or other constellations. Thus, the heuristic functioning of the current implicit representations must be interrupted so that construction of more adaptive self and other models and patterns of interaction can occur. As emphasized by Bucci (1997, 2003), subsymbolic knowledge can only be modified as a result of experiencing new information presented in the same code. In other words, implicit relational representations are transformed only when adaptive interpersonal information connects with individuals' subsymbolic experience.

Therapeutic interventions can connect with clients' subsymbolic affective cores and lead to transformation of implicit relational representations in two manners: indirectly, through affectively-ladened verbal communication and directly, through novel subsymbolic experience. Bucci's (1997, 2003) writing emphasizes the indirect reconstruction of attachment models through the articulation of unsymbolized experience. Such articulation connects individuals' unsymbolized sense of danger to the context in which their attachment assumptions were established, providing clients with the means to make sense of their emotional reactions toward others and to differentiate them from the current relationship with the therapist and God.

In addition to the verbal, indirect means of reconstruction, we propose that implicit relational representations can be directly transformed when clients experience novel interpersonal information presented in the subsymbolic code. In other words, contingent, nonverbal communication between therapist and client can create a shift at the level of implicit relational knowledge, even if it is never verbalized. For instance, a client recently experienced a positive shift in his sense of emotional connection and safety with one of the authors (T.H.) as a result of seeing the therapist's facial expression in response to his story of a painful experience. While negative implicit representations tend to skew how novel emotional experiences are interpreted, this process is not absolute. It seems possible that the level of trust within the therapeutic relationship and the process of symbolizing clients' negative, implicit models may enable clients to differentiate their therapists' responses from those of early attachment figures and to internalize these experiences directly.

Whether accomplished through indirect, verbal interventions or direct, subsymbolic experience, we would suggest that the development of adaptive, attachment-related neural networks largely occurs as a result of drawing clients' attention to their experiences that are felt to be dangerous and are, thus, avoided. In helping clients to experience their unsymbolized emotions, the therapist interrupts the dissociation and provides the insecurely attached with the novel experience of receiving contingent emotional responses to their emotions. Such emotional synchrony establishes neural networks corresponding to an experience of attunement to difficult feelings and, consequently, the expectation that others, including God, will be available during distress. As a result, believers begin to consolidate images of themselves as lovable and/or of God as loving. The association of attunement and soothing with the experience of difficult emotion is also the foundation of clients' abilities to autoregulate and, thus, decreases their need for defensive self-sufficiency or interpersonal affect-regulation to achieve a sense of felt security. With an internalized sense of themselves as safe and loved in the presence of God, believers are able to pursue a relationship with God vulnerably and for its own sake.

STRENGTHS AND WEAKNESSES OF THE CURRENT CONCEPTUALIZATION

All theories emphasize certain points of interest, while leaving other facets of the same phenomena underdeveloped or, sometimes, ignored. The current conceptualization of the formation, difficulties, and means of transforming believers' images of and relationships with God is no different. From our perspective, the combination of theories integrated in this chapter enables a crucial differentiation to be made between symbolic and subsymbolic levels of spiritual functioning. Symbolized, or explicit spirituality, refers to the beliefs and practices maintained by believers that they can verbally describe and over which they exert a considerable degree of control. Subsymbolic, or implicit spirituality, refers to the manner in which believers' nonverbal experiences, such as their internalized patterns of infant-caregiver emotional communication, automatically and nonconsciously impact how they perceive and relate to

God. This distinction clarifies that the quality of secure and insecure believers' perceptions of and interpersonal patterns with God correspond to the security of their implicit relational representations, not the frequency of religious behavior or the content of theological beliefs (see Hall et al., 2004). Lasting therapeutic change in believers' images of and relational patterns with God, thus, requires therapists to use the power of emotion, metaphor, and the therapeutic bond to access clients' subsymbolic experience of God. Providing more accurate explicit theological beliefs, in and of itself, will not lead to lasting change in clients' experiences of, and relational patterns, with God.

The current conceptualization emphasizes the impact that experiences with primary caregivers and therapists have on implicit relational representations and, as a result of generalization, on believers' relationships with God. Although we have not emphasized this, we view God as a legitimate external object with which believers relate. This religious/theological perspective suggests the importance of direct, affectively-ladened experiences with God to establish novel neural networks which then generalize to and transform implicit representations of human attachment figures. McDargh (1983) and Jones (1991) have similarly argued for a reciprocal interactionism model, in which interactions with God can impact our implicit relational representations. In this vein, Sorenson (2004) invites clinical psychoanalysts–religious and nonreligious alike–to "... take an interest in our patients' spirituality that is respectful but not diffident, curious but not reductionistic, welcoming but not indoctrinating" (p. 1).

Indeed, imagery-based inner healing exercises or intense spiritual experiences elicited through worship, for instance, can connect with believers' maladaptive implicit representations of God and provide reparative experiences that then transform general models of relating. Given the implicit, experience-based formation of implicit relational representations, however, the absence of physical interactions with God may impede the development of a secure attachment with Him when insecure attachment dynamics continue to operate within the individual. Therefore, it seems likely that the development of a secure attachment to God, in the midst of continued operation of insecure relational representations, is mediated at least to some extent by affiliative human relationships with a therapist, members of one's spritual community, and spiritual leaders. With this theoretical framework in place, we offer an extended case example below that illustrates our theoretical perspective on attachment and God image.

CASE EXAMPLE

Below, we present the case of Allison, a forty-two-year-old, African American, elementary school teacher who was seen by the first author (J.N.). A number of facets of Allison's case illustrate the model of God image and transformation presented above.

Client History

To Allison's knowledge, her parents' marriage was stable during her childhood. However, when Allison was seven, her mother suddenly reported that she and Allison's father were getting a divorce. Allison recalled that she responded blandly to the announcement of the divorce, deciding to color her mother a picture to help her feel better. Allison's mother moved out of the family home in New York that day. Although she shared custody of Allison and her older brother, Allison's mother, Judy, moved to Texas to be near her relatives soon after the divorce. Allison saw her mother on holidays and during the summer and reported that her mother responded to her more as a friend, rather than as a parent, after the divorce.

Allison described her mother as sociable, energetic, and fun. At the same time, Allison reported that her mother gave frequent advice and criticism about Allison's decisions and reactions, implying that Allison's ideas were inferior to her mother's. Allison also experienced her mother as a poor listener, describing her as filling up their conversations with stories and giving unattuned, simplistic advice to resolve Allison's troubling emotions. Allison described her father as gentle and loving but as constantly preoccupied with concerns about his plumbing business. Allison occupied a mediator role in her family. Her parents' divorce was highly conflictual, and they continued to be overtly disparaging of each other to the children. The parents communicated to each other by sending messages through Allison, which she often softened to spare her and the other parent's feelings. Her parents, particularly her mother, were competitive for the children's affection and attempted to induce guilt in the children when they spent time with the other parent.

With regard to religious up-bringing, Allison's parents attended an Evangelical, Christian church while they were married. After the divorce, Allison's mother felt angry at God for not protecting her from a difficult marriage and became disparaging of faith. The father also stopped attending church but was more indifferent toward God. Allison's father continued to send Allison to Sunday school.

Allison enjoyed her teachers and the students at Sunday school and made a personal commitment to the Christian faith at a summer camp during junior high school. In adolescence, Allison became more dedicated to her faith, continued her affiliation with the Evangelical church, and chose to attend a conservative, Evangelical college, against her mother's advice.

Presenting Problem

Allison pursued treatment due to vague reports of difficulties in her 16-year marriage. Allison had minimal insight into the impact of her familial experiences on her emotional functioning, except for a general awareness that she was distrustful that her marriage could last long-term. As we spent time together, it became clear that Allison was experiencing significant confusion about her identity. With exploration, we realized that she perceived her feelings and desires as "selfish" and organized her sense of self by suppressing her subjectivity and aligning herself with an esteemed authority figure, such as her mother, her husband, the principal of her school, or God. As a result, she was highly dependent on others to define the "right" or "holy" way for her to live and to assure her that she was valuable. In addition, while her dependence on others was evident, it became clear that Allison also experienced minimal intimacy and often felt alone and unknown by others.

Case Conceptualization

Research indicates considerable longitudinal stability of attachment (Hesse, 1999). Thus, a parent's pattern of interpreting and responding to emotional information would remain largely consistent over time, barring significant, schema-altering emotional experiences. Allison reported that her mother had never entered therapy and had not manifested any marked relational shifts as a result of reparative spiritual or interpersonal experiences. Thus, Judy's patterns of emotional communication during Allison's early childhood and adolescence can be assumed to be structurally similar to the manner in which she responded to Allison as an infant. It appears that Judy, Allison's primary attachment figure, experienced considerable anxiety when her emotional state was not mirrored or contained, indicating that Judy had difficulty with emotional separation and likely had a preoccupied attachment. Given her impaired ability to sooth herself, Judy appears to have been overwhelmed by emotion. As a result, it seems that she responded to Allison's cues but often in a noncontingent manner. Specifically, it seems likely that Judy's anxiety heightened her reactions so that she provided an accurate response in form but overwhelmed Allison with her uncontained intensity. It also seems likely that Judy's feelings of abandonment sensitized her to experiences of danger and uncertainty, leading her to over-control Allison's spontaneous movements and feeling states in order to contain her anxiety.

Judy's emotional response patterns regulated Allison's arousal by recruiting the same neural activation patterns in her daughter, resulting in a preoccupied attachment. Due to inconsistent provision of contingent emotional responses, preoccupied individuals develop a conscious, positive image of the elusive but gratifying nurturance that others have to offer and an image of the self as the impediment to its receipt. Specifically, Allison perceived her needs and feelings as overwhelming, leading her to become preoccupied with the expectations of others, including God, and to experience a foggy sense of self. Allison viewed others as possessing the right answers that she needed to define and direct herself. Yet at a subsymbolic level, Allison expected others, including God, to be critical and burdened by her emotions, which Allison resented.

In other words, Allison consolidated an implicit relational representation that her relationships with others persist only when she accommodates to their perceived wishes and suppresses her subjectivity. This image of others as insensitive and controlling and her corresponding reaction of anger, were dissociated from her benign, powerful view of others and her shameful, helpless view of herself in order to, initially, maintain her bond with her mother and with all others thereafter. Allison's mistrust and anger at others were evident, however, in the emotional distance she maintained from them, despite her reliance on their direction for maintaining a sense of self-esteem. In sum, Allison's experience of emotion elicited intense secondary anxiety, the trigger for which was dissociated, so that she interpreted her emotions as being inherently overwhelming.

To cope with the intense anxiety associated with her subjective experiences, Allison developed various affect-regulation strategies aimed at maintaining a moderated sense of felt security. As described above, those with a preoccupied attachment subsymbolically believe that closeness is desirable but tenuously available and, thus, develop a strategy that maximizes attachment-related affect and attention on the unpredictable relationship in order to attempt to achieve an interpersonal source of affect-regulation. Indeed, in addition to devaluing and suppressing her subjectivity, Allison preoccupied herself with pleading with God for guidance and asking others for advice in an attempt to draw others close and to find the "right" way to approach situations. In times of distress, however, Allison could not keep her true feelings at bay. Yet she was uncomfortable with the assertive act of owning her needs and directly asking for assistance. Instead, she would present as helpless in order induce the receipt of comfort.

Treatment Plan, Interventions, and Therapeutic Outcomes

Allison attended treatment for about a year and a half, twice a week for about half of the duration. Initially, the therapist gained the historical information central to understanding the development and maintenance of Allison's primary, maladaptive relational schema. Specifically, the therapist noted the role that the mother's critical, controlling communication style played in establishing Allison's visceral sense that her feelings are overwhelming and unimportant and the expectation that she will need to accommodate to others in order to maintain the relationship. In addition, it was noted that Allison's role as the mediator between her parents recapitulated this experience and supported her implicit relational schema. In order to begin establishing the therapeutic bond and challenging Allison's implicit relational expectations, the therapist identified and validated the affects that Allison was communicating subsymbolically at this time, namely feeling unseen, burdened, and parentified.

This period of treatment involved many interventions that indirectly connected with Allison's subsymbolic experience through the use of metaphors to capture her sense of feeling ignored and devalued, such as feeling invisible or reduced to a tool used to contain her parents' emotions. In addition, the therapist's nonverbal mirroring of Allison's sense of dejection helped directly usher Allison into her subsymbolic experience, confirmed by her statements that she often did not realize how sad she felt until she looked at the therapist's face. This process of articulating and validating Allison's painful emotions began the consolidation of a new implicit relational schema corresponding to the experience of being soothed by an attuned other, as evidenced by Allison's ability to access a significant degree of sadness and loneliness that she expressed across several sessions.

At this point in treatment, Allison began to distance herself emotionally from the therapist, to minimize her experiences, and to ask for tips on ridding herself of her painful emotions. Initially, the therapist was unaware that Allison was experiencing her emotions and the therapeutic relationship through the filter of her maladaptive implicit relational representation. In other words, at a subsymbolic level, Allison's genuine expression of sadness triggered considerable anxiety and shame associated with her implicit relational knowledge that others experience her feelings as unacceptable and that they distance themselves from Allison as a result. Thus, Allison returned to an emotionally-superficial, people-pleasing role.

The therapist began to have images of an interview and realized that this imagery expressed Allison's retreat into safe, polite roles. The therapist noted the affective shift and, in order to interrupt the heuristic functioning of the implicit relational schema, explained that her maladaptive relational model was helping her prepare for rejection. The therapist challenged Allison's implicit belief, using language resonant with her subsymbolic experience, that her feelings needed to be cut off or sanitized for the relationship to survive. Said another way, the therapist indicated that a broader range of emotional cues could be tolerated within their relationship than Allison had learned to emit with her mother. Allison responded with intense anxiety and curiosity, indicating that she doubted that others could be responsive to the full range of her emotional signals and that she could achieve a sense of felt security outside of her compensatory strategies of suppressing her feelings and mirroring others. Yet sufficient trust was established within the therapeutic relationship so that Allison struggled to remain hopeful that honest emotional expression would not end the therapeutic relationship.

Following this particular session, a shift occurred in the treatment in which Allison became acutely aware of how ashamed she felt when experiencing and expressing her ideas and feelings. In Bucci's (1997, 2003) terms, referential activity had occurred. Allison could now reflect on her visceral belief that others could not tolerate her subjectivity, relational knowledge that she would have previously been able to express only in action. Allison stated that verbalizing her needs to others felt selfish and that needing anything from anyone, except God, was sinful. These beliefs are examples of how religious ideas of self-sacrifice and the centrality of Christ are reshaped to correspond with the nature of, in this case, the invalidating implicit relational representation.

At this therapeutic juncture, the therapist noted that Allison had identified with her internalized maternal image and perpetrated the invalidation on herself. The therapist also noted that Allison experienced God as if He was fashioned in her mother's image, expecting Him to punish her if she honestly acknowledged her degree of spiritual development and

feelings toward Him. In this way, God was expected, like all other attachment figures, to reject her emotions. Furthermore, He functioned as
a means through which Allison criticized herself. The therapist noted
the discrepancy between these experiences of God and the Christian
tenets that humans, including their emotions, are created in the image of
God and that there is no actual condemnation in the Christian life. While
these interventions appeared to help Allison cognitively differentiate
her God image from her experience of her mother, the emotional shift
occurred when Allison and the therapist made eye contact. The earnest-
ness of the therapist's vocal tone and facial expression shifted Allison's
affective state and tears came to her eyes. She expressed that she felt
free in the moment to live as she truly was before God. It appears that
the therapist's ability to emotionally synchronize with Allison enabled
her to further consolidate a representation of others as able to attune to a
fuller range of her emotional experiences, allowing her to individuate
from her internalized critical dyad.

After this phase in treatment, the therapist became aware that the imagery she was using to connect with Allison's experience, such as feeling like a welcome mat, resonated with Allison's unsymbolized anger.
We explored Allison's conspicuous lack of anger at people's criticism
and expectations that Allison act according to their preferences. As a result, Allison realized that she had dissociated her anger at her mothers'
chronic criticism and her parents' mutual disregard for her subjectivity
because she feared that they could not tolerate their relationships with
her or with each other if she was emotionally genuine. She feared that
they would abandon her. At the same time, the therapist noted that
Allison was implicitly expressing her anger about feeling overlooked
and undervalued by maintaining emotional distance from people. It
seemed that, although Allison insisted that others draw close and give
her advice, she resented their intrusions.

The therapist noted that Allison's anger continued to impact her relationships, despite her desire to believe that she did not experience this
"sinful" emotion. Further, the therapist indicated that the dissociated
nature of her anger impeded Allison from bringing this emotion into relationship with herself, others, and God, where she would likely find
some form of resolution, affirm her ability to tolerate conflict, and
achieve a greater sense of connection with others.

As a result of integrating her experience of anger into her sense of
self, Allison individuated further from her identification with her maladaptive
relational schema and began asserting her feelings and ideas to others
and to the therapist. In addition, Allison began to make decisions, such

as whether to return to school, according to an intuitive sense of what she wanted and what was best for her, trusting that God would use and direct her regardless of the path she chose. Initially, if Allison was met with resistance from others, she would revert to interpreting the situation through her maladaptive schema, assuming that she had acted inappropriately by asserting herself. This reaction reveals both the development in Allison's ability to autoregulate and her continued need for interpersonal forms of affect-regulation to maintain a sense of felt security in times of stress.

Toward the end of treatment, Allison was often able to assert herself without a sense of shame or guilt, regardless of the recipient's reaction. For instance, Allison admitted to her elderly mother that she had always resented her for positioning Allison as the mediator between her parents. She disagreed with and, ultimately, did not follow her husband's demands that she put "practicality before fantasy" and continue teaching rather than return to school to earn a degree in ministry. Finally, she expressed irritation with the therapist when she focused on the consequences of Allison's assertive behaviors rather than on validating the risks Allison took, possibly indicating the therapist's momentary fear of and attempts to suppress Allison's anger. Aware of the enactment, the therapist observed Allison's ability to not only acknowledge her anger but to also maintain a realistic image of its validity and intensity, despite the therapist's anxiety. In other words, Allison's implicit relational schema of emotional attunement and repair had become firmly established and reinforced, enabling her to validate her experience in the midst of noncontingent emotional communication and to trust that the tension would not irreparably damage the relationship.

Termination

During the last few months of treatment, Allison began to notice more aspects of the therapist's dress and office and to refer more to the dynamics of the therapeutic relationship. The therapist understood this shift as indicating that Allison had established an implicit schema of her subjectivity, even its darker aspects, as acceptable. As a result, Allison relied less on interpersonal interactions for affect-regulation, freeing her to engage in more mutual relationships. In other words, she had developed what is termed an "earned secure" attachment and was becoming curious about and pursuing interpersonal interaction as an end in itself (Hesse, 1999). At the same time, Allison expressed a deeper understanding of the sinful, self-focused part of herself, communicating these reflections with a sober, rather than a frenzied, tone of voice. Indeed, as a result of the therapeutic work, the quality of Allison's primary implicit relational representation had transformed, producing changes in her characteristic approach to affect-regulation and, consequently, to interpersonal and intrapsychic interaction with God and others. As a result of having experienced and internalized a sense of feeling loved and safe in the presence of an other, Allison had become more embracing of the uniqueness of others and bolder about exploring the darker corners of her soul, signs of significant emotional and spiritual development.

CONCLUSION

In this chapter, we have outlined a theoretical framework for understanding God image that integrates attachment theory, emotional information processing theory, and affective neuroscience. The central idea is that repeated relational experiences with primary caregivers (attachment figures) are encoded in implicit memory as implicit relational representations-a gut level sense of "how to be with" significant others. These implicit relational representations then function as an "attachment filter" with God as one becomes attached to God, biasing an individual's experiences of God toward that of human attachment relationships. We proposed a model of transformation of the God image that involves both nonverbal relational information from the therapist and an integration of this code with the symbolic, verbal code. New relational experiences recruit new neural networks that lay down the neural basis for a different way of experiencing, representing, and being with God. We illustrated this model of transformation of the God image with a case study.

REFERENCES

Beebe, B. & Lachmann, F. M. (2002). *Infant research and adult treatment: Co-constructing interactions.* Hillsdale, NJ: Analytic Press.

Benner, D. G. (1988). *Psychotherapy and the spiritual quest.* Grand Rapids, MI: Baker Book House.

Brokaw, B. F., & Edwards K. J. (1994). The relationship of God image to level of object relations development. *Journal of Psychology and Theology, 22,* 352-371.

Bowlby, J. (1969). *Attachment and loss: Vol. 1. Attachment.* New York: Basic.

Bucci, W. (1997). *Psychoanalysis & cognitive science: A multiple code theory.* New York: Guilford Press.

Bucci, W. (2003). Varieties of dissociative experiences: A multiple code account and discussion of Bromberg's case of "William." *Psychoanalytic Psychology, 20(3)*, 542-557.

Byrd, K. R., & Boe, A. (2001). The correspondence between attachment dimensions and prayer in college students. *The International Journal for the Psychology of Religion, 11(1)*, 9-24.

Granqvist, P., & Hagekull, B. (2005). *Examining relations between attachment, religiosity, and new age spirituality using the Adult Attachment Interview*. Manuscript submitted for publication.

Hall, T.W. (2004). Christian spirituality and mental health: A relational spirituality framework for empirical research. *Journal of Psychology and Christianity, 23*(1), 66-81.

Hall, T.W., Halcrow, S., Hill, P.C., & Delaney, H. (August, 2005*). Internal Working Model Correspondence in Implicit Spiritual Experiences*. Paper presented at the 113th Annual Convention of the American Psychological Association, Washington, DC.

Hesse, E. (1999). The Adult Attachment Interview: Historical and current perspectives. In J. Cassidy, & P. R. Shaver (Eds.), *Handbook of attachment: Theory, research, and clinical applications* (395-433). New York: Guilford Press.

Jones, J. W. (1991). *Contemporary psychoanalysis and religion*. New Haven: Yale University Press.

Kirkpatrick, L. A., & Shaver, P. R. (1992). An attachment-theoretical approach to romantic love and religious belief. *Personality & Social Psychology Bulletin, 18*(3), 266-275.

LeDoux, J. (1996). *The emotional brain*. New York: Simon & Schuster.

Main, M., Kaplan, N., & Cassidy, J. (1985). Security in infancy, childhood, and adulthood: A move to the level of representation. In I. Bretherton & E. Waters (Eds.), Growing points in attachment theory and research. *Monographs of the Society for Research in Child Development, 50* (1-2, Serial No. 209), 66-104.

McDargh, J. (1983). *Psychoanalytic object relations theory and the study of religion*. New York: University Press of America.

Noffke, J. L. (2006). *Refining correspondent and compensatory relationships with God: A synthesis of object relations and attachment literatures*. Unpublished doctoral dissertation, Rosemead School of Psychology, California.

Pipp, S., & Harmon, R. J. (1987). Attachment as regulation: A commentary. *Child Development, 58*, 648-652

Schore, A. N. (2003). *Affect dysregulation and disorders of the self*. New York: W.W. Norton & Company, Inc.

Siegel, D. J. (1999). *The developing mind: How relationships and the brain interact to shape who we are*. New York: Guilford Press.

Sorenson, R. (2004). *Minding spirituality*. New York: The Analytic Press.

Sroufe, L. A., Waters, E. (1977). Attachment as an organizational construct. *Child Development, 48*, 1184-1199.

Stern, D. (1985). *The interpersonal world of the infant*. New York: Basic Books.

doi:10.1300/J515v09n03_04

Chapter 5

Time-Limited Dynamic Psychotherapy and God Image

Glendon L. Moriarty, PsyD

SUMMARY. Time-Limited Dynamic Psychotherapy (TLDP) is an empirically supported treatment that can be used to conceptualize and address God image difficulties. This article provides an introduction to TLDP and outlines how the God image develops and can be modified through this method of psychotherapy. A case study is also provided to practically illustrate the TLDP process, treatment plan, and technique.
doi:10.1300/J515v09n03_05 *[Article copies available for a fee from The Haworth Document Delivery Service: 1-800-HAWORTH. E-mail address: <docdelivery@ haworthpress.com> Website: <http://www.HaworthPress.com> © 2007 by The Haworth Press. All rights reserved.]*

This chapter conceptualizes the God image through the lens of time-limited dynamic psychotherapy (TLDP). TLDP was created and empirically tested by Hans Strupp and colleagues at the Vanderbilt University Center for Psychotherapy Research in the 1980s. Hanna Levenson (1995) defines TLDP as "an interpersonal brief psychotherapy. Its goal is to help the patient move away from replicating dysfunc-

[Haworth co-indexing entry note]: "Time-Limited Dynamic Psychotherapy and God Image." Moriarty, Glendon L. Co-published simultaneously in *Journal of Spirituality in Mental Health* (The Haworth Pastoral Press, an imprint of The Haworth Press) Vol. 9, No. 3/4, 2007, pp. 79-104; and: *God Image Handbook for Spiritual Counseling and Psychotherapy: Research, Theory, and Practice* (ed: Glendon L. Moriarty, and Louis Hoffman) The Haworth Pastoral Press, an imprint of The Haworth Press, 2007, pp. 79-104. Single or multiple copies of this article are available for a fee from The Haworth Document Delivery Service [1-800-HAWORTH, 9:00 a.m. - 5:00 p.m. (EST). E-mail address: docdelivery@haworthpress.com].

Available online at http://jsmh.haworthpress.com
© 2007 by The Haworth Press. All rights reserved.
doi:10.1300/J515v09n03_05

tional interpersonal patterns by facilitating new experiences and under-standings within the context of the therapeutic relationship" (p. 30). It is a brief, psychodynamic form of treatment that focuses on the hear-and-now relationship between therapist and client.

The primary assumptions that underlie TLDP are that interpersonal problems develop in past relationships, are continued in present relation-ships, and are acted out in the therapeutic relationship (Levenson, 1995). The client reenacts their problematic way of relating with the therapist by recreating a "microcosm" of their world in the therapy office (Yalom, 1985, p. 28). For example, a client who is dependent and pulls on others for overt guidance will also be submissive and pull on the therapist for direct guidance. Therapists are naturally and unconsciously "hooked" into acting in a manner that is similar to how other people respond to the client. So, the aforementioned therapist would respond to this client in an overly direct manner that reinforced the client's dependency pattern.

Psychotherapy consists of the therapist becoming aware of this problematic way of relating and offering a different, curative re-sponse. In the above example, the therapist would recognize that she feels pulled to tell the client what to do. She would then offer a heal-ing response by relating in a way that encouraged the client to be more independent.

TLDP also offers a practical framework to understand how the God image develops and how God image difficulties are maintained. From this perspective, the client's same interpersonal problem that was learned in the past, maintained in the present, and played out with the therapist is also going to be acted out in their relationship with God. That is, their interpersonal style not only colors their current relationships, but also colors the way that they emotionally experience God. Using the exam-ple from above, the client who feels weak and like others need to control her, will have a paralleled personal experience of God in which she feels weak and like God needs to control her.

TLDP therapists use techniques to both indirectly and directly change the God image (Tan, 1996). Indirect techniques focus on the client and do not explicitly address the God image. However, indirect techniques alter the self and, as a result, implicitly modify the way that clients expe-rience God. Direct techniques explicitly address the God image. This chapter discusses both indirect and direct techniques. In addition, a life example of "Debbie," a 39 year-old divorced, evangelical, Caucasian female, is used to illustrate how techniques are used to change the God image through the TLDP process.

BACKGROUND

TLDP has its roots in three main areas. The first is psychoanalytic thought. The second is the brief therapy paradigm and the third is empirical research.

TLDP has been heavily influenced by the spectrum of psychoanalytic theory that has spanned from Freud to the contemporary interpersonal theorists. Freud created drive theory and suggested that psychological problems occur because people repress threatening impulses originally experienced in childhood (Freud, 1923). He sought to correct these problems through free association and the analysis of the transference. Freud believed that it was possible to remain objective and keep a blank slate presence on which the patient would project their issues. Then, through the process of interpretation, the repressed drives would naturally surface and be integrated into the person's life in a healthier manner.

The process of psychoanalysis required a considerable personal and financial commitment. Analysands would meet with Freud multiple times a week for a number of years. This process was very expensive. Today it would cost approximately $16,000.00 a year. Freud predicted that psychoanalysis would one day be modified so that it was less intensive and more common, but he stuck to his core assumptions and despised attempts by others to change his dogma (Strupp & Binder, 1984).

Nevertheless, many theorists questioned his assumptions and sought to make psychoanalysis more effective and practical. Salvador Ferenczi and Otto Rank were some of the first dissenters (Strupp & Binder, 1984). They suggested that analyzing repressed impulses from childhood should be lessened and more of an emphasis should be focused on the client's experience of emotion in the therapeutic relationship. It wasn't necessary to spend days digging up the past when it could be captured in the here-and-now dynamics that occurred between client and therapist. They also differed from Freud in that they recommended a more active and empathic therapeutic stance. Clinicians should see the relationship as a two-way dialogue in which they impact the client rather than see it as a one-way dialogue where they remain neutral. In addition, they advised clinicians to avoid acting in a manner that exasperated a client's interpersonal difficulties (Strupp & Binder, 1984). For example, if a client had a distant parent, then they would advise them to be emotionally available rather than withdrawn. These differences would have significantly altered Freud's psychoanalysis. They were met with resistance from Freud and others. So, the technique of analysis remained the same despite these early attempts to more efficiently focus and resolve the client's transference neurosis.

Alexander and French (1946) revived Ferenczi's and Rank's idea by fleshing it out and making it more practical. They suggested that the core relational problem has to be alive and acted out in the therapeutic relationship for it to be resolved. Clients need to experience their problem in the therapeutic relationship and then experience a curative response from the therapist. For instance, if a client had a distant parent, then they would work through the transference of seeing the therapist as distant and then emotionally experience the therapist as close and caring. This cathartic experience would then be paired with a cognitive interpretation of what occurred; thus, the "corrective emotional experience" provided clients with a new affective experience and a new intellectual understanding (Alexander, 1956).

Alexander and French's ideas, like those before, were not celebrated (Strupp & Binder, 1984). Once again, the core dogma held sway over the minds of the majority of analysts. Nevertheless, these early attempts created space for future analysts to experiment with new techniques. They showed that progress only comes with change and laid a foundation for later clinicians to introduce, test, and practice new forms of psychoanalysis.

These innovative thinkers helped pave the way for what would be the second major influence that shaped TLDP–the brief therapy paradigm. TLDP was affected by the theory and research that supported short-term psychotherapy as a viable alternative to long-term treatment. A number of factors helped dismount long-term treatment as the only option. Although nowhere near an exhaustive list, these initial issues influenced the development of TLDP.

First, many clinicians were finding that they were doing "brief" therapy by default (Budman & Gurman, 1988). They did not plan to only go 20 sessions, but many clients opted out of therapy at around this time. This led many theorists to change their models so that therapy was brief by design, not happenstance.

Next, the rise of insurance companies and HMO's required more fiscal accountability. This business motivation drove psychotherapy models to develop treatments that could be measured, so that cost-effectiveness could be assessed. This required clinicians to prove that psychotherapy was worth healthcare dollars.

Another factor that contributed to the move towards a short-term model of treatment was that research comparing long-term and short-term models of treatment showed little difference in terms of symptomatic change. Clinicians found that many of the long-term curative factors could be condensed into short-term treatment (Davanloo, 1995, Malan 1979; Mann, 1973).

In addition to psychoanalytic thought and the emergence of brief therapy, TLDP was also heavily influenced by empirical research. Strupp (1958, 1980a, 1980b, 1980c) undertook numerous studies that helped shape and validate TLDP. He, along with fellow researchers, conducted the Vanderbilt I study to see if there were differences between specific therapeutic factors (i.e., particular techniques) and nonspecific factors (i.e., interpersonal factors; Strupp & Hadley, 1979). They divided a group of 30 patients who struggled with anxiety, depression and/or social introversion into two groups. The first group was seen by trained therapists and the second group was seen by empathic college professors. After treatment, there was not much difference between the two groups. However, there was a difference between the affect therapists and professors experienced towards non-challenging patients and challenging patients. The non-challenging patients readily aligned with the therapists and professors and also experienced greater amounts of change. The challenging patients had much more difficulty aligning with the therapists and professors and experienced little to no change.

Strupp and colleagues ran a number of other analyses and concluded that difficult clients are the ones that need psychotherapy the most, but are the most at risk of not receiving it because they tend to annoy, aggravate, or otherwise frustrate their therapists. They developed TLDP as a form of treatment that could help therapists quickly identify and treat ingrained, problematic, behavior patterns. They then conducted Vanderbilt II to see if training in TLDP affected how clinicians treated difficult patients (Henry, Strupp, Butler, Schact, & Bidner, 1993). The general finding showed that specific training did result in successfully teaching therapists to use TLDP techniques. Other findings led the authors to conclude that less experienced therapists will internalize TLDP strategies more efficiently than more experienced therapists, because they have less to unlearn. In addition, not surprisingly, the study displayed that specific focused feedback increased the internalization of TLDP more than general, vague, feedback (Levenson, 1995).

Levenson (1995), along with Bein, tested TLDP by using it in the VA Short-Term Psychotherapy Project. Many of the 101 patients had longstanding issues and characterological problems. They found that "60% . . . achieved positive symptomatic change . . . At termination, 71% of the patients thought their problems lessened [and] . . . 21% of the patients achieved clinically significant interpersonal improvement" (Levenson, 1995, p.

28). Long-term follow-ups showed that the majority of the patients maintained treatment gains. In addition, other analyses showed that patients valued TLDP congruent interventions over non-congruent TLDP techniques. For example, they perceived greater benefit from TLDP strategies that focused on here-and-now interpretations of problematic interpersonal patterns than they did on non-TLDP strategies like giving homework or direct suggestions.

ASSUMPTIONS

There are seven assumptions that underlie TLDP. Each assumption has its roots in psychodynamic thought with strong emphases from object relations, attachment therapy, and interpersonal theory. The first assumption is, "The patient needs an interpersonal therapy for problems stemming from disturbed interpersonal relationships" (Levenson, 1995, p. 30). The need to connect with others is seen as one of the primary drives in life. People often experience difficulties learning how to meet this need. They can avoid others, withdraw when it becomes too intimate, or emotionally suffocate people. TLDP posits that an interpersonal treatment is needed to solve these and other interpersonal problems. Cognitive, behavioral, or humanistic approaches may be helpful, but they will not be as direct in solving relational problems.

The next assumption is, "dysfunctional styles were learned in the past" (Levenson, 1995, p. 30). People learn how to relate to others based on their early experience of their caregivers or parents. The brain is fluid in childhood, so that it can quickly pattern itself after the environment that it is found in (Grigsby & Stevens, 2000). As the individual matures, the brain becomes less flexible and patterns become more rigid. John Bowlby (1969) and Mary Ainsworth (1978) masterfully showed how these attachment patterns develop and affect how individuals relate to others.

A third assumption is, "dysfunctional styles are maintained in the present" (Levenson, 1995, p. 30). People crave consistency. Some of the need for consistency occurs consciously, but most occurs on an unconscious level. People will maintain a sense of consistency even if it is painful. If feeling worthless marked one's childhood, then maintaining that sense will be an unconscious priority in adulthood. If a person had a distant parent that they conformed themselves to please, then they will find a distant partner who they will conform themselves to please. Familiarity is comfortable, so it is better to feel hurt and consistent, than healed and inconsistent.

Another assumption is, "the patient reenacts interpersonal difficulties with the therapist" (Levenson, 1995, p. 30). Patients unconsciously recreate their relational patterns with the therapist. They instinctively "show" the therapist their issues by acting them out in therapy. Patients may verbally state that they have a tendency of annoying others, but they will also display this annoying behavior in therapy, which will result in the therapist feeling annoyed with them. In this manner, therapists get a visceral experience of what other people feel when they relate to the client.

The fifth assumption is that "the therapist is a participant observer" (Levenson, 1995, p. 30). Harry Stack Sullivan (1963) coined this term to describe the two, simultaneous roles of the therapist. The first part involves actively participating in the relationship. This is a different stance from what early analysts held. TLDP therapists recognize that they impact the client, whereas early analysts believed that they were able to remain neutral. The second part involves observing the relationship as it develops. Therapists strive to be aware of the process that occurs in the relationship. The therapist is actively engaged, while, at the same time, observing how the dynamics unfold between them. The goal is to enter and genuinely engage in the relationship, so that it can be changed from the inside-out.

The next assumption is that, "The therapist becomes hooked in to reenacting difficulties with the patient" (Levenson, 1995). This assumption lies at the heart of TLDP. Therapists automatically get pulled into acting out the client's main interpersonal problems. This happens naturally and on an unconscious level. The countertransference is complementary to the client's transference. For instance, if the client is irritating, then the therapist will feel irritated. Once the therapist gets hooked, the therapist has to get unhooked. They have to recognize that they were unconsciously repeating the interpersonal problem that brought the client into treatment. Instead of reinforcing the problem, the therapist needs to offer a different response that encourages the client to act in a new manner. For example, the irritating client that annoys others will also annoy the therapist. The therapist needs to get unhooked by becoming aware of his or her annoyance. Then, the therapist should respond in a manner that is different from how other others respond. That is, if others distance themselves and get annoyed, the therapist has to stay close and work through that annoyance, so that the problem is resolved and not repeated.

The last assumption states "there is one identifiable, problematic interpersonal problem" (Levenson, 1995, p. 30). TLDP therapists practice "benign neglect." There are a variety of relational problems to focus on, but they instead focus on the core problem. Changing the larger problem will result in changing the other smaller problems. Once the primary problem is resolved the healing effects will trickle down and correct the secondary problems.

GOD IMAGE DEVELOPMENT
AND GOD IMAGE DIFFICULTIES

TLDP draws upon many different strands of psychoanalytic theory, so using this model to conceptualize God image development involves many insights originally gleaned from psychodynamic and object relations theory. Freud (1927) started it off by publishing many controversial, and arguably pessimistic, works on the God image and psychoanalysis. His central thesis was that the God image has its roots in projection and wish fulfillment. People have difficulty dealing with pain, so they project that there is a God who cares for them. D.W. Winnicott (1971) implicitly countered some of Freud's assumptions and provided a context in which positive aspects of the God image could be better understood. Ana Maria Rizzuto (1971) built upon Winnicott's work and developed the first, comprehensive, God image development theory by integrating object relations and Erik Erickson's developmental theory.

Dynamic theory views the person as developing through a number of stages. When the task of the first stage is adequately met, the person can move onto the next stage (Erickson, 1980). The successful resolution of each stage provides the person with a new of way relating to the world. The unsuccessful resolution of a stage results in fixation. In general, the earlier the fixation at a particular stage, the more challenging the problem is to overcome. Some theorists see these stages as more rigid, whereas others see them as more flexible. However, the easy majority hold to the main assumption that early relationships teach people how to relate to others and those ways of relating are carried on into future relationships.

The God image develops along with the changing self. Each developmental stage affects how the God image is experienced by the person.

There are a number of developmental stages; however, this chapter focuses on what this author considers to be the most important.

The first stage is trust vs. mistrust (Erickson, 1980, Rizzuto, 1979). This stage influences whether children learn to trust or mistrust others and God. The primary caregiver, usually the mother, plays the main role here. If the caregiver loves, accepts, and meets the needs of her infant, then the infant concludes that others, the universe, and God can be trusted. If the caregiver neglects or abuses her infant, then the infant will conclude that others, the universe, and God *cannot* be trusted.

When this stage is successfully resolved children move onto the separation-individuation stage (Mahler, Pine, & Bergman, 1975). This stage influences whether or not children learn to follow their internal drive and slowly psychologically separate from their caregivers. If they do not feel safe, then they will feel that they need to remain with their caregiver. They will not grow and emotionally separate from the caregiver, but will instead feel that growth is threatening. They may fear that if they separate from their caregiver, then bad things will happen.

This stage has a tremendous impact on the God image (Rizzuto, 1979). Children, later as adults, will play out this same pattern with God. If they can trust and separate from their caregiver, then as an adult they will experience God as mature and encouraging of their autonomy. If they cannot trust and separate from their caregiver, then they will later experience God as immature and possibly needy. They may not be aware of this, but their behavior will be characterized by a fear that if they grow too much or become too independent, then God will be unhappy and abandon them.

The next main stage of development is the Oedipal phase. It occurs between the ages of 4 to 6, and is marked by intense feelings for the parent of the opposite sex (Brenner, 1973). In a healthy family, the child is able to navigate this conflict with success. He will slowly come to the conclusion that he cannot have his mother all to himself. This is a great loss to the boy, but instead of facing this reality entirely, he unconsciously transfers all of his feelings over to his father. He no longer longs for his mother, because he sensed he could not safely win all of her attention; instead, now, he hopes to win all of his father's attention. Gradually, he becomes aware that this is not going to occur either. The boy then realizes that he will have to wait until he is older to have an adult relationship. At that point, he will see his parents from a more objective stance.

The child who grows up in a dysfunctional family has a much more difficult time with this conflict. Because his fundamental needs were never satisfied, he will not be able to let go of his desire to wholly possess another. As a result, he will constantly seek out others in an attempt to complete himself. This feeling of wholeness will never be captured. As he moves into adolescence, he will potentially lock onto his God image to satisfy this deep longing. His relationship with God may be "highly charged." Unfortunately, this relationship will not satisfy his inner needs.

Rizzuto's thoughts are helpful in understanding how the God image develops throughout the lifecycle. Her views are very traditional and emphasize that the self and God image are more or less solidified at age 6. Most dynamic theorists see these initial years as very important, but no longer believe that the self and God image are crystallized in early childhood. The self and God image are now seen as more fluid, adaptable and able to change.

Two recent studies support the shift towards thinking that the self and God image are not fixed in childhood, but can significantly change through therapy in adulthood. The first study, by Tisdale et al. (1997), focused on the effectiveness of an inpatient object relations based program on self-esteem, level of object relations development, and God image. The researchers found that treatment significantly improved the clients' view of themselves as well as their view of God. The second study, by Cheston, Piedmont, Eanes, and Lavin (2003) sought to test whether short-term psychotherapy (without explicit intervention to change the God image) would result in a decrease in symptoms and improvement of the God image. They found that the treatment did result in a decrease of symptoms and did improve the clients' God images. After therapy, the God image was experienced as significantly more loving and compassionate.

GOD IMAGE CHANGE

The self and the God image are closely interconnected; as the self changes, the God image changes. Clients learn to have a problematic sense of self and God image through early unhealthy relationships with their caregivers. Similarly, clients can learn to develop a healthy sense of self and God image through a healing relationship with their therapist. Maladaptive ways of relating result in God image problems, whereas corrective ways of relating result in the resolution of God image problems.

God image change occurs through internalization, which is the gradual process by which people learn to treat themselves as others treat them. If a client is raised by perfectionistic parents, then he will treat himself in a perfectionistic manner and also experience God as perfectionistic. TLDP utilizes the same process of internalization that occurs in the parent-child relationship to change the way a person treats themselves and to change the way that they experience God. The goal is for clients to internalize the character of the therapist to learn to treat themselves as the therapist treats them (Blatt & Behrends, 1987). Through this process, the harsh internal voice of the caregivers becomes replaced with the empathic voice of the therapist. This changes the way the person treats themselves and also changes the way that they emotionally experience God. The client's God image was initially shaped by the parent. As therapy progresses, the God image becomes patterned after the therapist. As a result, the God image becomes empathic and accepting, rather than disinterested and rejecting.

The first step the therapist takes to facilitate this process is to identify the client's cyclical maladaptive pattern (CMP; Strupp & Binder, 1984). The CMP outlines four quadrants of interpersonal information and helps identify the client's primary interpersonal problem. Levenson (1995) details each aspect:

1. Acts of the self–a patient's thoughts, feelings, wishes and behaviors of an interpersonal nature.
2. Expectations of others' reactions–this pertains to all statements having to do with how the patient imagines others will react to him or her in response to some interpersonal behavior.
3. Acts of others toward the self–this consists of the actual behaviors of other people, as observed and interpreted by the patient.
4. Acts of the self towards the self (introject)–this refers to the patient's behaviors or attitudes toward herself or himself–when the self is the object of the interpersonal dynamic. That is, how the person treats him or herself (p. 49).

Levenson furthered this model by adding a fifth component, which is Countertransference Reactions. Moriarty (2006) adds a sixth part, Experience of God image.

5. Countertransference reactions–includes the way you feel in relationship with the client. How do you feel being in the room with the client? What are you pulled to do or not do? (p. 50)

6. Experience of God image–refers to the thoughts and feelings the client experiences when relating to his or her personal experience of God.

After the therapist fills the client's information into the above six components, they analyze the relational data to determine the client's main interpersonal problem. There might be a variety of relational problems, but the therapist restricts their attention to the primary problem. If they change the one major problem, then the results will generalize and resolve the other minor interpersonal problems.

Once the therapist has identified the main interpersonal problem, they construct the 4 main goals of spiritually-oriented TLDP: (1) New experience of self and therapist (Levenson, 1995); (2) New understanding of self and therapist (Levenson, 1995); (3) New experience of self and God image; (4) New understanding of self and God image. The focus on experience and understanding has its roots in Franz Alexander's (1956) corrective emotional experience. His thesis is that client's need both an emotional experience *and* intellectual insight to achieve long-term change in their interpersonal patterns.

The emphasis on experience is important for a couple of reasons (Levenson, 1995). First, it allows clients to experience themselves in a different, more adaptive, manner. If a client usually experiences herself as weak with others, then it can be very empowering for her to experience herself as strong with the therapist. Second, it allows them to experience another person–the therapist–in a different, healthier, way. If a client usually experiences others as rejecting, then it can be healing for her to continuously experience the therapist as accepting.

The new experience of the therapist also translates to a new experience of the God image. If before she felt weak and rejected by her God image, she will now feel strong and accepted by her God image. Similarly, she will also experience her God image in a new way. It will no longer be rigid and inflexible, but will instead be fluid and flexible. The God image can be more than rejecting and demeaning. It can also be empathic and empowering.

The emphasis on a new understanding is also very important (Levenson, 1995; Strupp & Binder, 1984). A new experience is essential, but clients have to understand why that experience is significant. A new experience, without a rational understanding, results in change that quickly fades, whereas a new experience with understanding results in long-term change (Alexander, 1956). Cognitively framing the situation puts handles on the problem, so clients can more easily grasp it and guard against experiencing it again (McCullough-Vaillant, 1997).

If the client has this understanding, then they can more readily identify when they are experiencing their God image in a harmful manner. This map allows them to see how these difficulties originally arose and provides them with a means to correct painful God image experiences The intellectual framework, puts it in perspective and allows them to act on the situation rather than feel powerless to change it.

LIFE EXAMPLE

Presenting Problem

Debbie is a 52-year-old, divorced, evangelical, female who sought treatment for help with anxiety and feeling like God is mad at her. She worried about many things and frequently feared that others were going to reject her. She had a hard time making decisions for herself and would often get people to tell her what to do. In addition, she was a very devout Christian who regularly engaged in prayer and church activities, but continually sensed that God was displeased with her.

Client History

Debbie grew up in a working class family. Her parents had a very traditional relationship and often kept themselves separated from her. The boundary between her and her parents was wide. She often felt isolated and alone, even when they were with her.

Her father was a hard worker who spent most of his time in the machine shop. She thought they had a good relationship, but did not feel like she spent enough time with him. Her mother was very domineering and had rigid ideas as to how children should behave. There was not a lot of room for play and imagination. Instead, Debbie was expected to behave as a little adult. Her mother supplied her with a long list of chores each day and expected her to busily complete her duties.

Debbie's mother was very emotionally inconsistent. Sometimes she would be kind, but at other times she would become extremely angry for what seemed like no reason at all. She would then either lash out or emotionally withdraw. Debbie never knew what to expect. She learned to cope by doing all her chores, always smiling, and being as nice as possible.

People tended to like Debbie because she had a natural ability to tune in to what they wanted. She was quiet and friendly throughout her school years. Teachers thought she was well mannered and friends found her very trustworthy and eager to listen.

She met a man who was a little older than her after graduating from high school. He had a strong personality and was very controlling. Before she knew it, they had married and moved away from her childhood home. Shortly thereafter she realized that her new husband was unpredictable. There were times when he was happy, but other times in which he would get very angry. He did not talk a lot, but he still communicated exactly what he wanted. Debbie intuitively picked up on his desires and gradually shaped herself to please him. The only problem was that he, like her mother, could not be pleased. He eventually left her for another woman. Ironically, Debbie blamed herself for their unsuccessful marriage.

Debbie's active church life was one of the main things that helped her cope. She felt needed and respected at church. However, she also often felt overwhelmed because many people requested too much of her. She belonged to a very dogmatic church that clearly spelled out the "right" and the "wrong" way to believe. This structure fit her personality, because she craved direction and strongly desired the guidance of others. She loved her church, but she had an internal struggle that she did not often discuss. Her pastor always talked about a loving God, but this was not the God she encountered when she closed her eyes. Her God was harsh, critical, and very difficult to please. She tried desperately to make her God happy, but always felt like she failed God.

Debbie started therapy when she was at her "wit's end." She had been divorced for several years, but she still worried about her ex-husband. She enjoyed her work, but always felt like she was going to be "disciplined," even though her evaluations were consistently stellar. Debbie was also frustrated in her walk with God. She wanted to know the gracious and accepting God that she so often heard of and believed in, but seldom experienced.

Case Conceptualization

The best way to conceptualize Debbie is to use the CMP.

1. Acts of self–Debbie tends to please others at the expense of herself. She overworks and often does whatever people ask her to do,

even if she does not want to. She always "wears a smile," is often tired, feels anxious, worries frequently.

2. Expectations of others' reactions–Debbie expects to be rejected if she doesn't please others by being overly nice to them and doing what she feels they want her to do.

3. Acts of others toward the self–people ask her to do a lot of extra things, they frequently feel comfortable telling her what to do.

4. Acts of the self towards the self (introject)–Debbie criticizes herself for not accomplishing enough at work. She tells herself that other people do not like her.

5. Countertransference–Debbie acts out her people pleasing behavior with me. As a result, I feel idealized and pulled to tell her what to do.

6. Experience of God image–Debbie experiences God as demanding, critical, frustrated, and rejecting. Her God image expects a lot from Debbie and makes her feel guilty when she does not accomplish everything she sets out to accomplish.

Now that we have Debbie's CMP spelled out, the next step is to identify the one main interpersonal problem. Debbie's main problem is that she is skilled at getting others to tell her what to do. There are a variety of other problems that Debbie experiences, but the main theme that continually emerges is that she sacrifices herself to focus her efforts on pleasing others. She is driven to please others for she fears that if she does not they will abandon her. As a result, she ignores her own needs and invests considerable time and energy trying to please others by doing what she feels they want her to do.

Treatment Plan

TLDP utilizes a style of treatment planning that is flexible. In the age of HMOs most people think about treatment plans as containing specific interventions with measured outcomes. Most dynamic clinicians balk at this type of treatment planning because they feel that it defines the person and the therapy process in an unhelpful manner. TLDP therapists view treatment planning in a broader, less rigid, manner that is based on core goals. These goals are framed in response to the main interpersonal problem.

The first goal is a new experience of self and a new experience of the therapist (Levenson, 1995). This goal would be met if Debbie experienced herself as assertive (i.e., non-people pleasing) and me as caring for her when she is not trying to please me. This will be challenging because Debbie will repeat the same interpersonal pattern with me that she acts out with others. Remember, I cannot help but naturally react to what a person pulls for. What would Debbie's hook be? How would I feel pulled to respond to her? When Debbie first started therapy, she interacted with me in a manner that pulled for me to tell her what to do. I found myself making strong suggestions and being overly directional. I was too forward with my recommendations and saw Debbie as less strong and resourceful than she was. This is exactly what the CMP would predict. Debbie's main problem is that she is skilled at getting others to tell her what to do. That is what she was doing with me. She was replicating her main interpersonal problem by working hard to please me, just like she works hard to please others and God.

Once I realized I was hooked, I needed to get unhooked. I had naturally fell into her interpersonal problem and needed to get out of it to help her. Through discussing the dynamics of our relationship, Debbie was eventually able to see what was occurring. She recognized that she was ignoring her own real struggles to try to figure out what I wanted so that she could please me. After this realization, Debbie took risks and focused on her own needs. She allowed herself to be more assertive and confident. Debbie expected me to reject her and was shocked to find out that I still cared for her. She had a new experience in which she felt valued for being herself and not for pleasing me.

The second goal is a new understanding of self and therapist (Levenson, 1995). The new experience is essential, but it needs to be complemented with a solid cognitive understanding to result in lasting change. To cement this change, Debbie and I spent time talking about how her interpersonal problem developed in past relationships and is maintained in current relationships. We came to the conclusion that her tendency to get others to tell her what to do had its roots in her critical relationship with her mother. At that time, it served as a survival mechanism to help her remain connected to her mother. She had to bend and conform herself to his mother's wishes in order to keep a relationship with her. A painful relationship was better than no relationship. We also concluded that her interpersonal problem is maintained through her relationship with her colleagues. People ask too much of her and never seem to be pleased with what she does. As a result, she repeats the same problem with them that she learned with her mother. That is, she ignores herself and works doubly hard to please her colleagues. This problem is also maintained in her relationships with fellow church members. They have high expectations and she regularly sacrifices herself to take care of their wishes.

Debbie realized that she did not have a choice in her childhood relationship with her mother. She needed to repress herself in order to stay connected to her mother. However, she did have a choice as an adult. She did not have to ignore her needs in order to please others. Debbie could take steps to care for herself. She could abstract herself from being the caretaker and give other people the opportunity to learn to meet their own needs.

The third goal is a new experience of self and God image. This goal parallels the first goal in that the new experience of the self and therapist is the same as the new experience of self and God image. As Debbie took risks with me she was also able to take risks with God. She indicated that she more readily shared authentic thoughts and feelings with God. As a result, she felt her relationship with God became more genuine. She was no longer acting weak and passive, but was instead strong and active. This new experience of God loving her, even when she is genuine and confident, allowed her to learn to relate to God in a new manner.

The fourth goal is a new understanding of self and God image. Debbie needed a cognitive understanding of the dynamics that played out with her God image, so that she could monitor them and challenge negative relational experiences that occurred between her and her God image. We talked about the basic process of projection and Debbie readily understood how her negative experience of God helped her to maintain a sense of consistency with her past. She saw God as demanding and difficult to please, because she experienced her mother as demanding and difficult to please. Debbie was also more able to believe her evangelical theology. She became comfortable with the idea that she did not have to act passive and dependent to secure God's love.

Interventions

I used both implicit and explicit interventions with Debbie (Tan, 1996). Implicit techniques do not directly address the God image, but they still indirectly change the God image through changing the self. Explicit techniques directly address the God image and explicitly change it by incorporating the God image into the interventions.

One of the main explicit techniques I used was based on the work of Janis Morgan Strength (1998) who expanded Menninger's (1958) triangle to a square to offer interpretations addressing the person's relationship with God. She listens for the repetition of the same theme in a person's current relationship, past relationship, therapeutic relationship, and relationship with their God image. Each piece of information represents a side of the square, which she connects before she offers an interpretation:

Past Relationship ─────────────── Current Relationship

Therapeutic Relationship   God Image Relationship

Direct change of the God image occurs through calling attention to this and connecting each side of the square. For example, Debbie repeated a theme of letting people down and, as a result, feeling overwhelmed with guilt. I offered this interpretation to Debbie to bring this to awareness:

> It seems like you are frequently afraid that you are not doing enough to maintain your relationship with your co-workers (current relationship). When you recall your adolescence, you have expressed a similar regret surrounding your inability to accomplish enough to stay connected to your mother (past relationship). You also consistently experience God as upset with you because you feel you let God down when you do not achieve as much as you hope to (God image relationship). And, even today, you have indicated that you think I am disappointed with you because you are not making enough "progress" (therapeutic relationship). There appears to be a theme that runs through each of these relationships in which you feel guilty because you do not fulfill what you feel others expect of you.

TLDP interventions use immediacy to target how the client's dynamics unfold in the here-and-now relationship between therapist and client. To illustrate how this works, I have cataloged a number of TLDP interventions that I used with Debbie. Again, direct interventions incorporate the God image, whereas indirect do not.

One TLDP intervention, "encourages the patient to explore feelings and thoughts about the therapist or the therapeutic relationship" (Levenson,

1995, p. 241). In addition, it can also be modified to help clients explore their feelings about their God image.

Me: I wonder how you are feeling towards me?

Debbie: I really like you and I'm really glad to be working with you.

Me: I wonder if there is something you don't like about the therapy relationship. Something you are not crazy about or would like to change?

Debbie only allows herself to experience positive feelings toward others. This problem has its roots in her relationship with her mother who could not tolerate any form of negative feedback. Debbie quickly learned that she could only state things that made her mother feel good about herself. This problem was maintained with her husband before their divorce and is currently maintained with her friends and fellow churchgoers. Debbie experiences negative feelings and thoughts towards others, but she quickly denies them. She would never actually express them for fear that she would be immediately rejected. Debbie thinks that I will become enraged if she offers a slight criticism. When she took the leap and expressed negative feedback, she was shocked to find that I could hear and appreciate the feedback. That I was still connected to her and that our relationship was stronger because it is more honest and genuine. Providing Debbie with this new experience allowed her to begin to integrate negative thoughts and feelings.

Debbie was also afraid to express anything other than positive feelings towards God. Unconsciously, she saw God like her mother. After processing some of her frustration towards me, we were then able to process some of the things she is not too pleased about in her relationship with God. She gradually tolerated being able to be more authentic with God. She eventually recognized that God is not going to lash out at her for having non-plussed feelings or thoughts. She learned to value genuineness and reported feeling closer to God after she prayed and discussed things that she had unconsciously been keeping from God.

Another TLDP intervention, "encourages the patient to discuss how the therapist might feel or think about the patient" (Levenson, 1995, p. 241). Debbie projected that I felt the same way towards her that she imagines others feel about her. According to the CMP, Debbie expected rejection and believed she had to please me to gain my approval. My goal was to provide Debbie with a new experience in which she felt accepted and cared for regardless of her performance. Visualize how this intervention played out when she was late for a session:

Debbie: Sorry I'm late.

Me: How do you think I feel towards you?

Debbie: You are probably very frustrated with me for being late.

Me: What makes you think I am frustrated with you?

Debbie: Well, I'm late. I'm irresponsible. You cannot count on me to do things right. I feel really bad for letting you down.

Me: What do you think I want to say to you?

Debbie: Probably that you think I'm worthless . . . that you regret accepting me as a client (Notice the transference: it sounds like she is expecting me to respond as her mother would have).

Me: Have there been other people in the past or present who have told you that you are worthless for making a mistake? Have you ever experienced God in that way?

Debbie: Oh yeah, my mother was always telling me I'm worthless. I sometimes feel like God thinks I'm worthless too. I know He doesn't, but I feel this way especially after I feel like I've failed Him in some way.

Me: So, you learned from your mother that if you make a mistake you are worthless. You also experience God in this way too. Similarly, you expect me to be angry with you for being late. Can you see how that is a pattern?

Debbie: Yes I can. I do. I really expect you to be mad at me and reject me . . . just like my mother would have. Are you mad at me?

Me: No Debbie, I'm not mad at you. I like you just as much as I did before. How does it feel to hear that?

Debbie: It feels weird . . . weird, but good . . . different. I don't know if I've ever been accepted after making a mistake.

Me: Can you imagine God accepting you after you miss the mark?

Debbie: Yeah, yeah, I can. I just have to let myself feel Him in that way.

Debbie expects me to reject her for being late. Notice that I did not counter this right away, but instead allowed it to build up to get her in touch with her feelings. I then used the triangle of person to make connections to his past relationship with her mother, relationship with her God image, and transference with me. This allowed Debbie to recognize the interpersonal pattern. Then I offered her a different response by telling her I still cared for her. I stayed connected to her and helped her get in touch with that feeling. This provides Debbie with the new experience of feeling accepted after making a mistake.

Another TLDP intervention utilizes self-disclosure counter-transference reactions to help the client see how his or her behavior affects others (Levenson, 1995, p. 241). As mentioned earlier, clients evoke in the therapist the same feelings that they evoke in others. The therapist's goal is to become aware of this and then react in a manner that is healing. Through using Debbie's CMP, I predicted that she would sacrifice herself to please me. I was initially hooked into this by being very pleased with her, but then realized that she was neglecting herself in order to be the perfect client. I then gave her feedback, so that she could experience herself as being cared for even if she was not perfect.

Me: Debbie you are an excellent client. You work hard all the time, ask insightful questions, and are very committed. I find myself feeling very pleased with you, but I am wondering if this might be part of the problem.

Debbie: What do you mean? Problem?

Me: Well, you often sacrifice yourself to make others happy and I'm wondering if you are sacrificing yourself in here to make me happy. I know you have some real hurts and issues you are struggling with, but you seldom bring them up. You always give a positive report, but I'm wondering if you avoid these issues out of fear that I'd be displeased with you for discussing them?

Debbie: I realize that. I'm afraid that if I'm honest with how I really feel, you will grow tired of me. I want to open up about my real issues, but I'm scared you will grow frustrated with me if you knew the real me.

TREATMENT LENGTH AND THERAPEUTIC OUTCOMES

I saw Debbie for 20 sessions. We met one time a week for 50 minutes. Treatment progressed through the beginning, middle, and end phases of treatment.

The beginning stages of treatment were marked by building rapport and gathering information. Debbie experienced positive transference towards me and felt comfortable discussing her past and present relationships. In addition, she easily answered questions about her religious beliefs and readily shared about her emotional experience of God. She seemed very eager to make the most of her time and appeared willing to take steps to alleviate her anxiety and depression.

After our first few sessions, I felt I had a good understanding of her CMP and how the main interpersonal problem had developed, was maintained, and influenced her emotional experience of God. That is, I could trace the dependent pattern back to her unpredictable relationship with her mother, see how it was maintained with her ex-husband and current friends, and how it played out with her God image.

As therapy progressed through the middle stages of treatment, we began to explore how her CMP was played out in our relationship. How Debbie's tendency to please, repress her opinions, and be compliant impacted our relationship. I disclosed my feelings towards her. How I naturally really liked her and often felt good and validated when I was with her, but how this might be part of a larger problematic pattern. We explored how this tendency developed. How it was a great survival skill that helped her cope with difficult relationships. We also discussed how that underlying pattern affected her personal experience of God. She thus had experienced both emotional and cognitive change in her experience with me, others, and her God image. Debbie clearly saw this pattern and recognized that this way of relating served its purpose, but was now outdated. I used several TLDP interventions throughout this time to capture and work through this tendency in the here and now context of our relationship.

Throughout these repeated interventions, Debbie was gradually able to experience herself in a more assertive manner. She more readily expressed her opinions and began to put down boundaries in her relation-ships with people in her life. When others asked too much of her, she simply said "no" and indicated that she wasn't comfortable committing that much time and energy.

These treatment gains also translated to her God image. Debbie be-gan to see how she had unconsciously modeled her God image after her mother. She indicated that her spiritual life changed. She did not feel compelled to compulsively pray to "make things right with God." Her "operational theology"–the emotional underpinnings of her faith–had changed so that she could more readily believe in and experience her understanding of God's grace and forgiveness (Jordan, 1986). She be-gan to see God as a Being that she could share things with and not hide things from. Her God image became a source of encouragement rather than a source of perfectionism. In addition, she indicated that she felt that God had created her for a reason and that she could confidently follow her "calling" to fulfill that purpose.

The final stages of treatment were characterized by reinforcing the treatment gains she had made. We deliberately put cognitive frames on the relational changes she experienced. This provided her with an intel-lectual map to see how her interpersonal problems developed, were maintained, and consequently resolved. This helped her identify her triggers, so she could recognize situations that enervated her CMP. The end stages were also marked by discussions about termination issues like what it meant to say good bye. I let her know that I would be avail-able for future consultations if needed, and also explored the pro's and con's of her therapy experience.

STRENGTHS AND WEAKNESSES

There are a few key strengths and weaknesses of spiritually-oriented TLDP. The first strength is that it offers a practical framework to under-stand the relational dynamics and the God image. The facile use of the CMP enables clinicians to quickly identify transference, counter-trans-ference, and God image projections.

Another strength of the approach is that it has been empirically vali-dated. In the age of managed care, it is important for therapists to show that what they are doing works. A third, and related, strength is that TLDP works with a spectrum of clients. TLDP works well with adjust-ment issues as well as characterological problems (Levenson, 1995; Strupp & Binder, 1984).

A final strength is that TLDP interventions can be easily modified to address the God image. The techniques are based on analysis of the transference and relational dynamics. These issues play out with a person's God image, so the techniques can be used to explore this relationship in a meaningful manner.

TLDP also has a few weaknesses. One limitation is that there is a paucity of research on how TLDP can be used to affect the God image. There have been several studies that support the relationship between dynamic therapy and the God image (e.g., Tisdale et al., 1997), and studies to support non-specific treatment and God image change (Cheston, Piedmont, Eanes, & Lavin, 2003), but none specifically supporting TLDP and God image change. Despite this weakness, the case for TLDP as a useful model of treatment is buffered by these more general studies and theoretical support (Jones, 1991; McDargh, 1983; Spero, 1990).

Another weakness is that TLDP clinicians have to be fairly intelligent and patient to learn how to effectively use TLDP. Research has shown that it can be learned, but therapists need to overcome a few obstacles to fully grasp it (Henry et al., 1993). A final, and related, weakness is that clients also have to be of at least average intelligence to benefit from TLDP (Levenson, 1995).

SUMMARY

To sum up, TLDP is an empirically supported treatment that provides a practical framework to conceptualize and treat relational problems. In addition, it can also be utilized to understand and modify problematic God images. The main assumptions are that interpersonal issues develop in the past, are maintained in the present, played out with the therapist, and acted out with the God image.

Clients recreate their main interpersonal problem with the therapist and their God image. The therapist responds differently than other individuals in the client's life. This corrective emotional experience changes the client's self and God image. For example, the case of "Debbie" was used to illustrate how spiritually-oriented TLDP modified her sense of self and God image. Debbie's main problem was a dependent personality pattern in which she minimized her autonomy and maximized the control of others in her life. She had a parallel experience of God in that she felt God was domineering–

much like her mother, ex-husband, and colleagues. As treatment progressed, Debbie continuously experienced me as supportive and herself as increasingly independent. These experiences corrected her idea of herself and her emotional idea of God. As a result, she experienced herself as confident and autonomous and her God image as affirming and supportive.

REFERENCES

Ainsworth, M. D. S. (1978). *Patterns of attachment: a psychological study of the strange situation.* Hillsdale, N.J; New York: Lawrence Erlbaum Associates.

Alexander, F. (1956). *Psychoanalysis and psychotherapy, Developments in theory, technique, and training.* New York: W. W. Norton & Co

Alexander, F. & French, T.M. (1946). *Psychoanalytic therapy: Principles and applications.* New York: Ronald Press.

Baumeister, R. F. (1995). Self and identity: An introduction. In A. Tesser (Ed.), *Advanced Social Psychology* (pp. 51-98). Boston, MA: McGraw Hill.

Blatt, S. & Behrends, B. (1987). Internalization, separation-individuation, and the nature of the therapeutic action. *International Journal of Psychoanalysis, 68:2,* 279-297.

Bowlby, J. (1969). *Attachment and loss.* New York: Basic Books.

Brenner, C. (1973). *An elementary textbook of psychoanalysis.* New York: Anchor.

Cheston, S.E., Piedmont, R.L., Eanes, B., & Lavin, L.P. (2003). Changes in clients image of God over the course of outpatient therapy. *Counseling and Values, 47,* 96-108.

Danvanloo, H. (1995). *Unlocking the unconscious: Selected papers of Habib Davanloo.* New York: Wiley & Sons.

Erickson, E. (1980). *Identity and the life cycle.* New York: W.W. Norton.

Freud, S. (1927). *The future of an illusion. S.E. (Standard Edition),* 21:5-56. London: Hogarth Press.

Freud, S. (1923). *The ego and the id. S.E. (Standard Edition),* 19:12-66. London: Hogarth Press.

Henry, W.P., Strupp, H.H., Butler, S.F., Schact, T.E., and Binder, J.L. (1993). Effects of training in time-limited dynamic psychotherapy: Changes in therapist behavior. *Journal of Consulting and Clinical Psychology, 61,* 434-440.

Jones, J.W. (1991). *Contemporary psychoanalysis and religion.* New York: Yale.

Jordan, M.R. (1986). *Taking on the Gods: The task of the pastoral counselor.* Nashville, TN: Abingdon.

Levenson, H. (1995). *Time-limited dynamic psychotherapy: A guide to clinical practice.* New York: Basic Books.

Mahler, M., Pine, F., & Bergman, A. (1975). *The psychological birth of the human infant: symbiosis and individuation.* New York: Basic Books.

Malan, D.M. (1979). *Individual psychotherapy and the science of psychodynamics.* London: Butterworth.

Mann, J. (1973). *Time-limited psychotherapy.* Cambridge: Harvard University Press.

McCullough-Vaillant, L.M. (1997). *Changing character: Short-term anxiety-regulating psychotherapy for restructuring defenses, affects and attachments.* New York: Basic Books.

McDargh, J. (1983). *Psychoanalytic object relations theory and the study of religion: On faith and the imaging of God.* Lanham, MD: University Press of America.

Menninger, K. (1958). *Theory of psychoanalytic technique.* New York: Basic.

Moriarty, G. (2006). *Pastoral care of depression: Helping clients heal their relationship with God.* New York: Haworth.

Rizzuto, A.M. (1974). Object relations and the formation of the image of God. *British Journal of Medical Psychology, 47,* 83-99.

Spero, M.H., (1990). Parallel dimensions of experience in psychoanalytic psychotherapy of the religious patient. *Psychotherapy, 27,* 53-71.

Strength, J.M. (1998) Expanding Davanloo's interpretive triangles to explicate the client's introjected image of God. *Journal of Psychology and Theology, 26:2,* 172-187.

Strupp, H.H. (1958) The psychotherapist's contribution to the treatment process: An experimental investigation. *Behavioral Science, 3,* 43-67.

Strupp, H.H. (1980a). Success and failure in time-limited psychotherapy: A systematic comparison of two cases (Comparison 1). *Archives of General Psychiatry, 37,* 595-603.

Strupp, H.H. (1980b). Success and failure in time-limited psychotherapy: A systematic comparison of two cases (Comparison 2). *Archives of General Psychiatry, 37,* 708-716.

Strupp, H.H. (1980c). Success and failure in time-limited psychotherapy: A systematic comparison of two cases (Comparison 3). *Archives of General Psychiatry, 37,* 831-841.

Strupp, H.H. (1993). The Vanderbilt psychotherapy studies: synopsis. *Journal of Consulting and Clinical Psychology, 61,*431-433.

Strupp, H.H., & Binder, J.L. (1984). *Psychotherapy in a new key.* New York: Basic Books.

Strupp, H.H., & Hadley, S.W. (1979). Specific versus nonspecific factors in psychotherapy: A controlled study of outcome. *Archives of General Psychiatry, 36,* 1125-1136.

Sullivan, H.S. (1953). *The interpersonal theory of psychiatry.* New York: Norton.

Tan, S.Y. (1994). Ethical considerations in religious psychotherapy: potential pitfalls and unique resources. *Journal of Psychology and Theology, 22,* 389-394.

Tan, S.Y. (1996). Religion in clinical practice: implicit and explicit integration. In E.P. Shafranske (Ed.), *Religion and Clinical Practice of Psychology* (pp. 365-386). Washington, DC: APA.

Tisdale, T.T., Key, T.L., Edwards, K.J, Brokaw, B.F., Kemperman, S.R., Cloud, H., Townsend, J., Okamato, T. (1997). Impact of treatment on God image and personal adjustment, and correlations of God image to personal adjustment and object relations development. *Journal of Psychology and Theology, 25,* 227-239.

Winnicott, D.W. (1971). *Playing and reality.* New York: Tavistock.

Yalom, I. D. (1995). *The theory and practice of group psychotherapy* (4th ed.). New York: Basic Books.

doi:10.1300/J515v09n03_05

Chapter 6

Existential-Integrative
Psychotherapy and God Image

Louis Hoffman, PhD

SUMMARY. Existential therapy, rooted in the writings of May, and existential integrative theory, further developed in the writing of May and Schneider, provide a contribution to the psychological literature that emphasizes the role of paradox in the themes of freedom and responsibility, authenticity and isolation, and constrictive and expansive potentialities, among others. In this paper, these themes are applied to the development of the God image and how people experience God. This theory is illustrated in a case example which emphasizes case conceptualization and treatment approaches. Particular attention is given to the relational and experiential processes in psychotherapy. doi:10.1300/J515v09n03_06 *[Article copies available for a fee from The Haworth Document Delivery Service: 1-800-HAWORTH. E-mail address: <docdelivery@haworthpress.com> Website: <http://www.HaworthPress.com> © 2007 by The Haworth Press. All rights reserved.]*

Existential psychotherapy in the United States originates in the writings of Rollo May (1953, 1969). May's psychology, considered a branch of the third force of psychology or humanistic/phenomenological therapies, shares many similarities along with subtle distinctions from

[Haworth co-indexing entry note]: "Existential-Integrative Psychotherapy and God Image." Hoffman, Louis. Co-published simultaneously in *Journal of Spirituality in Mental Health* (The Haworth Pastoral Press, an imprint of The Haworth Press) Vol. 9, No. 3/4, 2007, pp. 105-137; and: *God Image Handbook for Spiritual Counseling and Psychotherapy: Research, Theory, and Practice* (ed: Glendon L. Moriarty, and Louis Hoffman) The Haworth Pastoral Press, an imprint of The Haworth Press, 2007, pp. 105-137. Single or multiple copies of this article are available for a fee from The Haworth Document Delivery Service [1-800-HAWORTH, 9:00 a.m. - 5:00 p.m. (EST). E-mail address: docdelivery@haworthpress.com].

Available online at http://jsmh.haworthpress.com
© 2007 by The Haworth Press. All rights reserved.
doi:10.1300/J515v09n03_06

humanistic psychology. In differing from humanistic psychology, existentialism puts greater emphasis on the need to deal with the darker realities of existence, such as suffering, evil, and human limitation. It shares with humanistic psychology a focus on subjectivity, experience, personal freedom, and human potential and dignity. In recent years, Schneider (in press, Schneider & May, 1995) introduced an existential-integrative approach which retains May's existential foundation while attempting to *critically* integrate other approaches to psychotherapy. The *critical* aspect of the integration recognizes that not all therapeutic approaches coherently fit with the existential approach. It is important that theories which are integrated are consistent with the existential foundation. This chapter will integrate ideas from contemporary psychoanalysis, humanistic psychology, and process-experiential therapy to an existential foundation. The goal of this integration is to illuminate one perspective on the God image[1] and how to work with clients struggling with painful and destructive God images.

EXISTENTIAL-INTEGRATIVE THERAPY: BACKGROUND AND PHILOSOPHICAL ASSUMPTIONS[2]

Freedom, Responsibility, and the Will

May's (1981) states, "that the purpose of [existential] therapy is to set people free" (p. 19). Implicit in this statement is the assumption that there are degrees of freedom which people can attain and that living freely is inherently good. Personal freedom, in this sense, is very different than political freedom. As Frankl (1984) asserts, personal freedom can even be attained in the confines of a concentration camp. Even though this context has removed political freedom, it cannot take away the freedom of how the individual faces his or her situation.

Freedom is not as simple as just living freely. In essence, *people are as free as they become*. Rank (1929/1936), the first to develop a psychology of the will, maintains that individuals are controlled by that which influences them of which they are unaware. It is by bringing these influences into consciousness that people become free. The challenge is that with freedom comes responsibility, which individuals often wish to avoid (Yalom, 1980). This *existential given* is one of the great challenges of contemporary times. The attempt to be free without being responsible is, by its nature, pathological and, arguably, immoral. The process of psychotherapy helps people embrace and enhance their freedom. By becoming free they become responsible for their lives and more moral.

This reality is illustrated beautifully by the resistant existentialist, Camus (1946/1989), in his novel *The Stranger*. The stranger lives his life passively, with no apparent will and no emotion. He is not a particularly moral or immoral person; he is just passive. Throughout the novel, the stranger just reports the events of his life with no emotion and no self-reflection. It is just as if he was a completely objective observer. Then, an event occurs in which he kills a person and is placed on trial. Through the process of the trial, the stranger begins to self-reflect, begins experiencing emotions, and becomes *response-able*. It is through this process that the stranger becomes a person, not just a product of his influences. The process is profoundly painful, but allows the stranger to become a genuine person for the first time.

The problem with the stranger for contemporary times is that most people are much more like the stranger than they would admit. Too often, the stranger is an existential reality in our own lives. Many psychotherapy clients are living their life as the stranger, or as "the living dead." In *The Stranger*, Camus illustrates the important existential conception of self-awareness. This plays a critical role in becoming free. As discussed by Rank, it is the process of becoming aware of what influences people that they become free. Without awareness freedom is limited. This is one of the great paradoxes of existential theory; *people are both necessarily limited in their freedom and at the same time condemned to be free*. It is not possible to escape the influences of biology, genetics, and the past. Furthermore, individuals can never become fully aware of the influences lurking in their unconscious. This is what Heidegger refers to as *thrownness*. Everyone is thrown into a particular life situation with a particular genetic makeup, with parents they have not chosen, and into a time and culture they are not able to control. A problem with much of contemporary psychology is that it assumes that these influences *are* the whole person. Existentialists respond stating this is only a partial understanding of being human. A fully human psychology must also deal with the freedom and the will.

Mendelowtiz (2006), in a beautiful illustration of the existential therapy process, reframes this in the context of the Oedipal complex. Beginning with May (1999) and Becker (1973), existentialists have reframed the Oedipal process, freeing it from Freudian sexuality. Instead, they interpret the Oedipal process as the individual's attempt to escape freedom through submitting to an authority figure. Initially, this is an internalized parent. However, as people grow older, they tend to replace the actual parent with other paternal objects, such as religion. This is not to claim all religion is oppressive, as Fromm (1941/1994) would suggest; however, it is a common for religious people to engage with religion as an Oedipal authority instead of genuinely engaging with religion. Existential therapy, in this context, seeks to help people overcome the unfreedom of Oedipal religion to genuine religion or faith. This does not change the content of religion as much as the way the individual engages with religion.

Relationships, Genuineness, and Authenticity

Existential psychology is often misunderstood as a being a cognitive, abstract, and individualistic approach to psychology. However, anyone who has had the opportunity to watch Rollo May, Jim Bugental, or Kirk Schneider demonstrate the existential therapy process recognizes that this misses the heart of existential psychology. Although existentialists tend to be well-read and interested in abstract thought, this realm is not directly brought into therapy sessions. Instead, this material is used to build a frame of reference that helps the therapist better see their clients.[3] Stated different, it is assumed that a broad understanding of what it means to be human, as illustrated in literature, art, and philosophy, influences how the therapist sees people. The existential therapy process focuses on the experience of the client, along with the intersubjective therapy process, while building a profoundly relational approach to therapy.

Another misconception about the relational process in existential-integrative therapy is the oversimplification of it as focusing primarily on empathy and reflective listening. Although these are part of the relational process, they only encapsulate one part of the experience. Stark (1999), from a contemporary psychoanalytic perspective, points out that empathy is not a complete relational process and significantly different than genuine engagement. She refers to this as a "one and a half person psychology" (p. 3). The therapist, when utilizing empathy, disengages from their subjective experience in the service of joining with what the client is experiencing. The disengagement from one's subjective self and experience is what makes it a one and a half person therapy. Both individuals are focusing on the client's experience and ignoring the therapists. Although this is healing, *it may not be fully healing*. This creates an artificial relationship which is not commonly experienced in the 'real world.'

A genuine relationship involves staying centered in one's own experience (Stark, 1999). *The therapist reacts to the client not from the client's experience, but from their own.* This involves a certain degree of risk for the therapist. He or she is no longer a disengaged observer and technician, but an active participant who can be genuinely hurt or rejected by the client. The therapist must take responsibility for their feelings and their mistakes, and cannot blame these on the therapeutic modality or technique. The more genuine, centered relational approach allows the development of what Yalom (1995) refers to as a "social microcosm." The client's relational problems are acted out in therapy allowing them to be more directly worked upon. Since, as Yalom indicates, existential therapy assumes that *it is the relationship that heals*, this allows for healing to occur.

Many therapy approaches assume that genuine relationships are impossible or highly limited. Individuals are believed to be so bound to the transference and projection processes that they are incapable of genuine relationships. Other approaches assume that genuine relationships can be built through learning social skills, having technically correct relationships, and overcoming distorted thoughts about the relational process. Although existential therapists agree that transference is a given and that the technique of relationship is necessary for healthy relationships, their primary interest goes beyond these limitations. They are more optimistic about the degree which transference can be overcome allowing for genuine relationships. Although acknowledging technique of relationship is necessary (to a degree), it is not sufficient for healthy, satisfying relationships.

The cultural obsession with the technique of relationship in Western culture may inadvertently serve to further isolate individuals. What is expected in relationships has been reduced to an impersonal, safe way of relating that is grounded in *correct communication*. This thin or shallow way of relating protects individuals from many relational risks and pains, but the true intimacy occurs in the "wild spaces" of relating (Olthius, 1999; 2001). Relationships of depth do not occur without risk, and do not develop without some pain and tension. There is more intimacy in a freely shared tear than in a million socially correct smiles, even if part of unconditional positive regard.

The healing process of therapy includes experientially teaching clients what healthy, satisfying relationships are like. Contrary to popular Western myth, healthy relationships are often messy, and this messiness is part of the beauty of the relationship. Until clients let go of idealized illusions of what relationships ought to be, they will not experience genuine intimacy to the depth they desire.

Constriction and Expansion: The Human Paradox

Paradox is another *existential given* in the human condition.[4] This is well illustrated in the constriction-expansion paradox, which occurs at various levels of experience. Everyone has the impulses, or drives, toward both constriction and expansion. For Schneider (1999), this is the basis of the human condition. This is a powerful understanding of the self for postmodern times. Although modernism focused on a reductionistic myth of self,[5] a common postmodernism view erred toward conceptualizing the self as fragmented (Hoffman, Stewart, Warren, & Meek, 2006). Schneider's conception of a paradoxical self allows for various conceptions of self to be integrated into a more holistic conception of the self. Many of the different conceptions of self developed in the modern, postmodern, and even premodern period may point toward different aspects of the self. Although each aspect can be interpreted as independent fragments, Hoffman and colleagues propose that a healthier, more sustaining myth of self conceives them as different aspects or tensions within the paradoxical self.

Most psychopathology falls into one of the extremes of the constriction-expansion paradox (Schneider & May, 1995). The denial, negation, or avoidance of the other extremity relegates it to the shadow, daimonic, or unconscious, inadvertently giving it more power within the psyche. Although this removes the tension at the conscious level, it remains with additional libidinal power through its negation. Many within the psychological community and contemporary thought believe greater psychological health is achieved through reducing tensions; however, existentialists see tension as a necessary and productive existential given. It is not the negation of tension which should be sought, but rather creative utilization of the tension and anxiety.

This balance of tensions should not be confused with the Stoic ideal of tempering, as this serves to squelch creative utilization of anxiety and genuine engagement with life. Stoicism encourages a form of balance which avoids the extremes; however, in doing so it falls prey to the extreme of emotional disengagement. Emotions, like paradox, should be embraced.

Engagement can be conceived of in a couple of ways to grant it special privilege in the world of paradox. First, engagement can be conceived of as falling outside of the givens of paradox (which is, in essence, a paradox!). In a sense, it is the backdrop for all the paradoxes and a necessary precondition for authentic experiencing of these paradoxes. In this way, engagement transcends the rules of the paradoxical condition. Alternatively, it can be seen as being granted an exception to the rules of paradox or even conceived of as a value choice or bias inherent in the existential theory. Regardless, full engagement, although it may be beneficial for it to be gradual or tempered at times, is something existentialists believe should be sought. Further, this engagement is necessary to authentically resolve the challenges of other paradoxes.

EXISTENTIAL INTEGRATIVE THERAPY AND THE GOD IMAGE

God Image Development

The early literature on the God image development focused on parental influences and wish-fulfillment as the basis for the experience of God. Contemporary theoretical investigations have critiqued the overreliance on these myopic perspectives (Hoffman, 2005; Hoffman, Grimes, & Acoba, 2005). Additionally, research suggests a variety of other factors impact the God image, including the God concept or cognitions about God (Hoffman, Jones, Williams, & Dillard, 2004), gender (Foster & Babcock, 2001; Krejci, 1989; Nelson, Cheek, & Au, 1985; Roberts, 1989), culture (Hoffman, Hoffman et al., 2005a), and therapy (Tisdale, Key, Edwards, Brokaw, Kemperman, & Cloud, 1997).[6] Hoffman (2005) proposed that a variety of other relational experiences, including experiences of the church, religious leaders, and the world, in general, are likely to impact how a person experiences God. Additionally, some attachment theorists have proposed that God may serve as an idealized attachment figure (Kirkpatrick 1997, 1998, 2004; Kirkpatrick & Shaver, 1990).[7] As should be evident, these varying experiences of God do not always fit coherently together creating further psychological unease or distress.

Hall and colleagues proposed that various factors may influence religious experience at different levels of processing (Hall, Halcrow, Hills, Delaney, & Teal, 2005; Hall & Porter, 2004).[8] It is possible, indeed probable, that parental and other relational or abstract experiences may impact the deeper levels of the unconscious, while various cognitive realms, such as the God concept, may be more impacted by conscious, rational thought. This literature provides strong evidence that the experience of God is very complex and often paradoxical. It is also important to keep in mind that little of this literature addresses the metaphysical question of the existence of God and rarely considers the possibility of mystical, transcendent, or transpersonal experiences as playing a role in the broader experience of God.

From an existential perspective, the God image can only be adequately understood by moving beyond reductionistic, over-simplified, and unified perspectives on the God image, which appear to dominant much of the literature. From an anthropological perspective, Geertz (1973) offers an extremely important critique of the use of research to understand culture and humanity, in general. He divided research into "thick" and "thin" categories. *Thin research* relies on quantitative measures, large samples, and tends to be more easily generalized. It is more interested in what is consistent across people. Conversely, *thick research* looks at people more in depth, focusing on the nuances of difference and individuality. Although this is not as generalizable, it says more about the individual.

Postmodern theory and research is rooted in an epistemological pluralism which suggests the best approach to knowing incorporates multiple ways of knowing (Hoffman, Hoffman et al., 2005b; Hoffman et al., 2006). The over-reliance on quantitative and reductionistic models (thin research) of the God image is major concern with the current literature. Future theory and research should utilize a more diverse epistemology and incorporate both thick and thin research methodologies. However, the integration of research methodologies still does not overcome Tillich's concern of scientism (Cooper, 2006). All science and research, according to Tillich, is still rooted in *faith* (epistemological) assumptions about knowing. Scientific explorations should not negate other approaches to understanding the God image. Instead, these approaches must be integrated and all conceptions need to show appropriate reverence for limitation in the ability to know, in general. This creates space for knowing related to transcendent or transpersonal experiences. Stated differently, this allows for God or other conceptions of the transcendent to have a role in how God is experienced.

Existential Perspectives on the God Image

Existential perspectives on the God image are informed by themes of (1) freedom and responsibility, (2) the human tendencies toward expansion and constriction, and (3) genuineness.

Freedom, Responsibility, and the God Image. Mendelowitz (2006) provides some important implications about the Oedipal conflict, or parental/authority figures, and religion. Although this is not the focus of his article, the implications are evident. Religion, religious experience, and the God image often function in the service of the Oedipal complex. In other words, they often serve as authority figures which are used in the service of escaping freedom. This Oedipal religion is the enemy of genuine religiosity, which often is conceptualized as "spirituality" or "faith." However, it is important to not judge religion too quickly as negative, or the enemy of faith. Religion can facilitate faith or, when connected with the Oedipal conflict, serve as a barrier to faith through creating a false sense of security in religious structures or content. Religion, to be healthy, involves risk and faith, not false security.

However, the securities of this religion should not be judged too quickly either. They may serve an important role in religious development. Stated differently, Oedipal religion is not counterproductive as a *stage*, but is dangerous as an *end*. It can provide security that allows individuals to delve into the more existential and ambiguous aspects of broader faith experiences. In this way, Oedipal religion serves as a transitional object facilitating the individuation process. However, just as it is not healthy for an adult to continue to carry their security blanket with them, the healthy adult must also move beyond the Oedipal religion to genuine faith or belief.

This is not, and should not, be an easy process. It entails deconstructing prior religious beliefs which offered security. It is not uncommon for this to illicit profound questioning of faith. Many individuals go through a period of a spiritual desert, or a "dark night of the soul," which may bring the concern of having lost faith. However, as Gerald May (2004) illustrates, the dark night of the soul is not a loss of faith, but a faith transition. The dark night is often misunderstood by religious individuals as any painful period that the religious person endures. At times, the dark night even sounds like a period of martyrdom where the individual endures tests of faith. However, May illustrates that this is not what St. John of the Cross intended. Instead, the dark night represents a period in which many religious rituals or symbols lose their practical meaning. This can appear as if one is losing faith; however, it is a process of spiritual development. In a Tillichian language, the individual is transitioning from dependence on the symbols to a deeper faith in what the symbols point toward. Put in Winnicottian terms, the individual no longer needs their transitional object because of a more personal, individuated faith.

Constriction, Expansion, and the God Image. Theology and religious thought is replete of examples of constriction and expansion projected as ultimate reality. This can be illustrated with the *sinner versus saint paradox* in Christian theology. Many theologies focus on the people as being bad (sinful) and God being good. By focusing excessively on the depravity of human nature, this becomes a constrictive theology which distorts the human image. Conversely, theologies of expansion focus on the saintly aspirations while negating the human potential for evil. By focusing on the expansive tendency exclusively, or nearly exclusively, the human image is again distorted.

Gnostic beliefs, which emerged in religious thought the several hundred year period following the life of Jesus, illustrate another way of dealing with the constrictive-expansion tendency. In these traditions, the flesh or body is associated with evil, sinfulness, and constriction. The soul or spiritual realm is associated with the good, saintliness, and expansion. In one sense, this provides an answer to humanity's paradoxical condition through reconciling how people contain both the potential for good (expansiveness) and for evil (constriction).[9] However, the problematic dualism remains, easily corrupting theologies into asserting that the body or flesh (human image) is wholly bad, which can be psychologically destructive.

Luther, who Tillich often thought of as an early depth psychologist, attempted to resolve this paradox through viewing people as both saint *and* sinner (Cooper, 2006). Although, at times, this has been developed in the direction of Gnosticism, Luther's thought can be interpreted as an early existential position incorporating a place for expansion and constriction, sinner and saint.

Genuineness and the God Image. Genuineness is not possible without freedom. When a person is free, they *chose* to be in relationship. Too often, relationships are built off of defenses, dependency, transference, and projection. This does not allow for genuineness and authenticity. However, genuineness is always at least partially limited. As with other relationships, the goal of existential therapy is to help clients attain a more genuine relationship with God and others.

A genuine relationship must entail the ability to fully engage with God. For many, they develop the false perception that relationships with God must always be positive. When the unpleasant emotions, including anger at God, are held back, then the relationship is no longer genuine. A genuine relationship with God requires the ability to trust God enough to share pain, anger, and hurt, even when it is directed at God.

CASE ILLUSTRATION

Client History

"Juliett?"

"Jules, I always go by Jules."

Seven words in and therapy was already off to an auspicious start. I knew by the tone in Jules voice and the accompanying look not to make that mistake again. It didn't take long to see that Jules was riddled in contradictions. Beautiful and seductive, yet sharp and self-controlled; Jules most often knew was she was doing.

Jules grew up a rebellious adolescent in a conservative religious home. Yet, she married a conservative minister who was now seeking a divorce from her on grounds approved by his church that adamantly opposes divorce. In their view, it was obvious that the divorce was her fault and thus appropriate. Not to mention, it would surely save the church much embarrassment down the line. She was asked not to return and he was given a sixth month sabbatical to a church retreat center to recover.

But who could blame the church? As the tensions in the marriage became more obvious to their congregation, Jules went on many suspicious trips to visit old friends, wore increasingly revealing outfits to church, and was seen drunk and flirtatious in a local bar. Jules never seemed to mind the rumors of infidelity or even that people at church seemed uncomfortable in her presence, but she was devastated that Rick was leaving her.

Childhood. From early on it was evident that Jules was daddy's little girl. The sparkle in his eyes when he first saw her each night when he came home led to her being called "daddy's jewel" and later just "Jules." She loved her dad's attention and always felt special when he showed her the affection he so loved to give.

The rest of her family was different. Her brothers resented the attention she received from her father and her mom was also jealous of the attention she received. As she grew older, the tension and distance became more obvious to Jules, so she focused on getting as much of daddy's attention as she could. He was happy to comply, always adoring his little Jules.

Things began to change when she was in high school. Jules was attractive and seemed to receive attention everywhere she went. Her father started becoming protective, afraid that someone would take advantage of his little girl. Jules sensed the change and didn't like it. She wanted to go back to the object of his affection, instead of the object of his protection. The protection felt distant and rigid, more like the relationships she was familiar with having with her mom and brothers. Starved for affection and warmer attention, she started to seek this out elsewhere. The boys at school were happy to oblige.

Fearful of the attention Jules was receiving from the boys at school, her father had a religious awakening. Their family had always been somewhat religious. They attended church on a regular basis, prayed before meals and bedtime, talked about God, and lived a pretty good life according to church standards. However, now things changed. Dad started "devotions" as a regular part of their family time. The devotions used scriptures to tell his children how to live and the topics were generally no drugs, no sex, and not much fun.

Jules two older brothers were almost out of the house and tolerated the changes, appearing to oblige their father. But they knew this was really for Jules and were able to get away with things as long as they were discrete. Maybe out of revenge for years of not getting as much attention, they seemed to enjoy being an extension of dad's new morality for Jules.

By her sophomore year, Jules had enough and had given up on returning to her father's spotlight of affection. She began rebelling against the rules and against religion. Her father, more afraid than ever, started to clamp down, often leading to yelling arguments. Jules was as smart as she was stubborn, quickly developing a way of getting her needs met. Her father closely monitored the clothes she would buy and wear, so she would get her many suitors to buy her more and more revealing outfits. Although she would keep these hidden, not putting them on until she left the house, she also had a way of letting her dad know about it. As her anger and the tension increased, she always retained a longing to go back to how it was. She knew that if he gave her the attention she craved, she would be happy to give up the boys and the parties.

By Jules senior year, her father had all but given up. Filled with guilt and feelings of being a failure, he focused his attention on his religious life and his wife. Jules mother, happy to have regained his attention, gladly became his perfect Christian wife. She also gladly reinforced perceptions of how bad Jules' turned out, solidifying her place in her husband's hierarchy.

Jules parents offered to pay for college only if she went to the Christian College of their choice. She strung them along her entire senior year, pretending to agree and gaining acceptance to their college. The day of graduation she announced to her parents that she secretly applied to the local state university and was attending there instead. Infuriated, her parents took away her car keys and refused any financial support at college. Jules' grades, however, were good enough for her to receive a full scholarship and she quickly found a part-time job on campus.

Jules barely survived her first year of college, drinking most nights and becoming very promiscuous. In her second year, after getting in trouble for under age drinking on campus several times, she was finally asked to leave. She stayed with her boyfriend for over a month before telling her parents. They again offered to pay for her to go to the Christian College which accepted her previously. Although the college was now hesitant, her parents were able to convince them to give her a chance. Jules agreed to attend feeling that she didn't have any other choice. Her first semester, she isolated herself and focused on her coursework, catching up to complete her sophomore year on schedule. Her junior year she gradually found other friends who were coerced into attending the college by their parents and began returning to her old patterns of behavior. After nearly getting kicked out of school her junior year and again early on in her senior year, she started to become anxious about what her life would be like after college. She knew that her current lifestyle would be difficult to maintain while living on her own.

Jules, relying on the skills she developed to get what she wanted, focused on a new plan. She started spending time with a different group of friends, finally meeting Rick. Rick was an intelligent and passive religious studies student who planned to become a minister. He was stable, secure, and very fond of Jules. Their relationship quickly became serious. When Jules took him home to meet her parents, she was very disappointed. She had hoped that her new found religious lifestyle and religious boyfriend would regain her place in her father's life. Although he was pleased with her choice of a boyfriend, he was not willing to give his affection back to his Jules who hurt him so badly. She became more determined to win her father's affection back, immersing herself in a highly religious life the next several years.

Rick, too, was very pleased with this. Initially, he had some reservations about Jules past, but he was convinced her newfound enthusiasm was a genuine religious conversion. They excitedly planned their first parish and how they would minister together. While Rick couldn't be happier, Jules knew her love for Rick was not real. However, he was safe and she knew she could trust him. They were married while Rick was in seminary and two years later began their first parish ministry. Jules began as a housewife, active in the church's ministries, but soon became bored and depressed. She started to talk about looking for a job.

Her passion was writing, particularly poetry and short stories, but thought she could find a job in journalism or as an editor. Rick, although disappointed, passively supported Jules.

Jules found a job as an editor at a publishing company that Rick didn't think looked the best for their ministry. They published some racy magazines and Rick worried it would offend his congregation. Jules was able to once again win his support, although it was with reservations. Gradually, Jules seemed to change the longer she worked at the magazine. She spent more time with her friends from work and less time involved in their ministry. Although Rick voiced his concerns, Jules seemed unrelenting in her excitement about her new job and life.

As the changes continued, Jules started to return to her more risqué dress and started going out to the bars with her friends from work. When his congregation started to voice concern, Rick finally "set his foot down." Incensed, Jules became enraged, saying he wouldn't allow her to express herself and be happy. She left to "take a break," quit her job, and spent a month with a friend from college. When she returned, she began focusing on writing and spending time with friends. When tensions mounted, she would go to stay with her friend. After several months of this, rumors began to surface that she was having an affair. Jules maintained that she just enjoyed the attention of men, but would never have an affair. Her flirtations were her way of getting the attention she no longer received from her husband, or from her father.

After another fight with Rick, Jules dressed up in a revealing outfit and went out dancing with some friends. A couple from the church saw Jules drunk, flirting with another man. They quickly left and called Pastor Rick. Devastated, Rick started to question Jules's fidelity for the first time. The next day, Rick went to his supervisors to confess about his wife. Having heard the rumors, they proceeded to suggest a separation and investigation into Jules behavior. Rick was sent to a retreat center while his supervisors led a quick investigation which they felt gathered sufficient evidence to justify Rick divorcing Jules. Rick returned home to tell Jules.

Jules was devastated and full of rage. She threw several pieces of glass at Rick while he calmly gathered his clothes and packed the car. With Jules still yelling, he calmly told her that he was leaving to a retreat center and would have the divorce paper sent. As he was leaving, he handed her a business card for a Christian therapist that he recommended she call. Jules tore up the card and threw it at him as he walked out the door. As soon as he drove away, Jules collapsed on the floor in tears. A couple of days later she called to set up her first appointment.

Presenting Problem

When Jules presented in the first session, there was no indication of distress other than the very evident anger. As she sat down on the couch she said,

> "I don't know why I am coming to see *you*. All the men in my life just screw me over."

> "Is that why you are here?"

> "Right to the point. I guess that's good. At least you are not a coward, like my husband. He never showed a bit of spine in his life until he left me."

> "That sounds like pretty fresh anger. Did he just leave you?"

> "Don't get too confident in your ability to figure me out, but yes, he left 4 days ago."

> "And that's why you're here."

> "I guess, in part. But I know it's more than that. I saw a therapist once before when my parents made me go my senior year in high school. He seemed pretty alright until he told my parents I was hysterical . . . no, no . . . a histrionic personality. After looking up what that was, I went back one time in my sexiest outfit to tell him off and then walked out."

Jules was angry, but insightful. She knew her problems were much deeper than the divorce. That was just the tip of the iceberg. However, it was also what pushed her to the point of thinking about suicide for the first time since she first realized she lost her dad's affection.

> "The divorce is just what got me here. I know my problems go way back. I've been messed up for a long time."

> "Your husband leaving you provided the motivation to deal with problems that have been there for a while."

"Yeah, I've never had good relationships with men. Women neither, for that matter, at least not until the last several years. Now I have some women friends who helped me get through the last few years."

"Most of your relationships have been difficult."

"Yeah, sometimes I think I'd be better off a complete loner. But that's not me. I need people, maybe too much. I wish I didn't sometimes. You know, like those monks or nuns, but without all the religion."

"Without the religion?"

"Don't get me started on religion. I hate the church, and God, too, for that matter. It seems like God and religion have screwed up all my relationships. I sound just like a minister's wife, huh? Maybe now you know why he left me."

"Your husband was a minister?"

"Yeah."

"You think that's why he left you? Because your not a good Christian?"

"That's what he tells me. He even thinks I had an affair, can you believe that? I mean, I used to be a little wild, but I've never been anything but faithful to him. And I've had the opportunities. So I like to flirt, big deal! I wouldn't have to if he gave me a little attention. I gave up everything for him and now he accuses me of cheating on him?! He was the first man I thought I could trust since my father; but he screwed me over, too."

"Your father also hurt you, betrayed your trust."

"Yeah, until high school I thought my dad was the greatest man in the world. He loved me, loved me so much, like I thought I'd never again be loved. But then the first time a guy looked at me in *that way*, dad turned into this religious freak and tried to make me into one, too . . . Hmmm . . . I guess he succeeded a bit, too."

"Because you married a minister."

"Yeah, and at first I played the role well, too. I never thought of that before . . . "

Although I generally assume that real presenting problem will not surface until several sessions into therapy, Jules gave me a lot of information from the start. The identified problem on the pre-therapy questionnaire was her divorce and associated depression. However, a long time ago I learned not to trust those forms too much. It didn't take long for Jules to add suicidal ideation to the list of presenting problems and, although not explicitly stated, a good deal of relationship problems dating back to her relationship with her father. I was also aware that her God image was very negative; however, Jules did not want to include issues of this sort in therapy.

As therapy unfolded, it became increasing evident that her religious problems, particularly her God image, were a primary contribution to some of her emotional difficulties and suicidal ideation. About 12 sessions into therapy, Jules began talking about her anger at God a lot more. Because she had indicated in the first session she didn't care to work on issues related to God, I was cautious in proceeding. However, after two sessions in a row where her anger at God was central in her session content, I revisited the issue.

"Jules, in our first session you indicated that you did not want to deal with your relationship with God in here. However, the last two sessions you've talked about being mad at God quite a bit. If you do not want to discuss religious issues in therapy, I want to respect your decision. However, it does seem like this is a pretty important issue."

"I don't know. I mean I am mad at God, but I am not sure I want to discuss that in here."

"Okay, but maybe we can explore some of your concerns about talking about this."

Jules was quiet, appearing hesitant to go forward. I suspected that she felt I was trying to trick her into talking about religious issues, especially concerned that I may use religion against her, as this has been her experience in the past.

"I can see that you're hesitating a bit. I don't want to force you to talk about religion, but I do think it would be helpful if I understood your concerns since it has been a common topic the last couple of weeks. If, while exploring your hesitation around these issues you feel uncomfortable, I want you to tell me to stop. Are you willing to give it a try?"

"Okay, I'll give it a shot."

At this point, I used a focusing approach, similar to some of Gendlin's (1998) work. We had used this in therapy previously, so it was not new.

"I'd like for you to close your eyes and take a couple of slow, deep breaths. Allow your gaze to fall downward, with your eyes still closed. I have suggested it could be beneficial for us to explore some of your anger toward God, but you voiced some hesitation. I want to see if you can identify where in your body you feel this resistance."

"In my chest, I feel my muscles tightening in my upper chest, and on up my lower neck."

"This tension is telling you something."

"I'm preparing for a blow. I feel like I'm going to get attacked."

"You feel like I am going to attack you."

"Yes, yes . . . I don't know why. I don't know what's bringing this up."

"Okay, open your eyes now. I think this is something significant, that you feel like I am going to use religion against you."

"This doesn't make sense to me. I've been mad at you before, but I've never felt like you were going to use something against me."

"Let's take a look at this. There is something I'm doing that is contributing to your fear."

"I don't know what it could be. You are approaching the topic slowly, even though you are persisting . . . (long pause) . . . maybe that is part of it. You are persisting with it, just like my father and Rick did. It was always about religion, and I was always in the wrong."

"You are worried that if we talk about religion, a topic you feel I have pushed on you today, that I will use it against you."

"(long pause) I guess so. Maybe I give religion a bad rap because of my dad and Rick."

"The tension in your chest and neck, is it still there?"

"Yeah, it's definitely there, but it's not so strong. I do think this is something I need to explore more, but I'm still scared."

"The tension is still telling you this is dangerous ground, but I think you are right, it does sound like an important issue for us to consider. But we need to proceed cautiously. Any time religion comes up, I want you to tell me if you feel like I am pushing to hard or if you feel like I may be using religion against you."

At this point, in the twelfth session, we had identified the presenting problems in a more explicit language and these would become the focal point of the rest of the treatment. The identified problems were (1) working through the grief and pain of her divorce, (2) addressing her depression and suicidal ideation (the suicidal ideation had fully subsided never to return by this time), (3) addressing her difficulty establishing healthy relationships, particularly with men, (4) increase self-awareness, which was agreed upon in the first session, (5) working through her anger and hurt associated with God and religion.

Case Conceptualization[10]

A number of issues had a profound impact on Jules experience of God, in particular her relationship with her parents, the church, and various men, including her husband. Early in life, she developed an experience of God based upon her father. Rizzuto (1979) points out that the God image can be based upon the experience of the father, the mother, or a combination of both. Jules experienced her father as safe and loving, providing a basis for a very positive experience of God. She described some memories of strong feelings of being loved by God at an early age. However, when her father withdrew his affection from her rather suddenly and without her understanding why, her experience of God also began to change. At this point, her experience of God became more diffuse. Although this is common in adolescence in general, it is likely that the abrupt change in her father's reaction to her also played an important role in broadening the experiences that influenced her God image.

When Jules began therapy, she had become aware that it was her developing sexuality and the attention from men which provided the impetus for father distancing himself from her. At the time this occurred, she was unaware of the reasons his affections were no longer there. Her initial experience was feeling a rejection from her father, but not being sure why it occurred. This created instability in her experience of God, never knowing when God may unexpectantly pull away or reject her. Later, when she realized the role her emerging sexuality played in the change in her relationship with her father, she began to feel as if her sexuality was dirty or sinful, and that God would reject her for being sexual. This realization occurred after Jules became sexually active, often using her sexuality to get the male affection she craved. This contributed to a very complex experience of God. In part, she still was afraid that God may reject her at any time for unknown reasons. However, she also had complex feelings about her sexuality related to God. In part, she felt guilty as if her sexuality would cause God to reject her. At the same time, sexuality became the way she kept people close to her and felt valued. In ways, her relationship with God felt sexual when it was intimate, further confusing her. She felt as if her beauty was something that God enjoyed, but also felt it could cause God to reject her. At the same time, there were some deeply hidden warm feelings about God, largely attributable to her early relationship with her father and some more recent relationships, which would provide a basis for a healing relationship later. Her God image was full of contradictions.

Over time, Jules continually felt in a double bind with her sexuality. She enjoyed it and it helped her keep male figures around, even though these were often hallow relationships. Her sexuality was a great defense against her loneliness and feelings of being small. At the same time, it felt expansive and powerful. This was something she could control. However, when she neared the end of college and began looking for security, she felt her expansiveness, mostly in the form of sexuality, was dangerous and needed to be contained. Here she returned to her Oedipal religion, using it to protect her from her fears of freedom and expansiveness. This created a very shallow, but safe primary religious experience. For many years, the security of the Oedipal religion kept her, and her sexuality, contained. For Jules, the libidinal energy became tied to sexuality in a very Freudian way.

After a few years of marriage, the repression was no longer working for Jules. She attempted to find creative outlets, even showing the inner wisdom to seek this through the creativity of writing instead of the familiar paths of sexuality. However, without insight and healing from her past wounds, the libidinal expression quickly took the familiar path of sexuality. She was now strong enough to contain it, preventing the promiscuous acting out which still tempted her. Nonetheless, it contributed to the demise of her already shaky marriage.

Her marriage to Rick was merely an extension of the Oedipal conflict. Rick was safe and secure, which protected her from her sexuality, fears of rejection, and her own expansiveness. He helped contain her, but she also felt small and alone. Even when their relationship was at its best, it never met her needs or desires. Because it was so closely tied to the Oedipal needs, it was doomed to problems from the start. Although Jules was committed to stay with it, even if it meant a rather bare existence, it had become so enmeshed with the Oedipal religion that one would not survive without the other. When Rick left, so did her religious beliefs.

Although divorce is not the desired end, it can, at times, provide the impetus for incredible growth and healing. In Jules case, this is what happened. In particular, Jules divorce helped her separate libidinal energy from sexuality. She learned to re-direct this energy into creative outlets through her writing and her relationships. At first, this was scary, as her expansiveness had become so intertwined with fears. The fears that she would be rejected because of her sexuality generalized to fears that she would be rejected because of her creativity. Over time, this connection gradually dissolved.

Jules relationship with God and religion took some difficult lumps along the way to healing. At first, she outright rejected God and wanted nothing to do with "him." If mentioned at all, it was in the pejorative. Gradually, she started to express anger at God, leading to some deep insights into her experience of God. However, understanding did not bring trust, and she still feared rejection from God. Her healing, which was associated with her expansiveness, was also associated with fears of being rejected by God. In an odd, distorted manner, Jules felt that God would reject her for healing, but her commitment was to healing and becoming whole. This would be something Jules would have to confront with God directly.

The change in her relationship with God began to occur when Jules began expressing her anger to God, instead of about God. This began a shift in which God became personal once again. However, it was not the loving intimacy she experienced as a child; it was a threatening and domineering force which Jules would often retreat from, only to return in with more invigorated anger. Through time, Jules began experiencing God as staying present no matter how much she pushed God away and no matter how much she vented her anger toward God. Finally, in the midst of a session of really letting God have it, she broke down crying. When processing this experience later all she could say is, "I'm mad at him, but I know he's still here."

Treatment Plan

Existential therapy often conceptualizes a treatment plan as unnecessary, and potentially problematically constraining. If the treatment plan is designed too narrowly or rigidly, then it does not allow the flexibility to adapt to emergent themes. For example, in the discussion of the presenting problem, it took twelve sessions before some of the issues were brought into the explicit goals of therapy. Oftentimes, it may take even longer than this. The concern is that developing a narrow treatment plan early on may work to prevent the therapist from recognizing emergent issues as they surface. When working with religious issues, this is particularly important as clients often will not broach these topics until sufficient trust has been established.

A second concern is that when treatment plans too narrowly define what a successful outlook will look like, it can become constraining. This is an issue that I address with clients early on in therapy. Jules was more than happy to agree to this, as she, like many clients, did not know what she wanted from therapy except for something different. She did, however, want to include being less depressed and having more satisfying relationships, to which I agreed.

If a treatment plan can be developed with sufficient flexibility, it can help provide some structure which allows the client to journey into the more threatening existential aspects of the presenting problem. Our treatment plan, which was agreed between Jules and myself, was to work towards a resolution to the identified problems stated above. We agreed to leave the specifics of that outcome open.

Interventions

The interventions employed were primarily aimed at (1) increasing insight, (2) processing past and recent experience, (3) providing experiential healing, and (4) providing new, healing relational experiences. In existential theory, cognitive change, insight, and experience are not sufficient on their own. Each, on their own, may be beneficial, but a more holistic healing and growth process requires all four. As will be demonstrated, these work together quite smoothly.

Increasing Insight. Insight generally came pretty easy for Jules. As already demonstrated, she was able to show proclivity for insight in the first session. Insight was facilitated through encouraging reflection, processing of experience, and interpretations made by the therapist.

Processing Past and Recent Events. Processing involves digesting past experiences. Generally, this entails cognitively and emotionally reviewing experiences in order to obtain some release, understanding, and insight. A good portion of therapy was spent processing events from Jules past. Each processed event helped free her from some of her repressed emotions and contributed to an understanding of her patterns and current feelings.

In addition to processing the more remote pass, we also processed many events which occurred during therapy. These experiences often related to transference processes. Because the same transference which was put onto God was also put onto me, working through transferences in this direct manner helped free Jules to work through her transferences with God. Two common transference processes occurred in our work.

First, Jules often had intense anger toward me. These most often occurred when she was unsure as to my response to her or when she felt rejected. She was not used to discussing her anger directly; instead, she acted it out or become passive aggressive. I encouraged Jules to stay with her anger toward me longer than she was accustomed. Although this was uncomfortable, it led to a greater depth of understanding of where the anger was coming from. It also provided an experience of her anger being safe.

Second, Jules would often work very hard to obtain my approval. At times, this was in the form of seduction, which primarily occurred early in the therapy process. On a couple of occasions, she began dressing more seductively in therapy and become flirtatious. Each time this occurred, I quickly addressed the behavior and Jules was able to make the insightful connections. At other times, primarily later in the therapy, her seductiveness was more subtle in the form of trying to please and impress me. During these periods, she would appear to work very hard in therapy, giving me the content she thought I wanted. She would bring dreams, profound insights, and talk about 'work' that she did between sessions. However, the insights lacked emotion and depth. In these situations, I relied strongly on my intuition to recognize the changes.

"Jules, something feels different today. You are saying the right things, but I'm not feeling it."

"What do you mean? *Are you saying that I'm not working hard?*"

"No, that's not it. It's evident you are trying, but I don't think we are connecting; something's missing. Let's try something. I want you to really focus on what you are experiencing in the session today. How are you responding to me?"

"Well, I guess I'm very conscious of what you are thinking of me, and I'm feeling a bit defensive in this discussion."

"That fits with what I've been experiencing. My sense is that you've been trying very hard to please me."

"I guess that's true. I am feeling toward you much like I often felt toward my dad when our relationship was falling apart. I wanted to please him, but didn't know if I could."

This abbreviated example was much easier than most of these conversations, but illustrates how a therapy segment can be processed.

Provision of Healing Experience. Some of the most important therapy work occurred through the provision of healing experience. Although many of these could be described as techniques, something existential therapy is often skeptical about, they emerged naturally in the therapeutic process. In other words, when they were used was dependent upon timing and were rarely planned.

The first experiential technique involved an approach to letter writing intended to help Jules bring emotions into the therapy process. First, Jules was asked to write a letter to her father, focusing on feelings toward him. I had her create a ritual around the letter writing in which she listened to music reminding of her father and created a special time and place to write the letter. After writing it, she was to seal it in a blank envelop and try to put it out of mind until the next session. When she brought the letter in to therapy, I asked her to read it aloud to me. Jules was surprised by the amount of emotion this prompted. This provided information for several weeks of processing and also provided important content for later conversations she had with her father.

Several weeks after the letter to her father, I recommended writing a letter to God. Initially, Jules was very resistant to this idea. I initially backed off, but returned to the idea a couple of weeks later. We agreed that Jules would keep the idea in mind, considering writing the letter at her own pace. To my surprise, the next week she walked in and handed me an envelope.

"Go ahead, it's what you asked for."

"The letter to God?"

"It wasn't easy. I'm still not sure what it's all about."

"Would you read it?"

"No way, I'm not touching that thing again. I'm already looking around for the lightening to strike. You read it."

"I think it's important for you to read the letter. If you'd like, it doesn't have to be today. We'll wait until you are ready."

"What's this supposed to do anyway? I don't see the point."

"It's an opportunity to express your feelings to God. In part, it allows you to free up emotions you've been keeping inside. But it also can help us understand more about your relationship with God."

Quietly, Jules reached for the letter and opened it. Before unfolding the letter, tears began to well up in her eyes.

"I don't understand; I was mad as hell when I wrote this. Why am I crying?"

I encouraged Jules to proceed. As she read the letter, about 3 handwritten pages, she often fluctuated from tears to anger and then back to tears again. When finished, she plunged her head into her hands, leaning forward, crying. After several minutes of silence, Jules began to speak.

"I guess I've always been afraid of being honest with God, well, at least since I was a kid."

"Afraid?"

"I don't know. Afraid he'd reject me? Be mad at me? I can never put a finger on it."

"But it was different as a child."

"Yeah," with a bit of a smile, "It was. I felt very free around God when I was a kid. I remember thinking of God as my friend, almost like a playmate. I thought God was fun and cool."

"But that changed."

"When I started to rebel against my parents, I guess I started thinking of God differently. Actually, I felt like God just went away."

"Much like your father."

"Yeah," tears welling up, "just like my dad. But it became more than that. I began feeling like God was out to get me at times, like God was more than just rejecting me, he was mad, especially about my sleeping around. But if I had to choose between God and sex, the choice was easy. When having sex, I knew where the guy stood, he was into me. But I never knew where God was."

The letters were an important part of Jules beginning to feel more open to expressing her feelings to God. As therapy progressed, I began to include using the empty chair technique with God in the empty chair, along with a variety of imagery techniques focused on exploring her feelings toward God. Each of these brought her feelings into the here-and-now, giving us more to work with. For Jules, beginning with the letter writing was important. She was very hesitant and frightened about expressing feelings toward God. The letter writing seemed less threatening, opening the door to expressing her emotions more directly. Additionally, explicitly giving her control to stop the process, as discussed earlier, was important for creating safety to engage in the experiential techniques.

Provision of Relationship. The therapy relationship provides the most important basis for all of therapy practice. In existential therapy, a genuine relationship is essential. If the client is not able to create a genuine relationship with the therapist, it is difficult to help them to engage genuinely with God or with others. Jules, like many clients, felt it more comfortable to deal with her therapist instead of "Louis" or "Dr. Hoffman." The title she used to refer to me provided a good gauge of where therapy was at on a given day, and also provided some fruitful territory to explore the relationship.

"I've noticed today that I'm 'your therapist' again."

"I know that bugs you, but its just easier right now to think of you as my therapist instead of Louis."

"What is going on today? Why do you need the distance?"

"We've been going into some really tough stuff lately. I guess I just needed some space."

"I think it's more than that. When you need space, you often are more direct in pushing me away. This is subtle."

"It's just easier if you are not a real person. Then I don't have to think about being hurt by you or hurting you. I don't have to worry about my feelings toward you. You're not real."

"But I am a real person, and it frustrates me when you treat me like an object and depersonalize me."

"See, just like that. It's so much easier if you just don't feel."

"Most relationships are easier if you don't have to worry about how the other person is feeling or going to respond. But that's not reality. Relationships are messy sometimes."

"I guess I do that with more than just you. I often wish I didn't have to worry about how people react. But I also just don't know where the boundaries are anymore; I don't want to cross the boundaries."

"In here, I am responsible for setting the boundaries and helping you learn from them. This is a real relationship, but the parameters are different. I will do my job to make sure that the boundaries are kept. Your job is to try to understand what you are feeling in relationships, including this one."

Conversations like these are common. Many therapists, as well as many clients, find it easier if the therapist hids behind their title, their role, and their therapeutic neutrality. In doing so, they often create artificial relationships. This felt all too familiar and very comfortable for Jules. God, her father, and Rick were all figures in her life that were cold and distant, playing out roles but not engaging. Her life was full of lifeless roles already, but what she was seeking was a real relationship. Were I to hide behind the therapeutic posture, lifeless and showing no emotion, it would have reinforced many of the unhealthy patterns already too prominent in Jules life. In offering a real relationship, Jules began learning what it meant to be in an intimate relationship. Later, she was able to use these skills in rebuilding her relationship with her dad, establishing a healthy romantic relationship, and developing an intimate relationship with God.

Duration of Treatment

Jules spent about a year and 5 months in therapy. I often tell clients at the beginning of therapy that it typically lasts from 6 months to 3 years, occasionally longer. When I told Jules this, she indicated that she would probably be my longest client ever; however, I anticipated that she would progress quickly because of her insights and openness to self-awareness. Additionally, I recognized that her statement of being in therapy a long time was connected to her need for security and stability at the beginning of therapy.

Termination

We made two attempts at the termination process. The first was at the end of approximately 14 months of therapy, which may have not been good timing on my part. This was around the anniversary of her divorce being final. The ending of therapy and year anniversary of her divorce was too many endings at one time; however, beginning the process of moving toward termination brought up new, fruitful material about her relationship with her father. During this time, she was able to confront her father on his pulling away and rejection of her. At this time, he still remained distant from her and evidenced some anger at her for the mistakes she made in life

Jules initiated two confrontations with her father over a period of one month which lead to profound healing in their relationship and some final healing in her God image. The first confrontation did not go well. Her father became defensive and she responded with anger. The conversation went downhill from there. After processing this in three therapy sessions, Jules came to believe that her anger played a major role in the first attempt not going well. She called her father and invited him to come to visit her and try again. Initially, he resisted, but when she said, "Daddy, please. I love you and I need this" he melted like he did when she was a little girl.

Her father arrived on Friday night, planning to stay until Sunday. That night, she prepared a nice dinner and said, "We are just going to enjoy ourselves tonight." They avoided talking about their problems, but shared a lot about their lives which they had not discussed in years. The next afternoon, Jules began the conversation. Her father quickly became defensive again. Jules, determined to remain vulnerable, not angry, persisted and soon found herself crying in front of her father for the first time since she was a sophomore in high school. Her vulnerability melted away his defenses allowing a long, sometimes difficult, conversation.

Existential therapists often make more than one run at termination. It is assumed that endings will often bring up new issues, just as with Jules. The initial run at termination brought up issues which led to a resolution to her over 15-year conflict with her father. In the second attempt, she was able to explore her difficulty saying goodbye to her therapist. For a long time she was resistant to seeing me as anything but a therapist. I pushed her to see me as a person with whom she shared a genuine relationship within different parameters than other relationships. When approaching termination, she again began referring to me as her therapist, which I recognized as her way of avoiding saying goodbye. Working through this was an important final issue. She often avoided engagement in relationships, because if she engaged, then it would hurt more when the relationship ended. Saying goodbye to me, as a real person whom she cared about instead of 'just her therapist,' was important in helping her to fully engage in relationships even though they might end.

Therapeutic Outcomes

Jules left therapy engaged with life. She still had periods of sadness, but she was not afraid of them and started to welcome these periods as friends who helped her reflect on where she was at in life. A couple of times, when these periods occurred, she would call me for a "touch up session." However, she would quickly realize that she didn't need the touch up; she just needed a reminder that some depression was okay. The last time we talked she talked herself out of the appointment before she ever scheduled it. A few weeks later I received an Email thank you saying she finally reached enough confidence to be fully on her own.

Jules did return to church, never attending regularly, but feeling it was an important part of her life. She believed that now that her relationship with God was genuine, she didn't need to prove it in weekly attendance. Often, skipping church was a reminder to herself that her relationship with God was not dependent upon being perfect. These Sunday mornings were when she felt closest to God, especially when hiking by herself in the mountains. She described walking along the trails, talking out loud to God, occasionally being embarrassed when another hiker would catch her 'talking to herself.' She would laugh and continue walking.

Jules never remarried that I know of; however, she had been in a significant long term relationship for over a year. She hoped to eventually marry and have children, but was not in a rush. She enjoyed her friendships and the freedom to spend time with her writing. Her goal was to "master solitude" before getting married. She was well on her way.

IMPLICATIONS AND CONCLUSION

Existential therapy, when working with religious issues, helps clients move from an Oedipal religion to a more genuine faith experience. This is not a change in what they believe, but how they believe. For some, changes in the content of faith occur. However, for many, their beliefs remain the same, but they are not as oppressive. This allows religion to move from a constraining source of guilt and anxiety to a source of freedom, security, and intimacy with God.

NOTES

1. Recently, I have discovered that references in my writing to "the God image" have been misunderstood as advocating for a singular God image. This has come as a surprise because a central focus of my writing on the God image has focused on

critiquing singular, unified, and oversimplified understandings of the God image while advocating for a more complex, diverse, and even contradictory understanding (i.e., Hoffman, 2005). Consistent with existential theory, the idea of the God image no more suggests a singular, non-contradictory experience than a reference to a person's general emotional experience indicates a simple, singular emotional experience.

2. For a more detailed account of Existential-Integrative psychotherapy, see Schneider (in press), Schneider and May (1995), Mendelowitz and Schneider (in press), or www.existential-therapy.com.

3. For a beautiful illustration of this, see Mendelowitz, 2006.

4. Paradox does not need to be interpreted in a dualistic manner, despite this being the common tendency. Though I utilize the metaphor of a continuum for simplicity's sake, this is not intended to mislead the reader into thinking that paradox necessitates two polar opposites, as dualism often suggests.

5. The idea of "myths of self" is developed in the paper *Multiple Selves in Postmodern Theory: An Existential-Integrative Critique* (Hoffman et al., 2006), which is available through www.existential-therapy.com. The authors suggest that the self is a socially constructed reality, but a construction of great importance. Myths of self provide a way for which people to understand themselves and their experience, which is essential for psychological health.

6. See chapter 13, *Diversity Issues and the God Image*, for a more complete discussion of some of these factors.

7. See also chapter 2, for a more complete review of the research.

8. See also chapter 4.

9. It is important to note that constriction and expansion is not just relegated to constriction as evil, and expansion as good. The potential for good and evil are just one way in which the constriction-expansion polarities can be illustrated. Other aspects of the constriction-expansion paradox can be more morally neutral.

10. With some hesitation, I will only address elements related to the religious/God image issues and some adjacent existential issues in this conceptualization. While this is limiting, as an existential approach is holistic and thereby somewhat distorted through such constraints, this is also necessary to work within the length constraints of the chapter.

REFERENCES

Becker, E. (1973). *The denial of death*. New York: Free Press.
Camus, A. (1989). *The stranger*. New York: Vintage. (Original work published in 1946)
Cooper, T. D. (2006). *Paul Tillich and psychology: Historic and contemporary explorations in theology, psychotherapy, and ethics*. Macon, GA: Mercer University Press.
Foster, R. A. & Babcock, R. L. (2001). God as man versus God as woman: Perceiving God as a function of the gender of God and the gender of the participant. *The International Journal for the Psychology of Religion, 11(2),* 93-104.
Frankl, V. E. (1984). *Man's search for meaning*. New York: Simon & Schuster.
Fromm, E. (1994) *Escape from freedom*. New York: Owl Books. (Original work published in 1941)

Geertz, C. (1973). *The interpretation of cultures.* New York: Basic Books.

Gendlin, E. T. (1998). *Focusing-oriented psychotherapy: A manual of the experiential method.* New York: Guilford.

Hall, T., Halcrow, S., Hills, P., Delaney, H., & Teal, J. (2005, April). *Attachment and spirituality.* Paper presented at the Christian Association for Psychological Studies International Conference, Dallas, TX.

Hall, T. W. & Porter, S. L. (2004). Referential Integration: An emotional information processing perspective on the Process of Integration. *Journal of Psychology and Theology, 32,* 167-180.

Hoffman, L. (2005). A developmental perspective on the God image. In. R. H. Cox, B. Ervin-Cox, & L. Hoffman (Eds.), *Spirituality and psychological health* (pp. 129-149). Colorado Springs, CO: Colorado School of Professional Psychology Press.

Hoffman, L. (in press). An existential-integrative approach to working with religious and spiritual clients. In K. Schneider (Ed.), Existential-Integrative psychotherapy: Guideposts to the core of practice. New York: Routledge.

Hoffman, L., Grimes, C. S. M., & Acoba, R. (2005, November). *Research on the experience of God: Rethinking epistemological assumptions.* Paper presented at the Society for the Scientific Study of Religion Annual Meeting, Rochester, NY.

Hoffman, L., Hoffman, J., Dillard, K., Clark, J., Acoba, R., Williams, F., & Jones, T. T. (2005a, April). *Cultural diversity and the God image: Examining cultural differences in the experience of God.* Paper presented at the Christian Association for Psychological Studies International Conference, Dallas, TX.

Hoffman, L., Hoffman, J. L., Robison, B., & Lawrence, K. (2005b, April). Modern and postmodern ways of knowing: Implications for theory and integration. Paper presented at the Christian Association for Psychological Studies International Conference, Dallas, TX.

Hoffman, L, Jones, T. T., Williams, F. & Dillard, K. S. (2004, March). *The God image, the God concept, and attachment.* Paper presented at the Christian Association for Psychological Studies International Conference, St. Petersburg, FL.

Hoffman, L., Stewart, S., Warren, D., & Meek, L. (2006, August). *Multiple selves in postmodern theory: An Existential-Integrative Critique.* Paper presented at the American Psychological Association Annual Convention, New Orleans, LA.

Kirkpatrick, L. A. (1997). A longitudinal study of changes in religious beliefs and behavior as a function of individual differences in adult attachment style. *Journal for the Scientific Study of Religion, 36,* 207-217.

Kirkpatrick, L. A. (1998). God as a substitute attachment figure: A longitudinal study of adult attachment style and religious change in college students. *Personality and Social Psychology Bulletin, 24,* 961-973.

Kirkpatrick, L. A. (2004). *Attachment, evolution, and the psychology of religion.* New York: Guilford Press.

Kirkpatrick, L. A. & Shaver, P. R. (1990). Attachment theory and religion: Childhood attachments, religious beliefs, and conversion. *Journal for the Scientific Study of Religion, 29,* 315-334.

Krejci, M. J. (1998). Gender comparison of God schemas: A multidimensional scaling analysis. *The International Journal for the Psychology of Religion, 8(1),* 57-66.

May, G. G. (2004). *The dark night of the soul.* San Francisco: Harper.

May, R. (1953). *Man's search for himself.* New York: Delta.

May, R. (1969). *Love and will.* New York: Delta.

May, R. (1981). *Freedom and destiny.* New York: Norton & Company.

May, R. (1991). *The cry for myth.* New York: Delta.

May, R. (1999). Oedipus and self-knowledge. *Review of Existential Psychology and Psychiatry, 24,* 10-16. (Originally presented in 1966)

Mendelowitz, E. (2006). Meditations on Oedipus: Becker's Kafka, Nietzsche's meta-morphoses. *Journal of Humanistic Psychology, 46,* 385-431.

Mendelowitz, E. & Schneider, K. (in press). Existential psychotherapy. In R. J. Corsini & D. Wedding (Eds.), *Current psychotherapies* (8th edition). New York: Wadsworth.

Nelsen, H. M., Cheek, N. H., Jr., & Au, P. (1985). Gender differences in images of God. *Journal for the Scientific Study of Religion, 24(4),* 396-402.

Olthuis, J. H. (1999). Dancing together in the wild spaces of love: Postmodernism, psy-chotherapy, and the spirit of God. *Journal of Psychology and Christianity, 18,* 140-152.

Olthuis, J. H. (2001). *The beautiful risk.* Grand Rapids, MI: Zondervan.

Rank, O. (1936). *Truth and reality* (J. Taft, Trans.). New York: Norton & Company. (Original work published in 1929)

Roberts, C. W. (1989). Imagining god: Who is created in whose image? *Review of Religious Research, 30(4),* 375-387.

Schneider, K. J. (1999). *The paradoxical self: Toward an understanding of our contra-dictory nature.* Amherst, NY: Humanity Press.

Schneider, K. J. (2004). *Rediscovery of awe: Splendor, mystery, and the fluid center of life.* St. Paul, MN: Paragon House.

Schneider, K. J. (in press). *Existential-Integrative psychotherapy: Guideposts to the core of practice.* New York: Routledge.

Schneider, K. J. & May, R. (1995). *The psychology of existence: An integrative, clini-cal perspective.* New York: McGraw-Hill.

Stark, M. (1999). *Modes of therapeutic action.* Northvale, NJ: Jason Aronson.

Tisdale, T. C., Key, T. L., Edwards, K. J., Brokaw, B. F., Kemperman, S. R., & Cloud, H (1997). Impact of God image and personal adjustment, and correlations of the God image to personal adjustment and object relations development. *Journal of Psychology and Theology, 5,* 227-239.

Yalom, I. D. (1980). *Existential psychotherapy.* New York: Basic Books.

Yalom, I. D. (1995). *Theory and practice of group psychotherapy* (4th ed.). New York: Basic Books.

doi:10.1300/J515v09n03_06

Chapter 7

A Neuroscientific Approach
and the God Image

Fernando Garzon, PsyD

SUMMARY. Recent neuroscientific discoveries are refining our understanding of what makes therapy work and how God image difficulties can be addressed effectively in counseling. This article discusses neural networks, implicit and explicit memory systems, hemispheric specialization and neurological aspects of trauma in regards to how these impact our assumptions about traditional psychotherapy and God image transformation. Given the varying levels of neuroscientific training in the pastoral and mental health professions, this discussion is written in an introductory fashion. Implications are highlighted through a case study demonstrating spiritually-based intervention strategies. doi:10.1300/J515v09n03_07 *[Article copies available for a fee from The Haworth Document Delivery Service: 1-800- HAWORTH. E-mail address: <docdelivery@haworthpress.com> Website: <http:// www.HaworthPress. com> © 2007 by The Haworth Press. All rights reserved.]*

[Haworth co-indexing entry note]: "A Neuroscientific Approach and the God Image." Garzon, Fernando. Co-published simultaneously in *Journal of Spirituality in Mental Health* (The Haworth Pastoral Press, an imprint of The Haworth Press) Vol. 9, No. 3/4, 2007, pp. 139-155; and: *God Image Handbook for Spiritual Counseling and Psychotherapy: Research, Theory, and Practice* (ed: Glendon L. Moriarty, and Louis Hoffman) The Haworth Pastoral Press, an imprint of The Haworth Press, 2007, pp. 139-155. Single or multiple copies of this article are available for a fee from The Haworth Document Delivery Service [1-800-HAWORTH, 9:00 a.m. - 5:00 p.m. (EST). E-mail address: docdelivery@haworthpress.com].

For you created my inmost being; you knit me together in my mother's womb. I praise you because I am fearfully and wonderfully made; your works are wonderful, I know that full well.

Psalm 139:13-14, NIV

Religious experience has always inspired a sense of awe. Over the centuries, the mysteries of our created design and ability to relate with God have stirred worship and adoration in every culture. Only recently have scientific investigations led to a substantial furtherance of our understanding of spiritual experiences from a physiological standpoint (e.g., Newberg & Newberg, 2005). Awe and understanding have begun to merge.

The field of neuroscience has exploded within the past ten years, prompting an examination of areas, like religious experience, once considered beyond the purview of science (Seybold, 2005). Indeed, progress in investigating religiospirituality has taken place so fast as to now lead to the subfield of neurotheology (d'Aquili & Newberg, 1999), which has been defined as an exploration of how the mind/brain operates in regards to one's relationship to God. One aspect of that relationship concerns our subjective emotional experience of God (i.e., our God image, Rizzuto, 1979) compared to our theological or knowledge-based conceptualizations of God (our God concept). People often come to therapy with maladies both in their interpersonal lives and in their God image. Neuroscientific findings can now inform our strategies in both areas. A person's God image can be impacted when it is seen to be maladaptive.

Certainly, worldview impacts how one interprets neuroscientific findings. Awe and understanding can lead to pride in thinking that religious experience can be explained entirely through neuroscience. Humility in seeking to synthesize these discoveries with other academic disciplines is another option. For myself, I adopt a nonreductionistic, critical realist epistemological framework. This means that I don't reduce spiritual experiences solely to the expression of neurological activity, and that I believe that God and the world exist independently of my brain/mind experience. Multiple levels of interdisciplinary understanding, analysis, and interpretation are present in the comprehension of religious experience and, in particular for this article, understanding how to impact God image in therapy. Each level has validity. A neuroscientific approach therefore is just one of many explanatory systems that await more integrative theoretical interaction and synthesis in the future.

In writing this article, I'm also aware that the variety of mental health professionals and pastoral counselors reading it will vary in their foundational knowledge upon which to build this discussion; therefore, I will endeavor to reduce the terminology down to a basic level. This includes minimizing the amount of brain anatomy discussion to a palatable level. Detailed resources are available for the reader who would like to explore general neuroscience related to counseling on a more in-depth level (e.g., Siegel, 1999, 2003; Schore, 2003a, 2003b).

What follows accordingly is an introduction to some of the basic concepts of neuroscience and how they influence assumptions about traditional psychotherapy as well as our strategies for influencing God image change. Neural networks, right and left brain functioning, implicit and explicit memory systems, and the role of trauma will be considered. Aspects of the transference and the unconscious will also be reflected on. We will discover that neuroscientific findings impact our assumptions about psychotherapy. As other articles in this volume have addressed God image intervention from a variety of traditional therapeutic frameworks (Gestalt, Psychoanalytic, etc.), the case study presented highlights the application of spiritual resources in God image treatment. The article concludes with the implications of neuroscience for our understandings of God concept and God image.

NEURAL NETWORK MODELS, TRANSFERENCE, AND GOD IMAGE

To bridge the gap between psychotherapy to neuroscience, one must be aware of the building blocks of neuroscience. These are neurons and neural networks. Neurons (or nerve cells) are the "electrical circuit" cells of the brain, spinal cord, and nervous system (Siegel, 1999). They provide the fundamental building blocks of neural networks.

The firing relationship of neurons leads to neural networks. Each neuron receives a variety of input signals from other neurons, some encouraging it to fire and some discouraging such activation. If a certain threshold level of positive input is reached for a neuron, then it fires in an all-or-none fashion. A circuit of interconnecting neurons which fire simultaneously leads to a unit of mental activity (emotion, thought, memory, perception, or behavior; Pally, 2000). This circuit of concurrently firing neurons that leads to a psychological or physical sensation is known as a neural network (Edelman, 1987). The more this network fires together, the more the developed connections between these neurons are strengthened (Hebb, 1949).

Hebb's (1949) concept that neural networks can be strengthened when they are fired together suggests that these neural networks can become "standardized" in the specific neurons that fire together (i.e., those that activate together essentially link together, according to Hebb's law). While linkage occurs, neural networks are also *modifiable* via the establishment of new connections with other neurons. In short, new wiring that impacts the neural network can take place under certain circumstances. The neurons must be connected to each other and they must start firing together (Schore, 2003b). This ability to form new network linkages is known as neuroplasticity (Siegel, 2006).

The time of much initial growth and development for the brain and nervous system is infancy and early childhood (Siegel, 1999). The intimate connection involved between caregiver and infant has the ability to initiate and modify the brain's wiring in certain regions (corticolimbic and orbitofrontal; Schore, 2003a). The modifiability of neural networks through environmental interactions reframes the nature versus nurture debate. We receive a genetically-based endowment of developing neural material in our brain and spinal cord, but our interactions with the environment can lead to different patterns of neural firing and thus different formations of neural networks. Gene expression can be modified; thus, "'nature versus nurture" arguments misrepresent this vital interaction (Kandel, 1998). While relationships in early development lay the groundwork for future interpersonal attachment, the neural systems involved continue to be modifiable throughout life (Cappas, Andres-Hyman, Davidson, 2005).

Another interesting feature of neural networks is the contexts in which they fire. The brain systems involved in using one's imagination are the same as made active through real perception (Cappas, Andres-Hyman, & Davidson, 2005). Perception and imagery processes use the same neural substrates (Kreiman, Koch, & Fried, 2000). For example, when one imagines someone's face, regions involved in the actual perception of faces become activated (O'Craven & Kanwisher, 2000).

Contextual stimuli are also involved in the therapeutic encounter. Neural network models inform both analytic and behavioral conceptualizations of the transference. Gabbard (2006) notes, for example, that the therapist represents an authority figure; thus, the neural networks associated with authority figures (parents, other significant caregivers, current bosses, etc.) become activated in the relationship. The therapist's specific appearance, office setting, etc. may also stimulate a variety of other networks. The initiated networks set off fears, expectations, and consequent defenses. As the transference is slowly worked through, new neural connections are established that modify the original neural networks triggered. From a behavioral perspective, transference represents a form of generalized learning (Rilling, 2000). The therapist, setting, etc., become the stimuli for classically conditioned activation of neural networks. Counter-conditioning builds new neural connections and extinction reduces the firing of the maladaptive components of pathologically triggered networks.

Implications for God Image

Neural transference explanations have pertinence for God image theories. When one thinks of "God," a variety of neural networks associated with authority figures, primary caregivers, etc. become stimulated. Consequently, one's subjective emotional experience of God (God image) may differ in negative ways from a more positive conceptual knowledge of God as loving, gracious, and caring. The therapeutic relationship in a positive counseling experience may change the composition of neural networks associated with authority figures and thus change one's God image even when God is not brought up directly. Truly, "the greatest of these is love" (I Cor. 13:13, NIV).

Indeed, while the therapeutic relationship is foundational, neuroscience does not imply that it is the only way God image transformation can take place in treatment. Given that neural networks can become activated via the imagination, Scripture meditation, for example, "living Scriptures" meditative practices of St. Ignatius Loyola (See Lonsdale, 1990) and other forms of contemplative prayer (e.g., Foster, 1988) become more understandable as potential vehicles of God image change. We can now hypothesize that new neural pathways are developed through these practices. Research on eastern forms of meditation (e.g., mindfulness) already has indicated their ability to produce neural pathway change (Siegel, 2006). Research is now needed on western forms.

NEUROSCIENCE AND THE UNCONSCIOUS

Neuroscience is informing our understanding of what is involved in unconscious processes. For example, the human brain is divided into right and left hemispheres, with each having generally distinct functions. Siegel (2006) notes that the right hemisphere develops first, rapidly from infancy to about three years old. After this period, the left hemisphere begins to alternate with the right in growth and development. This means that patterns of relationship learned through infant-mother and early caregiver interactions are stored primarily in the right brain. The right hemisphere perceives and encodes nonverbal aspects of communication (facial expression, eye contact, posture, tone of voice, gestures, posture, intensity of interaction, etc.). It is pivotal in stress response, spontaneous emotion, nonverbal empathy aspects, and autobiographical memory (Siegel, 1999). Relational attunement in therapy involves many nonverbal components and thus occurs primarily through right-brain to right-brain communication between therapist and client (Schore, 2003b). The left brain generally focuses on semantic language elements of communication (words themselves) and maintains a linear flow to reasoning. Cause-and-effect, logical syllogisms, and yes-no, right-wrong, on-off patterns of thinking predominate the left hemisphere (Siegel, 2006).

Cognitive neuroscience distinguishes several memory systems pertinent to the unconscious. Explicit (conscious) memory involves the recollection of autobiographical events, facts, and concepts or ideas. We are aware we are discussing these in therapy. Implicit memory is not in the client's awareness but can be observed in his or her behavior (Gabbard, 2006). Procedural memory, a form of implicit memory, is especially relevant to the unconscious. It involves "how to" knowledge, such as playing a piano or driving a car. Initially, one has to focus consciously on driving a car: Place the key in the ignition, turn the key, press the gas, put the car in gear, etc. However, soon this becomes automatic so we do it without thinking. We learn about how to be in relationships in analogous fashion, early in life.

Mother-infant and early caregiver interactions lead to our implicit procedural memory code for how relationships work. Our consequent psychological defenses that become automatic are based on these early experiences (Fosshage, 2003). Unlike explicit memory, which primarily is mediated through a brain structure called the hippocampus, implicit memory encodes these interpersonal learnings through the amygdala and related brain structures (Schore, 2003a). The quality of early life relational experiences and any traumas experienced at that time impact how the wiring of the amygdala and other structures involved in the implicit memory system progress (Schore, 2003a). Since the right brain develops much more rapidly during the first three years of life, much procedural memory coding for how relationships work takes place *without the benefit of language* and is encoded subsymbolically and nonverbally (Bucci, 1997). See Hall (2004, Hall & Porter, 2004; Chapter 3) for further in-depth discussion of attachment theory and memory system interaction.

At any age, severe trauma can impact memory systems. Solomon and Siegel (2003) propose one mechanism for how this occurs. Such trauma can lead to several rapid events: Secretion of high levels of stress hormones, the strong activation of the amygdala (the same organ involved in implicit memory), and the consequent temporary impairment of the hippocampus in its functioning (the same organ involved in explicit memory and the memory consolidation process). When these systems return to normal functioning after the episode, the neural encoding for the event can seem like unprocessed elements of bodily sensation, emotion, perception, and behavioral response. Because of the insufficient hippocampal consolidation of the memory, the person may feel these free-floating fragments as happening now when set off by environmental cues or internal emotional triggers. This is because of the "implicit memory predominant" encoding of the experience. Solomon and Siegel propose that flashbacks and other symptoms of Posttraumatic Stress Disorder (PTSD) occur via this mechanism.

The dynamics involved in implicit memory, along with awareness that the explicit memory system involved in autobiographical memory is malleable, lead to concerns over how to differentiate false memory production from recovery of traumatic memory in therapy. The debate goes on as to how research about false memory syndrome should be interpreted by clinicians (e.g., Madill & Holtch, 2004). The occurrence of recovered traumatic memories in treatment or other contexts that later were corroborated has been noted in case studies (e.g., Bull, 1999; Chu, Frey, Ganzel, & Matthews, 1999), including a prospective case study (Dougal & Stroufe, 1998). It appears that delayed recall of traumatic events poorly processed by the hippocampus does occur (Scheflin & Brown, 1996; van der Kolk & Fisler, 1995). Good clinical technique safeguards the creation of pseudomemories. Care must be taken not to be suggestive when clients report memory fragments that hint at the possibility of abuse but do not clearly indicate it. The fragments could also be a symbolic image (implicit memory driven) that encodes significant relational dynamics in the client's life. Statements such as "I think you might have been sexually abused" when no clear memory of abuse has emerged may plant the suggestion for such abuse to be reported. A nondirective, supportive, and empathic approach is best until the unclear memory fragments or symbolic images emerge sufficiently to indicate intervention direction.

Implications of the Neuroscientific Unconscious

Implicit memory processes further highlight the important role of the therapeutic relationship in promoting change. As clients experience the therapist relating in ways inconsistent with previous implicitly encoded patterns, new neural wiring takes place (Fosshage, 2003). Hall and Porter (2004) note that "it is not possible to separate implicit relational processes from 'spiritual processes,'... They are inextricably intertwined ... implicit experiences form the *foundation* [italics by original authors] of emotional appraisal of meaning in any aspect of spiritual functioning, including one's relationship with God" (p. 75). Thus, contrasts between one's conceptual knowledge of God as loving and a discrepant subjective emotional experience of that reality (a negative God image) have neurological underpinnings in the implicit memory coding system.

Some psychoanalysts and other therapists are now questioning the ability of insight and typical verbal processing to address sufficiently client relational issues that developed neurally before verbal coding could take place, or that involve significant trauma that occurs after such verbal ability develops (e.g., Hutterer & Liss, 2006; Neborsky, 2006). Therapy that is primarily focused on insight strategies mainly engages the left brain of the client. We've already seen that this is the hemisphere that processes in a linear, logical fashion. However, strong affective, implicit memory-based, and trauma-related aspects of the client's experience reside primarily in *the right hemispheric, amygdala-mediated neural pathways*. These areas produce the most prominent pathological components of the client's relational neural networks. The assumption therefore that these tremendously intricate, multidimensional neural mechanisms can be accessed sufficiently and processed primarily through the unidimensional verbal channel of the left brain is questionable. Perhaps this is one reason for the long term nature of some therapies (Hutterer & Liss, 2006). Eclectic, integrative treatment methods that engage the right brain and implicit processes, such as art therapy, psychodrama, gestalt therapy, emotion-focused, and experiential strategies have a much better opportunity to activate the centers of the brain most involved in the maintenance of the relational pathology. Many more recent approaches therefore are now intentionally considering the findings of neuroscience (e.g., Fosha & Yeung, 2006)

The above debate has direct implications for God image therapy. While the therapeutic relationship and insight-oriented techniques can produce God image change, such transformation may occur at an unnecessarily slow rate because of the principal strategies used. The relationship and verbal communication, however, are foundational to change; thus, the encouragement here is for incorporating strategies that more fully engage the right brain and implicit processes rather than deemphasizing the above two areas. Likewise, verbal theological clarifications around God image issues are worthwhile in dealing with God image issues.

With appropriate informed consent, assessment, and diagnostic considerations, spiritual interventions that are more affective and experiential in nature may be beneficial (Garzon, 2005). The case study that follows provides an example of an eclectic approach that includes affective experiential spiritual strategies.

CASE STUDY

The specific modalities described in this case were tailored for this particular client (i.e., a client with a conservative Christian background). Consequently, the exact interventions may not be appropriate for different Christian or religious backgrounds.

Presenting Problems

Rodrigo was an unmarried 25-year-old Latino male graduate student attending an evangelical Christian university who expressed great dissatisfaction in his current career path and social relationships. Specifically, Rodrigo lacked genuine friendships and believed he couldn't pursue areas of work that interested him. His rationale for maintaining an unsatisfactory career path involved the belief that God wanted him to do his current ministerial-related work versus developing in other areas of interest. Diagnostically, he reported symptoms consistent with Generalized Anxiety Disorder and Panic Disorder without Agoraphobia. He also exhibited Avoidant/Dependent personality features.

Rodrigo acknowledged the discrepancy between his God concept and God image. He knew theologically that God loved him, accepted him, and wanted him to develop his talents. He also knew the dichotomy between "sacred" ministerial work and "secular" work in other fields was artificial. His God image, though, consisted of a sense of harsh judgment if he did not involve himself in full time ministry. Guilt was his primary affect when considering alternatives. Regarding his social relationships, Rodrigo had good knowledge of assertiveness and general social skills through numerous previous psychological readings; however, interpersonally he had adopted a compliant, passive, and avoidant style. In his current work at a ministry, for example, he never talked with his boss about misgivings concerning assignments. He also would not suggest alternative tasks more to his liking. God image fantasized elements related to these behaviors involved a picture of God frowning at him and telling him to "turn the other cheek" and serve without "complaining." While he mentally recognized the exegetical and theological errors he was making in this fantasy, the affect-laden pictured reaction of God (his God image) motivated him.

Client History

Rodrigo's parents got divorced when he was five years old after a tumultuous, argumentative relationship. His mother never remarried and he grew up as the youngest of three brothers, with 10 years separating him from the second oldest sibling. His mother was very overprotective of him, perhaps unconsciously concerned he was going to leave home eventually like his brothers. For his brothers' part, they had moved out and were encouraging him to stay at home to "take care of mom." Some Latino cultural aspects were apparent in this emphasis on caring for mother; however, Rodrigo's siblings went beyond this emphasis in that they did not appear to take mutual responsibility in her care.

As a teenager, Rodrigo became a Born Again Christian and participated actively in an Hispanic Charismatic church and youth group. The church appeared legalistic from his description. His family moved from Venezuela to the U.S. when he was 22 and currently he attends a small Latino church that he described as "warm and supportive." My previous interactions with that church led me to concur with his appraisal. The pastor was supportive of Christian psychotherapy, and taught the Gospel in a balanced versus legalistic manner.

Case Conceptualization

A neuroscientific perspective of Rodrigo's distress proposes that his early development in an argumentative parental environment followed by paternal abandonment and subsequent maternal over-protectiveness had led to the formation of maladaptive neural networks regarding how relationships work. His pre-immigration experience with a legalistic church reinforced such negative associations. These pathological networks impacted how he related interpersonally and spiritually. As a result, his life revolved around themes like fear of rejection, inadequacy, and dependency. These entrenched network associations activated whenever a current interpersonal stressor occurred. His relationships, God image, and career aspirations were consequently adversely impacted.

Treatment

Initial psychoeducation helped normalize Rodrigo's distress concerning his panic attacks and general anxiety symptoms. To facilitate a reduction of his frequency of panic attacks, Rodrigo rapidly learned a Scripture meditation technique that utilized deep breathing (Benson, 1996). He would breath in slowly, hold his breath to a count of five, and then slowly breathe out quoting a comforting phrase from Scripture (Psalm 23:1), "The Lord is my shepherd."

Therapy focused on linking current stressors and Rodrigo's previously "read about" coping skills via role playing and imagery rehearsal of anticipated stressful events. To enhance the ability to address both implicit memory system and right hemispheric mediated emotional processes involved in his avoidant style, inner healing prayer based on Theophostic Ministry was used intermittently in treatment (see Smith, 2005, for a detailed description of this model).

Typical prayer sessions were scheduled for two hours instead of one. This permitted time both for the prayer itself and debriefing. Rodrigo would focus on anxiety-producing interactions that had occurred during the week. We would identify key affect-laden self statements in the events and he would close his eyes to imagine the most prominent scene. As noted previously, such imagination activates much of the same neural pathways as the original event; thus, his anxious affect increased more than would have occurred with a solely face-to-face verbal discussion. At this point, we would ask Jesus to take him to the source and origin that connects to the current fears. This was done in a nondirective fashion, such as "Lord Jesus, direct us to the source and origin of this pain . . . Rodrigo, report to me anything you see, sense, hear, or experience in your body. It doesn't have to make logical sense. If nothing is sensed, that's okay, too." The nondirective nature of the prayer petition permitted both symbolic content from the implicit memory system as well as trauma-based memories or combinations of memory and symbolic imagery to emerge.

Rodrigo frequently drifted to memories involving rejection from peers, his father's abandonment, or his mother scolding him for taking initiative. In these memories, we would identify the key maladaptive beliefs and do an "exposure protocol." Rodrigo would repeat the beliefs mentally and allow himself to feel the emotions around them without resistance. At this point instead of doing therapist-led cognitive restructuring, we would petition Christ to reveal his truth to Rodrigo regarding those beliefs in whatever manner He chose. Rodrigo would often have a deep sense of peace and hear the Lord's voice clarifying the distortions. When this interaction appeared at an end, we returned to the current situations that had been distressing Rodrigo, and he now rated them regarding their anxiety-provoking potential. After his rating was low, we explored his experience. Through the prayer form, affect-laden memories along with their encoded relational themes were processed. This further motivated Rodrigo to utilize the assertiveness skills he had previously known only by reading.

Example Prayer Intervention

One fascinating prayer time occurred in Rodrigo's twelfth session. He began the session noting his current frustration to change his passive stance at work. We prayed, asking the Lord to take us to the source of this frustration. After a pause, Rodrigo sensed a deep awareness of both his conscious desire to change and his unconscious desire to stay the same.

"Part of me wants to change and part of me doesn't."

[Pause] "Help me understand the part that doesn't want to change, Rodrigo. What's motivating this part?"

"I'm safe living a passive lifestyle. It's comfortable. There's no risk."

We continued to explore this gestalt-like deep awareness of two opposing forces. Unlike some prayer times, no memory or symbolic image accompanied it. Weeping, Rodrigo described how his lifestyle allowed him to blame others for his problems. It also protected him from potential arguments. Stunned surprise, sorrow, and grief were key affects.

"How would you like to respond to this awareness, Rodrigo?"

"I want to ask God to forgive me for choosing this lifestyle. I thought it was Him [requiring me to be passive]. It wasn't. It was me."

Rodrigo asked God to forgive him for unconsciously wanting to live a passive, "safe" lifestyle. He asked for God's help in expressing his needs and desires, and to live a life that expressed his gifts. "I choose a different life," he said. After Rodrigo's prayer of repentance, I asked God to fill all the areas of Rodrigo's heart that were opened up in this session with a sense of His Holy Spirit's presence. A calm, peaceful affect appeared on Rodrigo's face. When asked what was going on, he stated, "I'm forgiven. It's okay . . . He doesn't blame me . . . He loves me."

Prayer Analysis and Treatment Outcome

Rodrigo's spontaneous insights, powerful affective expressions, and sense of positive closure were likely based on increased access to his implicit memory system through amygdala-mediated right hemispheric processing. He had not been consciously in touch with the potent secondary gains he had received from his lifestyle. His response to these spontaneous insights permitted the building of new neural connections in his activated neural network. The new connections could potentially facilitate greater awareness of options and possibilities the next time he encountered a situation that triggered a formerly conditioned passive response. The prayer experience also transformed his maladaptive God image. Perhaps some of his new perception was based on enhanced neural linkages from his more positive left hemispheric-dominated God concept network and his more affect-based, right brain, and amygdala-mediated God image network. The supportive therapeutic relationship over the course of the earlier eleven sessions also may have been building new neural connections in his implicit memory system. As implied from my worldview description, this neuroscientific analysis does not minimize the work of the Holy Spirit in the awareness and repentance process.

After the prayer, we debriefed what happened. Rodrigo experienced the prayer as very helpful. As homework, he agreed to meditate on some biblical passages related to God's love and acceptance. Scriptural study and meditation can often augment insights gained from inner healing prayer (Sides, 2002). I also seized the opportunity afforded in this session to return to a hierarchy of current situations we had previously developed that necessitated assertive action. I proposed that we would begin with the least-threatening situations and work towards the most threatening (like talking with his boss about new assignments and job transfers). Rodrigo declined to do this and rather felt that he would like to try talking to his boss next week. Though I was cautious about such action, he persisted. At our next session, he had successfully discussed his needs with his boss and was awarded a job transfer. In addition, he verbalized more positive interactions with his peers. "I want to start taking responsibility for my life," he noted.

After three more sessions, Rodrigo's treatment ended. Fifteen sessions had taken place in all. At the end of therapy, Rodrigo reported no more panic attacks, greatly diminished anxiety, and a more active, assertive lifestyle. He also had changed churches to join one that was larger and had an active singles group.

CONCLUSIONS

The field of neuroscience continues to expand rapidly. Recent discoveries have spurred new considerations for God image theory and how therapy can be used to impact a client's God image problems. From the theoretical standpoint, while some clients may have both a negative God concept and a negative God image (or positive concept and positive image), others show a discrepancy, commonly being a disconnection between their positive theologically based concept of God as loving and caring, and their more affectively based negative experience of God as harsh and condemning. This is now more understandable. God concept and God image may be predominantly mediated through different neurophysiological pathways. God concept may be more left brain, hippocampally mediated and explicit memory dominant, and God image more right brain, amygdala-mediated, and implicit memory dominant.

Such a theoretical proposition leads to treatment implications. Interventions which facilitate dual processing of the neurologically distinct pathways of God image and God concept have a better chance to impact God image difficulties than those that appear primarily unidimensional and left brain oriented. A wide variety of both secular counseling and spiritually-derived techniques merit exploration. This article has focused on examples of spiritual techniques in its case study. Further neuroscientific research is needed to corroborate the proposed neural pathway differences between God concept and God image, and outcomes-based research on God image therapy interventions is also needed. In the future, neuroscientific research may dramatically impact the development of more efficient and effective psychotherapy and God image change strategies.

REFERENCES

Benson, H. (1996). *Timeless healing: The power and biology of belief.* New York: Scribner.
Bucci, W. (1997). *Psychoanalysis and cognitive science: A multiple code theory.* New York: Guilford Press.
Bull, D. (1999). A verified case of recovered memories of sexual abuse, *American Journal of Psychotherapy, 53,* 221-224.
Cappas, N., Anders-Hyman, R., & Davidson, L. (2005). What psychotherapists can begin to learn from neuroscience: Seven principles of a brain-based psychotherapy. *Psychotherapy: Theory, Research, Practice, Training, 42,* 374-383.
Chu, J., Frey, L., Ganzel, B., & Matthews, J. (1999). Memories of childhood abuse: Dissociation, amnesia, and corroboration. *American Journal of Psychiatry, 156,* 749-755.
d'Aquili, E., & Newberg, A. (1999). *The mystical mind.* Minneapolis: Fortress Press.
Dougal, S., & Stroufe, L. (1998) Recovered memory of childhood sexual trauma: A documented case from a longitudinal study, *Journal of Traumatic Stress, 11,* 301-321.
Edelman, G. (1987). *Neural Darwinism: The theory of neural group selection.* New York: Harper & Row.
Fosha, D., & Yeung, D. (2006). Accelerated experiential-dynamic psychotherapy: The seamless integration of emotional transformation and dyadic relatedness at work. In: G. Stricker, & J. Gold. (Eds.), *A casebook of psychotherapy integration.* (pp. 165-184). Washington, DC: American Psychological Association.
Fosshage, J. L. (2003). Fundamental pathways to change: Illuminating old and creating new relational experience. *International Forum of Psychoanalysis, 12,* 244-251.
Foster, R. J. (1998). *Celebration of discipline: The path to spiritual growth.* 25th anniversary edition. San Francisco: Harper.
Gabbard, G. O. (2006). A neuroscience perspective on transference. *Psychiatric Annals, 36,* 283-288.
Garzon, F. (2005). Interventions that apply Scripture in psychotherapy. *Journal of Psychology and Theology, 33,* 113-121.
Hall, T. W. (2004). Christian spirituality and mental health: A relational spirituality paradigm for empirical research. *Journal of Psychology and Christianity, 23,* 66-81.
Hall, T. W., & Porter, S. L. (2004). Referential integration: An emotional information processing perspective on the process of integration. *Journal of Psychology and Theology, 32* (4), 167-180.
Hebb, D. (1949). *The organization of behavior: A neuropsychological theory.* New York: Wiley.

Hunter, L., Entwistle, D., Monroe, P., Lehman, K., & Renn, B. (2005, April). Theoretical and ethical aspects of Theophostic Ministry. Panel discussion conducted at the international meeting of the Christian Association for Psychological Studies, Dallas, Texas.

Hutterer, J., & Liss, M. (2006). Cognitive development, memory, trauma, treatment: An integration of psychoanalytic and behavioral concepts in light of current neuroscience research. *Journal of the American Academy of Psychoanalysis and Dynamic Psychiatry, 34*, 287-302.

Kandel, E. (1998). A new intellectual framework for psychiatry. *American Journal of Psychiatry, 155,* 457-469.

Krieman, G., Koch, C., & Fried, I. (2000). Imagery neurons in the human brain. *Nature, 408,* 357-361.

Lonsdale, D. (1990). *Eyes to see, ears to hear: An introduction to Ignatian spirituality.* Chicago: Loyola University Press.

Madill, A., & Holtch, P. (2004). A range of memory possibilities: The challenge of the false memory debate for clinicians and researchers. *Clinical Psychology and Psychotherapy, 11*, 299-310.

Neborsky, R. J. (2006). Brain, mind, and dyadic change processes. *Journal of Clinical Psychology, 62,* 523-538

Newberg, A., & Newberg, S. (2005). The neuropsychology of religious and spiritual experience. In R. Paloutzian & C. Park's (Eds.) *Handbook of the Psychology of Religion and Spirituality* (pp. 199-214). New York: Guilford Press.

O'Craven, K., & Kanwisher, N. (2000). Mental imagery of faces and places activates corresponding stimulus-specific brain regions. *Journal of Cognitive Neuroscience, 12,* 1023-1034.

Pally, R. (2000). *The mind-brain relationship.* London, England: Karnac Books.

Rilling, M.(2000). John Watson's paradoxical struggle to explain Freud. *American Psychologist, 55,* 301-312.

Rizzuto, A. (1979). *The birth of the living God: A psychoanalytic study.* Chicago: University of Chicago Press.

Scheflin, A., & Brown, D. (1996). Repressed memory or dissociative amnesia: What the science says. *Journal of Psychiatry and Law, 24,* 143-188.

Schore, A. (2003a). *Affect dysregulation and disorders of the self.* New York: Norton.

Schore, A. (2003b). *Affect regulation and the repair of the self.* New York: Norton.

Seybold, K. (2005). God and the brain: Neuroscience looks at religion. *Journal of Psychology and Christianity, 24,* 122-129.

Sides, D. (2002). *Mending cracks in the soul.* Colorado Springs: Wagner Publishing.

Siegel, D. (1999). *The developing mind.* New York: Guilford Press.

Siegel, D. (2003). An interpersonal neurobiology of psychotherapy: The developing mind and the resolution of trauma. In M.F. Solomon & D.J. Siegel (Eds.), *Healing trauma: Attachment, mind, body, and brain* (pp. 1-54). New York: Norton.

Siegel, D. (2006). An interpersonal neurobiology approach to psychotherapy. *Psychiatric Annals, 36,* 248-256.

Smith, E. (2005). Theophostic Prayer Ministry: Basic Seminar Manual. Cambellsville, KY: New Creation Publishing.

Solomon, M., & Siegel, D. (Eds.) (2003). *Healing trauma: Attachment, mind, body, and brain.* New York: Norton.
van der Kolk, B., & Fisler, R. (1995). Dissociation and the fragmentary nature of traumatic memories: Overview and exploratory study. *Journal of Traumatic Stress, 8,* 505-525.

doi:10.1300/J515v09n03_07

Chapter 8

Rational Emotive Behavior Therapy and the God Image

Brad Johnson, PhD

SUMMARY. Rational Emotive Behavior Therapy (REBT) may be particularly well suited to the assessment and treatment of clinical difficulties related to the God image. REBT emphasizes helping clients to see how they create their own emotional reactions–including disturbed emotions related to God–by telling themselves certain things and how they can create more constructive and adaptive emotions by actively confronting absolutistic and evaluative thinking. This chapter summarizes a spiritually-oriented approach to REBT and then applies this approach to clinically-relevant concerns regarding God image. To illustrate God image change, a case example of treatment with a depressed and traumatized male is presented. doi:10.1300/J515v09n03_08 *[Article copies available for a fee from The Haworth Document Delivery Service: 1-800-HAWORTH. E-mail address: <docdelivery@haworthpress.com> website; <http://www.HaworthPress. com> © 2007 by The Haworth Press. All rights reserved.]*

Rational Emotive Behavior Therapy (REBT) is one of the earliest approaches to Cognitive Behavior Therapy (CBT). REBT posits that the

[Haworth co-indexing entry note]: "Rational Emotive Behavior Therapy and the God Image." Johnson, Brad. Co-published simultaneously in *Journal of Spirituality in Mental Health* (The Haworth Pastoral Press, an imprint of The Haworth Press) Vol. 9, No. 3/4, 2007, pp. 157-181; and: *God Image Handbook for Spiritual Counseling and Psychotherapy: Research, Theory, and Practice* (ed: Glendon L. Moriarty, and Louis Hoffman) The Haworth Pastoral Press, an imprint of The Haworth Press, 2007, pp. 157-181. Single or multiple copies of this article are available for a fee from The Haworth Document Delivery Service [1-800-HAWORTH, 9:00 a.m. - 5:00 p.m. (EST). E-mail address: docdelivery@haworthpress.com].

tendency to make devout, absolutistic evaluations rests at the heart of psychological disturbance (Ellis & Dryden, 1997). These absolutistic demands are often cloaked in dogmatic musts, shoulds, and oughts; such irrational thinking nearly always interferes with one's pursuit of personal goals and purposes. REBT has shown particular promise as a clinical approach with religious clients (Nielson, Johnson, & Ellis, 2001). A religious client's image of the divine-no matter how it may develop-can be a harbinger of basic self-image and a barometer of both psychological and spiritual adjustment. On occasion, a client's God image may be centrally linked to the reason for referral and thus a direct focus of intervention.

This chapter summarizes the primary philosophical assumptions and clinical interventions of REBT. It briefly considers the development of God Image and the nature of God image difficulties. The chapter gives in-depth consideration of the application of REBT to God image modification and the relative strengths and weaknesses of this approach are presented. Finally, the author offers a case example of REBT with a devoutly religious male client suffering from clinical depression and Post-Traumatic Stress Disorder (PTSD). In this case, the client's image of God was centrally connected to the irrational beliefs fueling his clinical symptoms.

BACKGROUND AND PHILOSOPHICAL ASSUMPTIONS

CBT is a broad term incorporating a wide array of therapeutic approaches that share three fundamental propositions: (a) cognitive activity affects behavior, (b) cognitive activity may be monitored and altered, and (c) desired behavior change may be affected through cognitive change (Dobson & Block, 1988; Hollon & Beck, 1994). All CBT approaches tend to favor cognitive interventions-those which attempt to produce change by influencing thinking (Mahoney, 1977). Aaron Beck, the architect of Cognitive Therapy (CT), described the process this way:

> In a collaborative process, the therapist and patient examine the patient's beliefs about himself, other people, and the world. The patient's maladaptive conclusions are treated as testable hypotheses. Behavioral experiments and verbal procedures are used to examine alternative interpretations and to generate contradictory evidence that supports more adaptive beliefs and leads to therapeutic change. (Beck & Weishaar, 2000, p. 241)

Taken together, most CBT approaches share several underlying assumptions and distinctive therapeutic activities (Blagys & Hilsenroth, 2002; Dobson & Block, 1988; Hollon & Beck, 1994; Propst, 1996; Tan & Johnson, 2005). These common features include: (a) the assumption that therapy is time-limited and that change will occur rapidly, (b) clients are seen as the architects of their own misfortune-they largely cause their own disturbances, (c) the therapist is active and directive, (d) CBT is explicitly educative and psychoeducational techniques are embraced, (e) CBT employs homework and outside-of-session activities, (f) CBT focuses on the impact of the client's irrational thoughts on both current and future functioning, and (g) to experience relief and prevent future dysfunction, clients must learn to work at correcting distortions and disputing faulty beliefs.

There is now substantial evidence that cognitive appraisals of events and irrational beliefs about self, others, and the world, can significantly impact one's response to those events and one's general level of symptom distress. There is also substantial outcome research supporting the efficacy and utility of CBT approaches in the treatment of unipolar depression, generalized anxiety disorder, panic disorder, agoraphobia, social phobia, posttraumatic stress disorder, childhood depression and anxiety, chronic pain, marital distress, and a number of other clinical problems (Butler, 2006; Hollon & Beck, 1994; Propst, 1996). Although CBT is characterized by a more active and directive stance on the part of the therapist, empirical reviews of the CBT literature reveal that a strong therapeutic alliance and the Rogerian variables of empathy, warmth, and positive regard tend to be present in effective CBT treatment relationships. It appears that an active-directive approach need not be incompatible with establishing an effective interpersonal relationship.

Rational Emotive Behavior Therapy (REBT)

Among the most widely practiced forms of CBT, REBT was developed by Albert Ellis on this simple premise: "This is what the rational therapist teaches clients to do: to understand exactly how they create their own emotional reactions by telling themselves certain things, and how they can create different emotional reactions by telling themselves other things" (Ellis, 1957, p. 38). The primary difference between REBT and other psychotherapies is REBT's emphasis on evaluative beliefs (Ellis & Dryden, 1997), or the "B" in the ABC model in which "A" is the Activating event and "C" is the negative emotional consequence (depression, anxiety, anger, and shame). REBT consistently targets fundamental irrational beliefs (e.g., "I must be loved by everyone I love, I should perform perfectly"), and has been described as a particularly "elegant" approach to psychotherapy because REBT therapists strive for a profound philosophic change or basic attitudinal shift in their clients (Walen, DiGiuseppe, & Dryden, 1992).

Before considering how REBT might be used with religious clients or with God image concerns in particular, it may help to review several of REBT's essential theoretical propositions (Ellis, 2000; Ellis & Dryden, 1997): (a) people are largely born with a potential to be both rational and irrational, (b) activating events and life circumstances contribute to but do not directly cause negative emotional consequences, (c) emotional and behavioral disturbances are largely created by the individual's belief system-even though most people wrongly attribute these disturbances to situations and events, (d) irrational beliefs-those which underlie emotional disturbance-tend to be logically inconsistent, inconsistent with empirical reality, absolutistic and dogmatic, and likely to block goal attainment, and (e) people will experience reduction in distress and long-term change only when they actively and consistently work against these irrational beliefs. Psychotherapy outcome research supports the efficacy of REBT with a number of mood, anxiety, relationship, and anger problems (c.f., Lyons & Woods, 1991).

Spiritually-Oriented REBT

At times, a religious client may be strictly interested in symptom relief or disposition of a problem. At other times, a client may introduce concerns which are spiritual in nature-related to experiences of transcendence and the search for the sacred-or specifically religious (Tan & Johnson, 2005). There are several reasons why CBT in general, and REBT in particular, is a particularly elegant therapeutic modality for religiously committed clients (DiGiuseppe, Robin, & Dryden, 1990; Ellis, 2000; Johnson, 2001; Nielsen et al., 2001; Propst, 1996). These reasons include: (a) REBT is highly belief-oriented and focuses on clients' foundational or core beliefs about themselves, others, the world, and their relationship to God; clients from various religious traditions are often quite comfortable with this emphasis on personal responsibility for transforming assumptions and beliefs, (b) REBT is quite flexible and eclectic and can easily accommodate elements of a client's spiritual journey or religious faith, (c) REBT is naturally existential and philosophical in nature, and (d) REBT's emphasis on teaching and education is familiar and comfortable to many religious clients who often appreciate homework assignments that integrate existing facets of spiritual or religious practice. It is also the case that there is considerable congruence between Holy Scriptures and many of the assumptions and techniques of REBT. For example, the Christian philosophy of grace is quite consistent with the REBT emphasis on self and other acceptance.

Further, Christian scripture supports the general CBT assumption that belief has tremendous implication for personal well being (e.g., Phil. 4:8-9: "Whatever is true, whatever is noble, whatever is right, whatever is pure, whatever is lovely. . . think about such things . . . and the God of peace will be with you;" "Prov. 23: "As a man thinketh in his heart, so is he"). A number of authors have described how REBT might be specifically accommodated to client religious faith (DiGiuseppe, et al., 1990; Ellis, 2000; Nielson et al., 2001; Johnson, 2001; 2003), and there is preliminary outcome research demonstrating the efficacy of REBT in the treatment of depressed religious clients (Johnson, DeVries, Ridley, Pettorini, & Peterson, 1994; Johnson & Ridley, 1992).

GOD IMAGE DEVELOPMENT

The vast majority of psychotherapy clients, whether identified with a religious denomination or engaged with a religious community, profess some faith in a divine being. One's image of God refers to how God is represented and experienced and comprises one component of a client's overall religious experience (Hall & Brokaw, 1995). Just as religious experience is highly idiosyncratic, God image can be quite personal and variable. Concept-mapping research indicates that God image is a multidimensional construct; the most common images produced by adult subjects include, creator, healer, friend, father, redeemer, ruler, judge and mother (Kunkel, Cook, Meshel, Daughtry & Hauenstein, 1999). Americans appear more likely to view God as a creator (82%) and healer (69%) than judge (47%) or mother (25%: Roof & Roof, 1984). Images of God can be reduced to the fundamental dimensions of nurturing and punishing (Kunkel et al., 1999), and over time, American's images of God have moved significantly in the direction of nurturing; God is less likely to be seen as judge and more likely to be seen as supportive (Nelson, Cheek, & Au, 1985).

The God Image appears to be influenced by and intertwined with early experiences with significant caregivers and thus highly correlated with images of mother, father, and self (Hall & Brokaw, 1995; Spilka, Armatas, & Nussbaum, 1964). Writing from a psychoanalytic perspective, Rizzuto (1979) concluded that God image forms in the earliest period of life, and that both parents–particularly the mother–contribute to God image formation: "God is a special type of object representation created by the child in that psychic space where transitional objects–whether toys, blankets, or mental representations–are provided with their powerfully real illusory lives" (p. 177). Unlike psychoanalysis, REBT does not promulgate a unified theory of personality or psychosocial development; REBT is an approach to conceptualizing and addressing dysfunction. In the next section, I show how REBT might approach God image difficulty.

GOD IMAGE DIFFICULTIES

Initially skeptical about the possibility of health-facilitating religiousness, Ellis has softened his rejection of religion over the years–largely in response to thorough literature reviews which support numerous positive correlations between religious commitment and mental health (c.f., Bergin, 1983; Donahue, 1985; Gartner, Larson, & Allen, 1991). Nonetheless, there is evidence that certain forms of religiousness are more likely to correlate with negative mental health outcomes (Johnson & Nielsen, 1998; Lovinger, 1994). Religious people, like all others, are prone to making irrational absolutistic demands of themselves, the world, and God. From a cognitive perspective, human behavior is often maladaptive because human beings frequently make thinking errors or produce dysfunctional, idiosyncratic interpretations of events and experiences (Beck & Weishaar, 2000; Ellis, 1962). A cognitive psychotherapist remains vigilant to dysfunctional schemas–complex cognitive/emotional grids that contain a person's perception of themselves, others, and even God (Beck & Weishaar, 2000), and dysfunctional beliefs–deeply embedded views of self, others, and God which are not supportable by logic, empirical reality, or even religious/scriptural evidence (Nielsen et al., 2000).

God image may become relevant in psychotherapy when a client is religiously or spiritually committed and when the God image appears linked to the presenting problem or primary emotional disturbance. Specifically, when a person holds a wrathful, controlling, or distant image of God–often a byproduct of negative experiences with primary caregivers in childhood–then both emotional health and spiritual maturity may be impacted (Hall & Brokaw, 1995; Rizzuto, 1979). In contrast, people who experienced loving, nurturing parental relationships tend to view God as loving, accepting, and forgiving (Richards & Bergin, 1997).

It is the strong connection between God image and self image which may be of greatest interest and concern to the psychotherapist. The positive correlation between God image and self-esteem is now well established in the psychology of religion literature (c.f., Benson & Spilka, 1973; Francis, Gibson & Robbins, 2001). Religious beliefs and images of God which construe God as judgmental, wrathful, and demanding predict lower self-esteem than God images and doctrinal beliefs which emphasize God's loving and forgiving nature. Benson and Spilka (1973) used Cognitive Consistency Theory (CCT) to explain the God image/self-esteem correlation. According to CCT, it is self-image or self-esteem that determines God image, not the reverse;

> negative or positive God images may be used in part to maintain or preserve one's level of self-esteem . . . a theology predicated on a loving, accepting God is cognitively compatible with high self-esteem, but it would be a source of discomfort for a believer low in self-esteem. (p. 298, 308)

CCT is particularly relevant to the practice of REBT with religious clients. Specifically, when a client-for whatever reason-holds a particularly damning, wrathful, or disengaged God image, it is quite likely that the client also engages in self-downing irrational beliefs which should become one focus of psychotherapy. Benson and Spilka (1973) note that a self-downing religious client would work to avoid the discomfort associated with dissonant cognitions about God (e.g., loving, accepting) and may therefore engage in selective perception, distortion, and denial to keep theological beliefs consonant with self-image; such distortions and irrational beliefs would become natural targets for the REBT therapist's primary intervention-cognitive disputation.

GOD IMAGE CHANGE

Change in REBT always begins with a careful assessment of the presenting problem–typically some form of emotional disturbance (the C), followed by a careful exploration of the activating event (situation, loss, problem) or A (Ellis & Dryden, 1997; Walen et al., 1992). Although most clients believe that A directly causes C, the REBT therapist assumes that it is some irrational belief–the B–which actually causes C.

Because clients do not easily or immediately articulate irrational beliefs, ferreting out these dysfunctional and irrational beliefs constitutes the heart of the REBT assessment process. REBT therapists often employ strategies such as inference chaining (e.g., "yes, and that would mean?"), and hypothetical questioning (e.g., "and after A, what might you have been thinking or saying to yourself that caused C?").

It is always useful to include a religious-spiritual component in standard client assessment procedures (Richards & Bergin, 1997). Understanding a client's religious commitments and beliefs may allow the clinician to better understand any connection between religious belief and the presenting complaint. Such an integrative assessment also provides an opportunity to consider how the client's spiritual or religious commitment might be leveraged as a resource in therapy (Johnson & Nielsen, 1998; Richards & Bergin, 1997). When assessing the religious dimension of a client's experience, it is essential that the therapist communicate openness and respect. Rather than communicate that certain beliefs or practices are irrational or inappropriate, the REBT practitioner engages in collaborative empiricism (Beck & Weishaar, 2000) with the client, a pragmatic exploration of the ways in which religious beliefs seem connected to both emotional upset and emotional support. For instance, the therapist may seek to understand how the client employs religious beliefs, how the client conceives of God, and whether specific beliefs or practices seem salient to the primary emotional disturbance (Johnson et al., 2000). When religion is more than merely important to a client, but also clearly intertwined with the client's emotional disturbance, then religion may be regarded as clinically salient and subsequently an appropriate focus of spiritually oriented REBT.

When the time comes to explore a client's God image and other religious experiences, it is imperative to maintain an attitude and approach characterized by what Bergin (1980) termed *theistic realism*. From this perspective, the therapist honors the client's views about God, the relationship of humans to God, and the possibility that spiritual forces influence behavior. At the same time, the therapist knows that clients must come to understand how their thoughts and beliefs strongly influence their emotions and well-being (Ellis, 1962). Religious clients can be offered religion-congruent rationale for exploring the scriptural support for their core beliefs about God (Nielsen et al., 2001). Rather than insist that an image of God is incorrect or biased, the religiously sensitive REBT therapist will guide the client through a process of exploration and clarification of views about God–preferably with support from the client's own faith community. It may be entirely appropriate to seek the client's permission in consulting with a relevant clergyperson (American Psychological Association, 1993; Johnson et al., 2000). By engaging a theologically sophisticated and respected member of the client's own religious community, there is an increased probability that idiosyncratic images of God–those that would not be congruent with the theological tenants governing one's faith–will be detected and corrected.

REBT Disputation and Client God Image

Although REBT incorporates a wide range of cognitive, emotive, and behavioral techniques (Ellis & Dryden, 1997), REBT's primary intervention is the cognitive disputation–a debate or challenge to the client's irrational belief system. There are several key disputational strategies, each of which can be tailored to a client's religious concerns: (a) *logical disputation* involves helping clients to understand the unreasonable, arbitrary nature of their irrational beliefs ["Help me understand how the sovereign God *should* or *must* ensure that the world be as *you* insist it should"], (b) *empirical disputation* involves helping clients see that the facts of the world (or scripture) do not support their irrational beliefs ["you say that God wants to punish you, but the Bible says God is 'gracious, compassionate, patient, and abounding in kindness,' which is correct?"], (c) *functional* or *pragmatic disputation* helps clients to see that irrational beliefs, in and of themselves, create a wide range of harmful consequences ["remind me how it is that rating your situation as awful is helping you to keep your focus on God and serve Him more effectively"], (d) *heuristic disputation*, or disputation by cognitive dissonance, proceeds by helping clients see that they have previously challenged and abandoned irrational beliefs in a range of situations and have benefited from doing so ["The Prodigal son squandered his father's inheritance and lived a sin-filled life. Still, his father loved him just as much as the older ("good") son. What does this say about you?"], and (e) *disputation by rational (or scriptural) alternative* involves introducing rational alternatives to the client's irrational beliefs to help clients experiment with the effects of dropping irrationality ["Well, I understand that you think God has damned you, but perhaps you need to memorize this verse: 'all have sinned and fall short of the glory of God, Rom. 3:23'"]. Finally, each REBT practitioner must adopt a disputational style (e.g., didactic, Socratic, humorous, self-disclosive) that best fits his or her personality and the clinical context (Ellis & Dryden, 1997; Nielsen et al., 2001; Walen et al., 1992).

When a client's God image appears linked to his or her clinical disturbance, the REBT therapist can select between two broad approaches to religiously-sensitive disputation (Johnson, 2001, 2003; Johnson & Nielsen, 1998). Using a *General Disputation* approach, the therapist attacks the client's evaluative and demanding beliefs without challenging or disputing the specific content or the religious client's world view or doctrinal beliefs. Specifically, the therapist will question and confront the client's absolutistic demands (God *should* give me what I want. I *must* perform perfectly to please God), and corollary irrational beliefs such as frustration intolerance (I *can't stand* not knowing whether God will save my soul), awfulizing, (it is absolutely *catastrophic* that I have sinned), and human worth rating (I am utterly worthless; God could care less about me). General disputes on the part of the therapist might include Socratic questions such as "I wonder how it is God's will for you to be depressed?" or "I'm not familiar with that scripture in the Bible that says God hates sinners and damns them for all eternity."

In contrast to this general approach, *Specialized Disputation* may be appropriate when a client's specific religious beliefs or practices are highly dysfunctional and idiosyncratic, or incongruent with the larger body of a client's identified religion. This approach assumes that the therapist has more than cursory knowledge of the client's identified religious culture or faith. It is imperative that the therapist avoids disputing core religious beliefs–especially those espoused by the client's broader religious community. Instead, the clinician asks: To what extent is the disturbing quality of this client's religious belief related to an incomplete or clearly idiosyncratic grasp of scripture or doctrine?

It is not uncommon for religious clients to make incomplete or inaccurate interpretations of scripture. DiGiuseppe et al. (1990) referred to such interpretive errors as *selective abstractions*; "people do not become disturbed because of their belief in religion: rather, their disturbance is related to their tendency to selectively abstract certain elements of their religion to the exclusion of attending to others" (p. 358). Thus, when a client holds a particularly malignant or distant view of God, the REBT therapist should be alert to the possibility that the primary disturbing belief is quite incongruent with other components of the client's larger religious affiliation. When an REBT therapist has sufficient familiarity with a client's religious doctrine or scripture, he or she might attempt to combat disturbing images of God–typically the result of a selective abstraction–by highlighting incongruent or discrepant information about the divine from scripture. By raising such incongruities, the therapist may create a state of *cognitive* or *orthodoxy dissonance* in the client; because dissonance creates unpleasant internal arousal, clients are often motivated to reduce dissonance by modifying their beliefs or changing their behavior. Scripture can be used to create dissonance and stimulate modification in a client's God image. Christian clients, for example, who pay selective attention to Biblical portrayals of the divine as wrathful (e.g., Numbers 11:1; Luke 12:47; Romans 2:5) might be asked how they account for the following scriptures:

- [God is] Gracious and compassionate, patient, abounding in kindness and faithfulness, assuring love for a thousand generations and forgiving iniquity, transgression and sin and granting pardon (Exodus 34: 6-7).
- If God is for us, who is against us? Who will bring any charge against God's elect? It is God who justifies. Who is to condemn? It is Christ Jesus who died, yes, who was raised, who is at the right hand of God, who indeed intercedes for us. Who will separate us from the love of Christ? (Romans 8: 31-34).
- For you know the generous act of our Lord Jesus Christ, that though he was rich, yet for your sakes he became poor, so that by his poverty you might become rich (2 Corinthians 8:9).
- In him we have redemption through his blood, the forgiveness of our trespasses, according to the riches of his grace that he lavished on us (Ephesians 1: 7-8).

If a client can be convinced to relinquish an image of God which is both inaccurate from within the person's own religion and which contributes to emotional disturbance, then it is quite likely that disturbance related to one's image of the Divine can be reduced.

Although REBT therapists often attempt an *elegant solution*–helping a client make a profound philosophic change or fundamental attitudinal shift in the way he or she thinks about a problem or an inference about a problem (Ellis & Dryden, 1997; Walen et al., 1992), this approach may be less effective in the case of a God image problem. Many religious clients will have great difficulty shifting their belief to something like, "well, God may hate me and damn me to hell but if that is true, there's not much I can do about it; I might as well just life my life and do the best I can in spite of God's intentions." Such a doctrinal shift in the salience or meaning of God might be both too difficult for many religious clients, and disrespectful of the meaning of God in the life of the religious client. The therapist is likely to get more mileage from disputing selective and inaccurate images of the divine.

Strengths and Weakness of REBT

CBT approaches, including REBT, enjoy considerable empirical support for use with a wide range of clinical disorders and syndromes (Dobson & Block, 1988; Hollon & Beck, 1994; Lyons & Woods, 1991). At present, there are very few disorders or types of emotional disturbance for which CBT interventions are not considered appropriate (Tan & Johnson, 2005). This is also true in the case of religious clients. Studies employing REBT (Johnson & Ridley, 1992; Johnson et al., 1994) and CT (c.f., Propst, 1996; Worthington, Kurusu, McCullough & Sandage, 1996) suggest that CBT treatments can be effectively accommodated to the worldview of religious clients. Like most psychotherapies, REBT is less likely to be efficacious with clients who present with multiple problems, those with serious mental illnesses such as Schizophrenia, or those who are not prepared to work hard at overcoming their disturbance (Ellis, 2000).

Perhaps the most salient source of concern when employing REBT with religious clients is the ethical risk inherent in challenging elements of a person's religious worldview. There is ethical risk involved in either ignoring a client's religious beliefs altogether–especially when they are clinically salient–or uncritically disputing a client's religious beliefs (Bergin, 1980; DiGiuseppe et al., 1990; Johnson et al., 2000). Because an REBT clinician can never rule out the truth or falseness of most religious beliefs (Meissner, 1996), it is prudent and ethical for the REBT therapist practicing a general approach to REBT to focus clinical interventions on the demanding and evaluative nature of the client's religious beliefs. In the case of more specialized disputation, the therapist, with appropriate training and familiarity with the client's religion, may address the negative effects of idiosyncratic religious views or the incongruence of such beliefs with the doctrine or scripture of the client's own religious community. Ethical and practice guidelines appear to enjoin all clinicians to avoid ignoring and trivializing a client's image of the divine when this image is related to the presenting problem (APA, 1993; 2002). Yet, these same guidelines serve to caution therapists about deliberately pathologizing or attacking an image of God. Efforts to disabuse a client of the existence of God would always be unethical, and God image modification should only be attempted collaboratively and with due appreciation for the salience of religion and spirituality in the life of the client.

CASE EXAMPLE

Client History

Jeff was a 24-year-old single white male. Jeff's history was remarkable for two reasons. First, although his parents had formally divorced when Jeff was 10 years old, his father was a violent alcoholic. During the years preceding and the year immediately following the divorce, his father threatened, stalked, and generally menaced the entire family– including Jeff, his mother, and two younger siblings. On more than one occasion, his father assaulted Jeff's mother and then either struck Jeff or threatened harm to him and his siblings should Jeff make any effort to call for assistance. After the divorce, the family lived in constant fear of his father breaking into the house and lying in wait for them. A particularly vivid memory involved coming home and discovering that his father had been hiding upstairs. When Jeff chanced upon him, his intoxicated and enraged father chased him down the stairs and seriously assaulted both Jeff and his mother before the police were summoned. Jeff did not see his father after the age of 11 and his father died a few years later.

The second remarkable thing about Jeff's history was his mother's inappropriate use of Jeff as a buffer between herself and her estranged husband. Jeff had vivid memories of his mother screaming for him to call the police while Jeff's father threatened to "kill" him if he did. On some occasions he would attempt to summon help–often receiving a beating from his father for his efforts–and on other occasions he would "freeze up" and just huddle with his siblings. Later, his mother would chastise and humiliate him for being "such a baby." In addition, during the years when his parents were separated and divorcing, his mother would often make Jeff, at age 10 or 11, enter the home first when the family returned from an outing, and go through the entire home alone to ensure that his father was not once again hiding and waiting for them to return. Even as a 24-year-old, trembling and tears accompanied Jeff's description of these searches. He had experienced abject terror at the prospect of discovering his drunken and belligerent father waiting to assault him.

His disturbed parental relationships aside, Jeff had developed normally and had graduated from high school with average grades. He had enlisted in the Navy at the age of 18 and had risen to the rank of E-4 or Petty Officer third class, signifying only modest advancement after six years of service. Although Jeff was intellectually capable and exceptionally hard working, he frequently turned down opportunities for leadership, advancement, and promotion–preferring instead to remain in the background. He had very few friends and had rarely dated in spite of the fact that he was a reasonably attractive young man. Navy comrades knew Jeff for his reticence and social isolation. He had no criminal or substance abuse history. Jeff was devoutly religious and a long-time member of a mainline protestant denomination. Throughout his childhood, Jeff's mother and siblings were involved in church activities several times during the week. Church acquaintances were among his only friends in high school.

Presenting Problem

A Navy chaplain accompanied Jeff to a Navy hospital emergency room where I happened to be the on-call psychologist for the weekend. Dressed in his enlisted uniform, Jeff was somewhat disheveled, fatigued, and dysphoric. He made poor eye contact and had recently been tearful. I spoke with the chaplain alone and learned that he had been "working" with Jeff, both as a pastor at the base chapel for approximately a year, and during the previous two to three months as a pastoral counselor in weekly counseling sessions. During the preceding two weeks, Jeff's affect had become increasingly depressed and Jeff had acknowledged feeling hopeless about ever "fitting in" in life. During a counseling session earlier that day, Jeff had also admitted suicidal ideation, which had precipitated the emergency room visit.

The chaplain noted that whether on board ship or stationed ashore, Jeff was punctilious about attending worship services on Sundays and that he participated in various forms of service through the Navy chapel such as ministries to local homeless men. Jeff was known for excessive devotion to work and seemed to use work to avoid being alone and as a cover to avoid social outings. It was only on the weekends that Jeff had down time. Notably, this was when Jeff would become more depressed. Over the course of Jeff's 6 years in the Navy, he had been drawn to military chapels, when not at sea, as though by an internal magnet. Chapels and chaplains had afforded an important connection with his childhood, yet he appeared to harbor genuine ambivalence about his own faith. The chaplain observed that he had rarely encountered a young man with such "horrendous self-esteem," and noted with some frustration that Jeff had seemed almost entirely resistant to the pastor's suggestions that Jeff was "worthy" and loved by God. The pastor seemed to genuinely like Jeff and easily agreed to collaborate with me in managing Jeff's mental health care.

In the intake interview, Jeff was cooperative but had great difficulty making eye contact. He spoke in soft tones and grimaced at times when describing himself and his isolative lifestyle. His mood was quite depressed but there was no evidence of psychosis or other serious psychiatric disturbance. Jeff admitted to occasional suicidal thoughts dating back to his sophomore year in high school. He had never before received mental health care and had never formulated a suicide plan. He admitted that he thought few people would be concerned about his death.

Jeff admitted with some trepidation and obvious shame that the specific precipitating factor for his current depressive state was financial difficulty related to his habit of spending one or both evenings on the weekend at one of several "hostess bars" located outside the gates of the Navy base. Hostess bars catered to lonely servicemen by offering attractive, usually foreign, women who would sit with them and offer flirtatious conversation in exchange for extremely expensive "drinks." Much like an escort service without the sexual implication, Jeff was frequently paying exorbitant prices for companionship with women who feigned strong interest in him. He denied that these hostess bar encounters ever resulted in a date outside the bar or any kind of sexual relationship.

During the emergency room interview, Jeff demonstrated remarkably poor self-esteem. He spoke in disparaging terms about his aptitude as a sailor, his charisma, his appeal to women, and his general opinion of himself. His language and demeanor were indicative of both the automatic negative cognitions that often accompany depression and a more fundamental sense of worthlessness. When asked about the chaplain and his connection to chapel activities, Jeff again appeared burdened and ashamed. He reported feeling ashamed that he had taken so much of the chaplain's time, embarrassed that the chaplain would now think he was "lame," and convinced that his suicidal thoughts were clear evidence that he would be a colossal disappointment to God. Although Jeff had a difficult time articulating a view of God, he clearly felt drawn to church, and was clearly seeking something in his relationship with the base chaplain. Finally, Jeff admitted difficulty sleeping as a result of nightmares, occasional intrusive thoughts of abuse–both his own and that of his mother–from childhood, and a general pattern of avoidance of male authority figures who reminded him of his father.

Case Conceptualization

Jeff was a depressed and socially avoidant 24-year-old white male with a history of child abuse and current symptoms of posttraumatic stress disorder (PTSD). Diagnostically, I conceptualized Jeff in the following terms:

Axis I	296.33 Major Depressive Disorder, Recurrent with Moderate Severity
	309.81 Posttraumatic Stress Disorder, Chronic
Axis II	Avoidant Personality Traits
Axis III	No Diagnosis
Axis IV	Social isolation, Occupational Stress
Axis V	GAF = 50 (current), 70 (last year)

I saw Jeff's depression and trauma-related anxiety as equally severe, and I thought that some of his avoidant behavior could be explained by his mood and anxiety disturbance, thus I did not diagnose a personality disorder. During the triage intake session, the only formal assessment beyond the interview and mental status exam involved administration of the Beck Depression Inventory (BDI; Beck, Ward, Mendelson, Mock, & Kendall, 1980). The BDI is a 21-item self-report scale for measuring clinical depression. Jeff's BDI score at intake was 32, indicating moderate to severe clinical depression. Although Jeff's symptoms of PTSD were mild compared to many clients with this disorder– primarily involving nightmares and avoidance–I thought his anxiety and depression were highly intertwined and both fueled by his early experiences and his remarkably poor self-esteem.

In terms of religious functioning, I would describe Jeff's faith as powerfully ambivalent. On one hand, he was reasonably well-versed in protestant Christian scripture and doctrine, loved the church, and felt a comforting connection between going to worship and positive childhood experiences, including those with his mother. On the other hand, Jeff admitted having difficulty with prayer or other personal communication with God. In his mind, God was intermittently distant, disappointed, and vengeful. Although drawn to images of the divine as loving and forgiving, Jeff felt unable to genuinely reconcile these with his horrifically low self-image.

Treatment Plan

At the conclusion of the initial emergency room intake, I decided not to admit Jeff to the psychiatry unit. He was not imminently suicidal, had formulated no suicide plan, and had no history of previous attempts or suicide models. He readily agreed to return two days later to commence twice-weekly intensive outpatient psychotherapy for depression. Jeff agreed to attend chapel services the following day and to check in with the chaplain afterward. He appeared encouraged and slightly more hopeful.

During the first outpatient session, Jeff and I discussed his diagnoses of depression and trauma-related anxiety in greater detail and he agreed that he had suffered episodes of serious depression several times during his life. Because these episodes often involved significant biological symptoms and suicidal thinking, I encouraged Jeff to consider a consultation with a psychiatry colleague for an assessment of the potential value of an antidepressant as an important part of the overall approach to his depression. After some education about these medications and assurance that they would not interfere with his fitness for sea duty, Jeff agreed and a medication consultation was scheduled.

I then offered a brief description of CBT with emphasis on this approach's established effectiveness with depression and gave Jeff a short introduction to the basic REBT model and how his very active involvement in our sessions-and between sessions with homework-would be essential to ensuring a successful outcome. We also continued our discussion of Jeff's religious faith and agreed that Jeff's faith was a genuine strength and something we would both work to incorporate in our approach to tackling his mood and anxiety difficulties. Further, Jeff agreed to continue religious counseling with the chaplain and regular attendance at services.

Finally, because PTSD is often best approached with exposure techniques and group formats, and because social reticence was a key component of Jeff's loneliness, I asked him to consider committing to an ongoing therapy group. At the time, the Navy clinic did not have a group focused on trauma; however, I worked with the chaplain to locate an ongoing group for adults from alcoholic homes led by two respected civilian social workers. The group was held weekly on base and Jeff was scheduled for an intake with one of the leaders.

Treatment Interventions

I met with Jeff for a total of 7 individual sessions spread over 4 months. In most cases, psychotherapy in military settings is necessarily brief and problem-focused, and REBT is a particularly parsimonious approach to anxiety and depression. In addition, Jeff's treatment was interrupted twice by brief deployments in which his ship got underway. These periods allowed him the opportunity to actively practice many of the cognitive and emotive interventions we covered in our individual sessions.

During the initial individual session, Jeff described several common activating events (As) or occurrences that he later attributed to depression. These include being alone yet afraid to initiate interactions with women or male friends, interacting with superior officers on his ship and believing he had failed or performed poorly, and going to chapel services or praying yet feeling inwardly ashamed or estranged from God. I then asked Jeff to articulate his experience of emotional distress in the wake of these experiences. Although depression was the most enduring emotional consequence (C), he also acknowledged that his immediate experience was shame, followed by depression. Although Jeff had no specific preference regarding which A he wished to focus on first in therapy, we agreed that given his immediate financial problems, it might be good to start with his dilemma related to women, dating avoidance, and his frequenting of hostess bars.

As is customary in REBT, I began by helping Jeff understand the ABC model of disturbance by applying it to one of his problems and letting him experience the process of ferreting out offending irrational beliefs (Bs) first hand. Although Jeff was familiar with several eligible women at work and through the chapel, and in spite of the fact that more than one had shown considerable interest in him, he avoided asking any of them on dates for fear of the rejection he assumed was a certainty (A), and then felt both ashamed and depressed afterward (C). I asked Jeff what he was telling himself about avoiding women that caused him to feel depressed and pointed out that other men might avoid dates but *not* become depressed–therefore he must be telling himself something to get depressed. When he had difficulty describing any thoughts or beliefs, I used an REBT technique known as *inference chaining* to help him articulate irrational beliefs. I asked, "let's assume the woman you ask out says no, what would that mean?" Jeff responded, "that she really doesn't like me!" I continued, "and if she doesn't like you, which you never actually find out, what would that mean?" He tried to laugh and said, "it would just prove that I'm a loser!" Looking for more specificity, I queried, "loser is a strong word, but what exactly does it mean for you?" He was quiet for awhile and more somberly said, "that I'm an idiot, that I'm weak ... that I don't have anything to offer." This statement was followed by silence. When I asked Jeff if he would agree that this might be a belief that caused him to feel depressed, he nodded.

It soon became clear that Jeff's primary irrational beliefs were self-downing or self-rating beliefs. Unfortunately, beliefs about self-worth are often the most difficult to change (Walen et al., 1992). I began using a range of spiritually oriented cognitive disputes with Jeff's self-downing thinking, and tended to employ both a Socratic and humorous style. Some of the general disputes that Jeff seemed to find most useful included:

- Jeff, if you believe it when the Bible says that you are God's creation, then how does it follow that you are a "worthless idiot?"
- On one hand, you say that if you didn't want to go out with a woman who asked you for a date, you would not necessarily think she was an "idiot" or "worthless," on the other hand you would say this about yourself if the situation were reversed. I'm confused; this doesn't seem fair does it?
- Help me understand how calling yourself worthless and idiotic helps you to either get dates or feel closer to God?
- Instead of the clearly unbiblical notion that you are no good or less than human, what is a more truthful or biblically correct thing you could tell yourself?

During the first three sessions, these and other disputes were used to vigorously attack Jeff's entrenched irrational self-downing. During the 4th session, Jeff noted that he had begun attending the adult survivors group and in the previous session had disclosed the following dream to the group: "I'm a little boy going up the stairs in my house. My mother is waiting outside with my little brother and sister and I'm going in alone to make sure my dad's not there. The next thing I know, there's this huge fireball coming down the stairs right at me. It's blinding and I'm terrified but I'm too scared to move, I freeze. Then I'm crying and explaining to my mom what happened but I can tell she's disgusted with me and I'm disgusted with me too."

Jeff clearly grasped the imagery of an angry and dangerous father in this dream and after some discussion, agreed that he had great difficulty not seeing God as this metaphorical ball of fire; God and father were dangerous, distant, and either disinterested in Jeff or disappointed–like his mother. The focus of therapy changed for two sessions to address Jeff's selective abstractions–irrational beliefs–about God. Using a Socratic style, I asked Jeff to help me understand how the following scriptures were remotely congruent with his current view of God:

- How great is the love the Father has lavished on us that we should be called children of God! (1 John 3:1).
- Your Father in heaven is not willing that any one of these little ones should be lost (Matthew 18:14).
- Never will I leave you; never will I forsake you (Hebrews 13:5)
- Your Father knows what you need before you ask Him (Matthew 6:8).
- He knows the number of the hairs on your head and not one sparrow falls down without being cared for by your Father (Luke 12:7).
- You are his beloved child (1 John 3:1).

By far the Bible story with the greatest impact on Jeff was the story of the prodigal son. In fact, after some initial disputing using the verses above, it was Jeff who mentioned this scripture: "But while he was a long way off, his father saw him and was filled with compassion for him; he ran to his son, threw his arms around him and kissed him" (Luke 15:20). Jeff understood that the Prodigal Son story was a metaphor for how God responds to wayward human beings. In spite of the fact that this son had had squandered his inheritance and engaged in all manner of sin and debauchery, his father rejoiced and celebrated at his return. I asked Jeff to help me understand what this parable said about his, Jeff's, worth in God's eyes. Jeff became tearful at this point and acknowledged the incongruence between the Biblical view of God and his own. This discrepancy clearly created some measure of cognitive dissonance for Jeff who admitted he was unable to reconcile or account for the strongly discrepant beliefs that God could be loving father *and* distant, angry, and disgusted. We began to distinguish between Jeff's image of his own father and the biblically-supported image of God.

One of the common problems in cognitive disputation is what some have called the "head-gut" issue (c.f., Walen et al., 1992) in which a client seems to understand the logical, empirical, or in this case, biblical evidence against a strong belief and yet are unable to really relinquish it. To help Jeff internalize a more biblically coherent image of God, I asked him to do two things. First, Jeff agreed to try "teaching" the image of God conveyed in the verses and parables referred to earlier–first to the chaplain in their counseling sessions, and later to other acquaintances in his chapel activities. Second, I asked Jeff to engage in brief imagery focusing on what it would be like for him and how he would feel if he really believed that God loved him and that like the prodigal son's father, God was always delighted to see him and unconditionally pleased with who he, Jeff, was. Jeff developed some insight regarding how really internalizing these more thorough images of God would impact his mood and his self-worth.

Many REBT clients benefit from rational-emotive imagery exercises (Ellis & Dryden, 1997). In two of our final sessions, I asked Jeff to practice changing inappropriate negative emotions (e.g., shame, depression) to appropriate ones while maintaining a vivid image of a negative or difficult activating event (A). Jeff chose an event in which two male co-workers made disparaging comments about him in front of a female sailor whom he very much wanted to impress. This event had been followed by intense shame and depression even though his object of interest had shown little regard for the derogatory comments. I asked Jeff to conjure up this scene with eyes closed and to raise a finger when he had gotten himself very ashamed and depressed. When he did, I asked him to then try to change his emotional state while keeping this scene in full and vivid detail. Jeff had some good success with this experience and he discovered that changing his self-defeating emotions was most easily accomplished by changing his beliefs about his own value–regardless of his coworkers' comments. Jeff found that imagery was also quite helpful in combating his negative images of God. In this case, he found it both calming and reassuring to imagine Jesus standing behind him (smiling) and laying his hand on Jeff's shoulder while Jeff practiced meditating on some of the scriptures noted above and new ones such as, "'For I know the plans I have for you,' declares the Lord, 'plans to prosper you and not to harm you, plans to give you hope and a future. Then you will call upon me and come and pray to me, and I will listen to you. You will seek me and find me when you seek me with all your heart'" (Jeremiah 29:11-13).

Treatment Termination

Our seventh and final session took place a full four months after his emergency room intake. Jeff's short deployments had helped spread out the final three sessions. Jeff had begun a trial of an SSRI antidepressant, was very active with the chaplain and chapel activities, and perhaps most important, had become a surprisingly avid member of the adult survivors group on base. This group had proven remarkably helpful to Jeff-both as a source of emotional support and as an opportunity to expose himself to his own history of child abuse in a contained holding environment. Jeff was often able to weave his REBT self-talk and cognitive disputation work into his new discoveries about the distinctions between his father, his God, and his image of self. But there was an equally important and highly unanticipated outcome of this group. The group was made up of several female members, a female leader, and Jeff. He began thriving in this rich environment of female attention and respect. Jeff received constant positive reinforcement from the group and his view of self relative to woman began to change dramatically as a result. He noted that he had stopped frequenting hostess bars and had begun to date one of the women in the group.

Because Jeff's ship was preparing for a longer deployment and because Jeff was experiencing significant symptom relief, was active in the chapel, and getting support from several different sources, we agreed to terminate psychotherapy sessions. In the final session, we discussed the importance of Jeff continuing to actively dispute self-downing thoughts and beliefs when these occurred, as well as the significance of maintaining a more theologically complete picture of God and his relationship to God.

Therapeutic Outcomes

The final BDI was collected during Jeff's sixth session, roughly 3 months following his intake. His score of 12 was in the borderline range between sub-clinical and mild depression. It is important to note that REBT psychotherapy was only one of several therapy modalities and that Jeff's antidepressant medication, group therapy, and pastoral counseling were probably all important in his symptom reduction. Jeff reported with some satisfaction that he had entirely stopped seeking companionship in hostess bars, that his finances were in order as a result, and that his self-esteem had improved rather dramatically-fueled to some extent by his first sustained dating relationship and ongoing reinforcement from women in his group and at chapel activities. Jeff demonstrated the ability to detect and dispute his own irrational beliefs related to self-worth, to differentiate his image of his father and his image of God, and to use disputation, imagery, and meditation to change mood states defined by depression or shame. In the end, it appeared that integrating Jeff's Christian faith with the REBT interventions was essential in making the treatment more meaningful and relevant to Jeff's presenting concerns.

REFERENCES

American Psychological Association (1993). Guidelines for providers of psychological services to ethnic, linguistic and culturally diverse populations. *American Psychologist, 48,* 45-48.

American Psychological Association (2002). Ethical principles of psychologists and code of conduct. *American Psychologist, 57,* 1060-1073.

Beck, A. T., Ward, C. H., Mendelson, M., Mock, J., & Erbaugh, J. (1961). An inventory for measuring depression. *Archives of General Psychiatry, 4,* 561-571.

Beck, A. T., & Weishaar, M. (2000). Cognitive Therapy. In R. J. Corsini & D. Wedding (Eds.), *Current psychotherapies* (6th ed.; pp. 241-272). Itasca, IL: Peacock.

Benson, P., & Spilka, B. (1973). God image as a function of self-esteem and locus of control. *Journal for the Scientific Study of Religion, 12,* 297-310.

Bergin, A. E. (1980). Psychotherapy and religious values. *Journal of Consulting and Clinical Psychology, 48,* 95-105.

Bergin, A. E. (1983). Religiosity and mental health: A critical reevaluation and meta-analysis. *Professional Psychology: Research and Practice, 14,* 170-184.

Blagys, M. D., & Hilsenroth, M. J. (2002). Distinctive activities of cognitive-behavioral therapy: A review of the comparative psychotherapy process literature. *Clinical Psychology Review, 22,* 671-706.

Butler, A. C. (2006). The empirical status of cognitive-behavioral therapy: A review of meta-analyses. *Clinical Psychology Review, 26,* 17-31.

DiGiuseppe, R. A., Robin, M. W., & Dryden, W. (1990). On the compatibility of rational-emotive therapy and Judeo-Christian philosophy: A focus on clinical strategies. *Journal of Cognitive Psychotherapy: An International Quarterly, 4,* 355-368.

Dobson, K. S., & Block, L. (1988). Historical and philosophical bases of the cognitive-behavioral therapies. In K. S. Dobson (Ed.), *Handbook of cognitive-behavioral therapies* (pp. 3-38). New York: Guilford.

Donahue, M. J. (1985). Intrinsic and extrinsic religiousness: Review and meta-analysis. *Journal of Personality and Social Psychology, 48,* 400-419.

Ellis, A. (1957). Rational psychotherapy and individual psychotherapy. *Journal of Individual Psychology, 13,* 38-44.

Ellis, A. (1962). *Reason and emotion in psychotherapy.* New York: Lyle Stuart.

Ellis, A. (2000). Can rational emotive behavior therapy (REBT) be effectively used with people who have devout beliefs in God and religion? *Professional Psychology: Research and Practice, 31,* 29-33.

Ellis, A., & Dryden, W. (1997). *The practice of rational-emotive therapy* (2nd ed.). New York: Springer.

Francis, L. J., Gibson, H. M., & Robbins, M. (2001). God images and self-worth among adolescents in Scotland. *Mental Health, Religion & Culture, 4,* 103-108.

Gartner, J., Larson, D. B., & Allen, G. D. (1991). Religious commitment and mental health: A review of the empirical literature. *Journal of Psychology and Theology, 19,* 6-25.

Hall, T. W., & Brokaw, B. F. (1995). The relationship of spiritual maturity to level of object relations development and god image. *Pastoral Psychology, 43,* 373-391.

Hollon, S. D., & Beck, A. T. (1994). Cognitive and cognitive-behavioral therapies. In A. E. Bergin & S. L. Garfield (Eds.), *Handbook of psychotherapy and behavior change* (pp. 428-466). New York: John Wiley.

Johnson, W. B. (2001). To dispute or not to dispute: Ethical REBT with religious clients. *Cognitive and Behavioral Practice, 8,* 39-47.

Johnson, W. B. (2003). Rational emotive behavior therapy for disturbance about sexual orientation. In P. S. Richards & A. E. Bergin (Eds.), *Casebook for a spiritual strategy in counseling and psychotherapy* (pp. 247-265). Washington, DC: American Psychological Association.

Johnson, W. B., Devries, R., Ridley, C. R., Pettorini, D., & Peterson, D. R. (1994). The comparative efficacy of Christian and secular rational-emotive therapy with Christian clients. *Journal of Psychology and Theology, 22,* 130-140.

Johnson, W. B., & Nielsen, S. L. (1998). Rational-emotive assessment with religious clients. *Journal of Rational-Emotive and Cognitive-Behavior Therapy, 16,* 101-123.

Johnson, W. B., & Ridley, C. R. (1992). Brief Christian and non-Christian rational-emotive therapy with depressed Christian clients: An exploratory study. *Counseling and Values, 36,* 220-229.

Johnson, W. B., Ridley, C. R., & Nielsen, S. L. (2000). Religiously sensitive Rational Emotive Behavior Therapy: Elegant solutions and ethical risks. *Professional Psychology: Research and Practice, 31,* 14-20.

Kunkel, M. A., Cook, S., Meshel, D. S., Daughtry, D., & Hauenstein, A. (1999). God image: A concept map. *Journal for the Scientific Study of Religion, 38,* 193-202.

Lovinger, R. J. (1984). *Working with religious issues in therapy.* New York: Jason Aronson.

Lyons, L. C., & Woods, P. J. (1991). The efficacy of rational-emotive therapy: A quantitative review of the outcome research. *Clinical Psychology Review, 11,* 357-369.

Mahoney, M. J. (1977). Reflections on the cognitive learning trend in psychotherapy. *American Psychologist, 32,* 5-13.

Meissner, W. W. (1996). The pathology of beliefs and the beliefs of pathology. In E. P. Shafranske (ed.), *Religion and the clinical practice of psychology* (pp. 241-267). Washington DC: American Psychological Association.

Nelson, H. M., Cheek, N. H., & Au, P. (1985). Gender differences in images of God. *Journal for the Scientific Study of Religion, 24,* 396-402.

Nielsen, S. L., Johnson, W. B., & Ellis, A. (2001). *Counseling and psychotherapy with religious persons: A rational emotive behavior therapy approach.* Mahwah, NJ: Lawrence Erlbaum.

Propst, L. R. (1996). Cognitive-behavioral therapy and the religious person. In E. Shafranske (Ed.), *Religion and the clinical practice of psychology* (pp. 391-407). Washington, DC: American Psychological Association.

Richards, P. S., & Bergin, A. E. (1997). *A spiritual strategy for counseling and psychotherapy.* Washington DC: American Psychological Association.

Rizzuto, A. M. (1979). *The birth of the living God: A psychoanalytic study.* Chicago: University of Chicago Press.

Roof, W. C., & Roof, J. L. (1984). Review of the polls: Images of God among Americans. *Journal for the Scientific Study of Religion, 23,* 201-205.

Spilka, B., Armatas, P., & Nussbaum, J. (1964). The concept of God: A factor-analytic approach. *Review of Religious Research, 6,* 28-36.
Tan, S. Y., & Johnson, W. B. (2005). Spiritually oriented cognitive behavioral therapy. In L. Sperry & E. P. Shafranske (Eds.), *Spiritually oriented psychotherapy* (pp. 77-103). Washington, DC: American Psychological Association.
Walen, S. R., DiGiuseppe, R., & Dryden, W. (1992). *A practitioner's guide to rational-emotive therapy (2nd ed.)* . New York: Oxford University Press.
Worthington, E. L., Jr., Kurusu, T. A., McCullough, M. E., & Sandage, S. J. (1996). Empirical research on religion and psychotherapeutic processes and outcomes: A 10-year review and research prospectus. *Psychological Bulletin, 119,* 448-487.

doi:10.1300/J515v09n03_08

Chapter 9

Theistic Psychotherapy
and the God Image

Kari O'Grady
P. Scott Richards, PhD

SUMMARY. Assessing and working with issues of God image in therapy are often an essential part of successful treatment. God image development is a complex process that may include influences from family,
peers, culture, gender, age, religious theology and tradition. From a theistic perspective, individuals' actual relationship with God can have the
greatest impact on God image development. According to this perspective, it is important that therapists help clients explore their image of
God and the ways it impacts their spirituality and presenting concerns.
Encouraging clients to engage in spiritual practices such as prayer, meditation, scripture study, and spiritual reflection can help them create a
more genuine relationship with God, and promotes a healthier, more mature God image. doi:10.1300/J515v09n03_09 *[Article copies available for a
fee from The Haworth Document Delivery Service: 1-800-HAWORTH. E-mail
address: <docdelivery@haworthpress.com> Website: <http://www.HaworthPress.com>
© 2007 by The Haworth Press. All rights reserved.]*

[Haworth co-indexing entry note]: "Theistic Psychotherapy and the God Image." O'Grady, Kari, and P.
Scott Richards. Co-published simultaneously in *Journal of Spirituality in Mental Health* (The Haworth Pastoral Press, an imprint of The Haworth Press) Vol. 9, No. 3/4, 2007, pp. 183-209; and: *God Image Handbook
for Spiritual Counseling and Psychotherapy: Research, Theory, and Practice* (ed: Glendon L. Moriarty, and
Louis Hoffman) The Haworth Pastoral Press, an imprint of The Haworth Press, 2007, pp. 183-209. Single or
multiple copies of this article are available for a fee from The Haworth Document Delivery Service
[1-800-HAWORTH, 9:00 a.m. - 5:00 p.m. (EST). E-mail address: docdelivery@haworthpress.com].

Available online at http://jsmh.haworthpress.com
© 2007 by The Haworth Press. All rights reserved.
doi:10.1300/J515v09n03_09

Theistic psychotherapy is an integrative approach in which therapists use spiritual interventions in a treatment-tailoring fashion, combining them with a variety of standard mainstream techniques, including psychodynamic, behavioral, humanistic, cognitive, and systemic approaches (Richards & Bergin, 1997; 2005). The conceptual foundations of theistic psychotherapy are grounded in the worldview of the major theistic world religions, including Judaism, Christianity, and Islam (Smart, 1994). The foundational assumptions of this approach are "that God exists, that human beings are the creations of God, and that there are unseen spiritual processes by which the link between God and humanity is maintained" (Bergin, 1980, p. 99). Perhaps the most distinctive contribution of the theistic orientation is that it assumes that clients who have faith in God's healing power and draw upon the spiritual resources in their lives during psychological treatment will receive added strength and power to cope, heal, and grow (Richards & Bergin, 2005).

Table 1 summarizes some additional characteristics of theistic psychotherapy. According to this perspective, therapeutic change and healing can be facilitated through a variety of means, including physiological, psychological, social, and educational, but complete healing and change may require a spiritual process. Therapeutic change is often more profound and lasting when people heal and grow spiritually through a relationship with God. Theistic psychotherapists encourage their clients to explore how their faith in God and personal spirituality may assist them during treatment and recovery. They may also encourage their clients to examine their understandings and perceptions of God during treatment and to engage in spiritual practices that may help them grow in their relationship with God and in their personal spirituality. They may also implement spiritual interventions designed to assist clients in their efforts tap into the resources of their faith in order to cope and heal emotionally and spiritually. Examples of such interventions include encouraging clients to pray, discussing theological concepts, making reference to scriptures, using spiritual relaxation and imagery techniques, encouraging repentance and forgiveness, consulting with religious leaders, and recommending religious bibliotherapy. There is growing evidence that spiritual practices and interventions can assist clients in their efforts to cope, heal, and change (Benson, 1996; Richards & Bergin, 2000, 2005).[1] Much more has been written about the implications of theism for therapeutic change and psychotherapy and we refer readers to other sources for more information about this topic (e.g., Bergin, 2002; Miller & Delaney, 2005; Richards & Bergin, 2005; Richards, Hardman, & Berrett, 2007).

TABLE 1. Distinguishing Characteristics of Theistic Psychotherapy. (© 2005. "Spiritual Strategy for Counseling and Psychotherapy, Second Edition." American Psychological Association. Printed with permission.)

Goals of Therapy	Therapist's Role in Therapy	Role of Spiritual Techniques	Client's Role in Therapy	Nature of Relationship
Spiritual view is part of an eclectic, multisystemic view of humans and so therapy goals depend on the client's issues. Goals directly relevant to the spiritual dimension include the following: (a) Help clients affirm their eternal spiritual identity and live in harmony with the Spirit of Truth; (b) assess what impact religious and spiritual beliefs have in clients' lives and whether they have unmet spiritual needs; (c) help clients use religious and spiritual resources to help them in their efforts to cope, change, and grow; (d) help clients resolve spiritual concerns and doubts and make choices about role of spirituality in their lives; and (e) help clients examine their spirituality and continue their quest for spiritual growth.	Adopt an ecumenical therapeutic stance and, when appropriate, a denominational stance. Establish a warm, supportive environment in which the client knows it is safe and acceptable to explore his or her religious and spiritual beliefs, doubts, and concerns. Assess whether clients' religious and spiritual beliefs and activities are affecting their mental health and interpersonal relationships. Implement religious and spiritual interventions to help clients more effectively use their religious and spiritual resources in their coping and growth process. Model and endorse healthy values. Seek spiritual guidance and enlightenment on how best to help clients.	Interventions are viewed as very important for helping clients understand and work through religious and spiritual issues and concerns, and for helping clients draw on religious and spiritual resources in their lives to assist them in better coping, growing and changing. Examples of major interventions include cognitive restructuring of irrational religious beliefs, transitional figure technique, forgiveness, meditation and prayer, Scripture study, blessings, participating in religious services, spiritual imagery, journaling about spiritual feelings, repentance, and using the client's religious support system.	Examine how their religious and spiritual beliefs and activities affect their behavior, emotions, and relationships. Make choices about what role religion and spirituality will play in their lives. Set goals and carry out spiritual interventions designed to facilitate their spiritual and emotional growth. Seek to use the religious and spiritual resources in their lives to assist them in their efforts to heal and change. Seek God's guidance and enlightenment about how to better cope, heal, and change.	Unconditional positive regard, warmth, genuineness, and empathy are regarded as an essential foundation for therapy. Therapists also seek to have charity or brotherly and sisterly love for clients and to affirm their eternal spiritual identity and worth. Clients are expected to form a working alliance and share in the work of change. Clients must trust the therapist and believe that it is safe to share their religious and spiritual beliefs and heritage with the therapist. Clients must know that the therapist highly values and respects their autonomy and freedom of choice and that it is safe for them to differ from the therapist in their beliefs and values, even though the therapist may at times disagree with their values and confront them about unhealthy values and lifestyle choices.

THEISTIC PERSPECTIVES OF GOD

Because of the potential important influence of religious theology and tradition on the development of God concept and God image, which we will discuss in more detail later in this chapter, in Table 2 we summarize some of the theological perspectives of God found in the theistic world religions. Table 2 shows that there are many theological differences among the theistic world religions in how they view God, but there are also a surprising number of similarities. For example, most theistic world religions teach that God is all-knowing, all-powerful, and all-loving. God has revealed himself to human beings and has provided teachings and commandments to help them live moral and happy lives. Human beings can communicate with God through prayer and other spiritual practices, and thereby receive strength and guidance from God to assist them in coping with life challenges. God wants human beings to live in harmony with his will and choose to do good rather than evil–in so doing they will be blessed in this life and in the afterlife. The theistic religions teach that God is an active God–a being who created the world, who has remained involved in the history of the world, and who continues to influence, guide, and bless members of the human family. However, as discussed below, such theistic conceptions of God have not yet been adequately considered in psychological theory and research about God image.

NATURALISTIC INFLUENCES ON THE STUDY OF GOD IMAGE

To date, God image research has primarily been conducted from a psychoanalytic orientation focusing mainly on an object relations perspective of God image formation. Most of the early literature in this area of study suggests that individuals' primary representation of God is projective of their relationship with their parents (Dickie, Ajega, Joy, & Kathryn, 2006; Dicki, Ajega, Kobylak, & Nixon 1997; Rizutto, 1979). More recent research has also considered culture, sense of identity, gender, class, age, religiosity, and personal experience as contributing factors in God image development (Bassett & Williams, 2003; Dickie et al., 1997; Francis, Gibson, & Mandy, 2001; Krejci, 1998; Lee & Early, 2000; Rowatt & Kirkpatrick, 2002).

The earliest psychoanalytic assertions concerning the idea of a God image can be traced back to the founder of psychoanalytic psychology,

TABLE 2. Major Western (Monotheistic) Religious Traditions' Perspectives of God. (© 2005. "Spiritual Strategy for Counseling and Psychotherapy, Second Edition." American Psychological Association. Printed with permission.)

	Judaism	Christianity	Islam
God's Characteristics	God is the only Supreme Being. He is called Elohim or Jehovah. He is the creator of all things. God is eternal, all-powerful, and all-knowing. Most modern Jews believe God does not have a physical body, but they believe God is real.	Most Christians believe in the Holy Trinity: God the Father, God the Son, and God the Holy Ghost. Some Christians believe that the Holy Trinity is one in essence, but other Christians believe they are one in purpose but not in essence. God is a personal God. He is the creator of all things. God is eternal, all-powerful, all-knowing, and all-loving.	God, also called Allah, is the only true God or Supreme Being. Allah is the creator of the universe and of human beings. God is all-powerful, all-seeing, all-hearing, all-speaking, and all-knowing. God does not have a body, but is real. God is eternal.
How God Reveals Himself to Humans	God revealed Himself and His law through Moses, as recorded in the Torah (the Pentateuch or first five books of the Old Testament). God revealed His law at Sinai.	God has revealed Himself and His words in Jesus Christ, of whom the Bible bears witness as the Son of God.	God has revealed his eternal speech and words to human beings in the Qur'an (the holy book of scripture).
God's Relationship to Humans	Human beings are made in God's image; humans are the high point of God's creations. The Jewish people are God's chosen people.	Human beings were created by God. Some view God as the Father. Many Christians believe that there is something basically evil in human nature because of the fall of Adam and Eve, which can be corrected only by God's grace, God wishes to have a relationship with human beings.	Human beings are God's creations. Some believe God determines human actions, whereas others say that humans have agency to choose, particularly those actions on which they are judged.
God's Expectations for Humans	Human beings have a mission to help make the world a better place morally and spiritually. Individually, each person needs to obey God's commandments and to develop morally and to qualify to live in a place of peace and eternal progress in the world to come. There are 613 commandments or religious duties (Mitzvat). Charity, good deeds, respect for human dignity, humility, truthfulness, controlling one's anger, and not being envious are examples of other morally good behaviors and qualities.	God created people to enjoy his divine presence forever. Human beings are to glorify God by having faith in Jesus Christ and by repenting of their sins and following the teachings of Jesus. Human beings must learn to choose good over evil. Accepting Jesus as Savior and following His teachings is the path to righteousness and morality. Morality includes behaviors and qualities such as love, service, honesty, family devotion, and abstinence from behaviors such as drunkenness, adultery, and fornication.	Human beings must learn to submit to God's will, obey His law, and do good. They must give up worldly things and overcome their vices. There are five classes of moral actions: those that are obligatory, recommended, prohibited, disapproved, and indifferent. Examples of prohibited behaviors include drinking of alcohol and immodesty of dress. Fasting and prayer, payment of alms, and devotion to the family are examples of expected behaviors. The path of spiritual growth involves overcoming vices such as arrogance, greed, and dishonesty.
How God Communicates with Humans	Humans can communicate with God through prayer and worship. God responds to people reaching out to Him.	Through prayer and the influence of the Holy Spirit, human beings can communicate with God and receive God's help, influence, and grace.	Humans can communicate with God through prayer, meditation, and repetition of set phrases or the name of God.
God's Rewards	Obedience to God's laws and worshipping Him leads to character development (acquisition of qualities such as goodness, humility, and holiness). Eventually the bodies of the dead will be resurrected, although many Jews believe only in the immortality of the soul. The righteous will go to a place of peace, where they will continue to progress and enjoy a nearness to God.	Accepting Jesus Christ as Savior will lead one to good works, a moral life, and devotion and worship. This will allow one to receive the influence of the Holy Spirit and partake of other fruits of the spirit (e.g., love). Those who do so will receive God's grace, be forgiven, and be welcomed into God's presence (Heaven) in the hereafter.	Obeying God's law as revealed in the Qur'an leads to higher levels of religious experience and union with God. There will be a judgment at the final hour of the world. The dead will be resurrected. Those who worship Allah and obey His laws will be rewarded in the hereafter (Heaven).
God's Punishment	There will be a judgment in which people will be judged for what they did with their lives Those who were evil will not enjoy a nearness to God.	There will be a judgment in which people will be judged for what they did with their lives Those who have done evil and who have not accepted Jesus will be banished to hell, outer darkness, or extinction.	There will be a judgment in which people will be judged for what they did with their lives The wicked will be punished by God being sent to hell, and the good rewarded in heaven.

This table was adapted from Richards and Bergin (2005). Used by permission of the authors and publisher.

Freud. Freud maintained that individuals created the idea of a God in reaction to the Oedipus complex. He asserted, "Psychoanalysis has made us familiar with the intimate connection between the father-complex and belief in God; it has shown us that a personal God is, psychologically, nothing other than an exalted father" (quoted in Rizzuto, 1979, p. 15).

Freud considered the development of a God image from an evolutionary perspective as well as its development within the individual (Rizutto, 1979). His evolutionary theory traces all human male's reaction to the Oedipus complex back to the primeval man's struggle with the first father. He asserts that the primeval people developed an intense animosity towards father and his representation of power. In reaction to this ambivalence, the primeval individuals murdered the father which produced a profound sense of object guilt. In an effort to reconcile their feelings of guilt, the primeval individual split off the favorable aspects of the murdered father and transmitted those aspects into the sacrificial totem meal. Years later, Moses of Egypt offered back to the people the repressed love of the father in the presentation of a personal God image. According to Freud, God is simply a fantasy image or *illusion* created by humans to help them deal with their childlike wish for a parental figure to rescue them from life's difficulties. He assumed that human maturity is marked by an individual's ability to overcome the need for a surrogate father figure. Freud described himself as having obtained this level of developmental maturity (Freud, 1923/1989). Freud's explanations of God image are clearly grounded in an atheistic-naturalistic worldview which assumes that God is not real.

Rizutto (1979) carefully studied Freud's work and elaborated upon it in her seminal, comprehensive study of twenty psychiatric patients and their development of a God representation. Her findings as well as her theoretical thinking have made important contributions to later studies of the God image and the field of object relations in general. Her study was designed in part to investigate some of the assumptions put forth by Freud's theory. Rizutto rejected Freud's assumption that a belief in a personal God is indicative of emotional immaturity; however; she concluded that Freud's assertions that God has his origins in "parental imagino," and evolutionary processes, and is formed in reaction to the Oeidpal complex, is accurate.

Although Rizzuto avoided taking a position concerning the question of God's reality, she adopted methodological naturalism in conducting and interpreting her findings. Methodological naturalism assumes that "human beings and the universe can be understood . . . without including God or divine influence in scientific theories or in the interpretation of research findings" (Richards & Bergin, 2005, p. 32). Rizutto made her position clear early in her book, *The Birth of a Living God,* when she stated, "Questions about the actual existence of God do not pertain here. My method enables me to deal only with psychic experiences . . . as a researcher I will not make pronouncements appropriate for philosophers and theologians" (1979, p. 4).

Perhaps as a consequence of her decision to not take a position about the actual existence of God, Rizutto consistently referred to God as a non-real or imagined object used by humans as a transitional object and as a means for coping with challenges. In our view what is missing in Ritzutto's work is exploration of the possibility that a real God may be having a real relationship with the individuals that participated in her study. One possible explanation for the development of individuals' images of God could be that there is a God there that they are experiencing (Hall & Brokaw; 1995; Porpora, 2006; Owen, 2004).

Much of the current literature on God image has sprung from Rizzuto's work. Although the topic under discussion is God, the atheistic-naturalistic assumptions of scholars in this domain seem to have narrowed the spectrum of study to only those questions that assume God is not real. Many measures created to assess the experience of the God image neglect to include items that inquire about individuals' actual relationship or experience with God (e.g. Francis, Gibson, & Robbins, 2001; Janssen, De Hart, & Geradts, 1994). This neglect seems to come from an underlying atheistic presupposition that because God is not real, a real relationship with him could not possibly be part of the explanation of God image formation. For instance one recent article explained the difference between a "representation" or "image" of a *real* being and that of God in the following terms,

> A representation of "mother" is formed from one's experiences of mother, and so forth. The God representation differs from other representations, however, in several ways. First, it is not based directly on experiences of God .... Further, the God representation, because it is not tied to direct personal experiences, can be more freely adapted by the individual as needed. (Lawrence, 1997, p. 214)

Research from an atheistic-naturalistic view of God tends to frame individuals' emotional experiences with God as a projection intended to meet internal needs (Kunkel, Cook, Meshel, Daughtery, & Hauenstein; 1999). Furthermore, God is frequently referred to in the God image literature as a "transitional object," "compensatory figure," or "substitute attachment figure" generated to help people cope with developmental challenges (Dickie et al., 2006; Dickie et al., 1997; Lawrence, 1997).

A THEISTIC VIEW OF GOD IMAGE DEVELOPMENT

There is a relatively large body of research demonstrating correlations between people's relationships with their parents, self image, cultural or social contexts, biological factors and the way their image of God develops. Most of the literature discusses these relationships in terms of maturational patterns, such as suggesting that children's God image is relative to the role their parent's play at various developmental stages throughout their lives (Dickie et al., 1997; Kreji, 1998; Rowatt, & Kirkpatrick, 2002). Consistent with these findings, our theistic view of the development of God image is that it is a complex process that may include influences from religious theology and tradition, popular culture, family and peer influences, gender, and age.

Our view is also grounded in the assumption that God is real, and that many people have genuine experiences with God. Further, individuals' faith in God's reality may be central to their worldviews and lifestyles (Bergin, Masters, Stinchfield, Gaskin, & Sullivan, 1988; Owen, 2004; Poll, 2005; Richards & Bergin, 2005). One of the most distinctive contributions of a theistic perspective to our understanding of God image development is the view that experiences with God can have a powerful influence on individuals' representations of God (Hall & Brokaw, 1995; Parker, 1998). According to this view, part of the change in people's perceptions of God over time may result from getting to know God better; analogous to the ways people's understanding of other significant others in their lives develops over time and with added experiences (Hall & Brokaw, 1995; Levinas, 1981). God is not merely a representation to be perceived but also a reality to be experienced first hand. Individuals may experience God as a compensatory figure because God really did help fill in the gaps left by inadequate parenting.

There is research suggesting that individuals who experienced emotionally disruptive childhoods may have a greater number of compensatory spiritual experiences than those who experienced less traumatic childhoods (Bergin et al., 1988). One interpretation of this finding could be that God helps make up the difference. This theistic interpretation can be very healing for theistic clients who have experienced neglect or abuse in their childhood and are trying to deal with feelings of injustice and abandonment.

Recent polls have suggested that a large number (41%) of Americans report having had religious or spiritual experiences that have "changed the direction of their lives" (Gallup, 2003, p. 7). Although naturalistic explanations for spiritual or mystical experiences have been proposed, a theistic perspective takes seriously the possibility that these phenomena represent genuine experiences with God (Poll, 2005; Richards & Bergin, 2005).

Although many psychological researchers are more comfortable talking about God image naturalistically, the study of anomalous experiences is a legitimate area of study for many serious scholars, including William James who assumed that individuals who reported experiences with God were having genuine experiences with God, as well as more recent scholars who begin their study of religious experiences based on the premise that individuals may be having actual experiences with a real being (Kunkel, Cook, Meshel, Daughtry, & Hauenstein; 1999; Miller & Delaney, 2005; Owen, 2004; Poll, 2005; Porpora, 2006; Richards & Bergin, 2005). Addressing the hesitancy of many scholars in discussing religious experiences as if they may be real, Porpora (2006) suggested that "there seems no more warrant to prejudge the reality or nature of objects of religious experience than any other object of experience" (p. 73).

Recent studies have provided some evidence that individuals can move beyond their childhood projections to develop a mature understanding of God based upon their own experiences with Him (Hall & Brokaw, 1995; Owen, 2004; Poll, 2005). Thus, according to our theistic perspective, not only do cultural and personal factors influence the development of God image, but individuals' experiences with God may have an impact on their God image development and on their psychological and social functioning (Bassett & Williams; Krejci, 1998; Owen, 2004; Parker, 1999; Poll, 2005; Richards & Bergin, 2005; Tisdale et al., 1997).

According to our theistic perspective, one marker of spiritual maturity is a God image based primarily on real experiences with God in which the individual's "relationship with God moves from socially constructed and consensual to authentically personal" (Kass & Lennox, 2005, p. 187). Spiritually mature individuals seek to develop and maintain a relationship with God through living in harmony with God's will for them and inviting God to be a central part of their lives (Kass & Lennox, 2005, Maloney, 1985, 1988). Spiritually mature individuals also tend to view God as loving, powerful, and nurturing (Tisdale et al., 1997; Parker, 1999).

Some studies suggest that spiritually mature individuals typically enjoy greater emotional well being, increased life satisfaction and greater psychological resistance (Plante & Sherman, 2002; Rowatt & Kirkpatrick, 2002; Schaap-Jonker, Eurelings-Bontedoe, Verhagen & Zock, 2002). Additionally, individuals with a positive God image are more likely to have a positive view of themselves and a greater sense of purpose or meaning in their lives; therefore a mature relationship with God can contribute significantly to clients' healing and growth (Hall & Brokaw, 1995; Francis et al., 2001; MacKenna, 2002). Both because a relationship with God can serve as a healthy pattern for other relationships and because a relationship with God can bring emotional and spiritual benefits to people, individuals who feel a sense of closeness and connectedness to God have an increased capacity to enjoy loving, affirming relationships with others (MacKenna, 2002; Owen, 2004; Parker, 1999; Poll, 2005; Richards & Bergin, 2005; Tisdale et al. 1997).

From a theistic perspective, individuals' representation of God may be generated much like their representation of other significant beings in their lives (Hall & Brokaw, 1995). For instance, individuals develop an "image" or representation of what a spouse is like and the role he or she will play in their marriage relationship partly from experiencing their parents and others in their role as a spouse. They also may form a representation of a spouse from teachings offered in cultural and religious communities about what it means to be a spouse. In addition they likely generate their sense of a spouse from their own sense of self. However, no one is likely to overlook that one important influence on individuals' representation of what a spouse is or ought to be comes from their personal experience with their spouse in the marriage relationship.

GOD IMAGE DIFFICULTY

As opposed to spiritually mature individuals, spiritually immature individuals tend to have God concepts that are based primarily on other's accounts of God, projections carried over from their childhoods, or projections of their personality disorders or other pathologies (Plante & Sherman, 2002; Richards & Bergin, 2005; Rowatt & Kirkpatrick, 2002). Spiritually immature individuals often view God as punitive and distant (Hall & Brokaw, 1995). In particular a study conducted by Schaap-Jonker et al. (2002) found that personality disorders are characterized by a negative and distorted perception of God. They found that when symptoms of cluster A (e.g. paranoid, schizoid, and schizotypal personality disorders) were present, God was viewed as detached and passive. When cluster C (e.g. avoidant, dependent, and obsessive-compulsive personality disorders) symptoms were present, individuals described God as a "harsh judge."

Distorted God images can be destructive to individuals' emotional health and often correlate with other unhealthy lifestyle concerns (MacKenna, 2002; Francis, Gibson, & Robbins, 2001; Rowatt & Kirkpatrick, 2002). For instance, some studies have found that psychiatric patients seem to view God as more punitive and wrathful than nonpatients and that longer psychiatric hospital stays seem to be associated with more distant and unloving God images (Tisdale et al., 1997). Perhaps these correlations are a consequence of not only a distorted image, but also due to a disengaged or distant relationship with God

Harsh God images can disrupt individuals' ability to form genuine relationship with God, which in turns prevents them from developing a truthful view of Him based on their experiences with Him. It appears that some individuals have trouble developing a relationship with God because they have not been able to overcome their childhood associations with his image (Parker, 1999). This prevents them from trusting in or desiring to have a relationship with God. In addition to childhood distortions, difficulties in developing a relationship with God can occur when people sin and do not repent or do not believe they can be forgiven for their failures. Sin makes it difficult for people to connect to God because it fosters a distorted view of self. When individuals lose touch with their true spiritual identities, they seem to lose touch with their relatedness with God (Brown & Miller, 2005; Parker, 1999; Evans, 2005). They no longer feel worthy of God's love and concern. When individuals are able to see themselves as both fallible and loveable, and God as forgiving and loving, they can resume a more honest view of themselves, and experience a deeper more fulfilling relationship with God.

When people neglect their spiritual growth and relationship with God and consistently ignore the influence of God's spirit and do evil, they are more likely to suffer poor mental health and unfulfilling interpersonal relationships (Parker, 1999; Richards & Bergin, 1997; 2005). Since a relationship with God is important in and of itself and also because it supports healthy emotional and social functioning overall, addressing God image distortions or difficulties should be a major area of concern for thoughtful therapists and counselors (Kass & Lennox, 2005; Richards & Bergin, 2005).

GOD IMAGE CHANGE

We think all possible influences on God image development should be explored during assessment and treatment planning; however, the noumenal as well as the phenomenological should be considered (Kunkel et al., 1999; Porpora, 2006). Because the theistic perspective assumes that a real relationship with God may play a significant role in individuals' psychological experience with God (Poll & Smith; 2003; Owen, 2004; Parker, 1999; Hall & Brokaw, 1995; Hood, 1989), we think the influence of experiences or lack of experiences with a personal and real God should be explored along with other possible influences.

In our view, clients' images of God can be altered by a variety of influences, but the most powerful influence of change in God image comes from experiencing God first hand. Individuals who have a relationship with God often gain added insight into the difficulties in their lives (spiritual struggle) and increased courage to make the changes necessary for healing and attainment of their fullest potential. From a theistic perspective, humans "need a relation to God to be all they were intended to be" (Evans, 2005, p. 84).

Assessment. Theistic psychotherapy assumes humans are multisystemic (e.g., social, behavioral, cognitive, educational, spiritual, intellectual, etc.) and therefore a multisystemic assessment, including spiritual assessment, can be helpful in understanding our clients (Richards & Bergin, 2005). If it appears that clients want to explore their spiritual life, one important area of inquiry includes a client's relationship with God. Therapists can help clients develop an honest view of God and a personal relationship with Him by examining the nature of the client's God image relative to an accurate and positive representation of God's attributes (Tisdale et al., 1997). There are a number of standardized research instruments that measure people's concepts and images of God that could be useful for clinical assessment, including the Adjective Rating Scale (Gorsuch, 1968), God Image Inventory (Lawrence, 1997), Loving and Controlling God Scales (Benson & Spilka, 1973), Spiritual Well-Being Scale (Pauloutzian & Ellison, 1982), and Spiritual Assessment Inventory (Hall & Edwards, 1996). Copies of all of these measures are provided in *Measures of Religiosity* (Hill & Hood, 1999).

An exercise that could help clients explore their conception of God and how it may have been influenced by projections of others in their lives is to ask clients to list attributes of their parents and to list attributes of God. Therapists and clients may then wish to consider together any similarities and differences that exist between the lists (Richards, Hardman, & Berrett, 2007). Another activity that can be used both for assessment purposes and to help facilitate therapists in their efforts to help their clients develop a meaningful relationship with God involves asking clients some or all of the following questions:

1. Is God there for me? How do I know?
2. Do I believe that my God image corresponds to a being that actually exists?
3. Am I good enough for God's love?
4. How much can God control me and I control God?
5. Do I believe God wants to have a relationship with me and will help me develop a relationship with Him?
6. Do I believe that God will comfort me in times of trial?
7. Do I believe that God will help me heal emotionally?
8. Am I afraid to surrender control to God?
9. What does God's love feel like in my life?
10. What can I do to foster a relationship with God? (Lawrence, 1997; Richards et al., 2007).

Therapists may also want to examine whether clients seem to exhibit a healthy or unhealthy dependency on God. Clients may express faith in God, but the faith may manifest in unhealthy ways. For instance, some clients with a strong faith in God expect God to guide them in every decision they make, and they can become paralyzed when they are unable to discern the direction God may want them to take at a particular moment. On the other hand, some clients may view God as unconcerned and uninvolved in their lives. Some scholars have suggested that a spiritually mature individual recognizes his or her own agency while affirming the need for God and others (Baumeister, 2005; Kass & Lennox, 2005).

Pargament et al. (1988) outlined three religious problem solving styles: self-directing, deferring, and collaborative and constructed the Religious Problem-Solving Scale (Pargament, Kennell, Hathaway, Grevengoed, Newman, & Jones, 1988) to assess these styles. Self-directing individuals see God as removed from the problem solving process and consider themselves independently responsible for solving their problems. People with a deferring style take little or no responsibility for solving their problems and rely completely on God to provide the solutions to their problems. Both self-directing and deferring styles inhibit individuals from having a healthy relationship with God. Individuals with a more satisfying relationship with God are more likely to engage in a collaborative problem solving style. They believe that "the problem solving process is held jointly by the individual and God. . . . Both . . . are viewed as active contributors working together to solve problems" (p. 92). Therapists may wish to assess their client's level of dependency on God to better understand how the individual functions in their relationship with God and also to help the therapist determine the appropriate approach (nondirective, directive, collaborative) in working with their client (Richards & Bergin, 2005). A copy of the Religious Problem-Solving Scale is available in Hill and Hood (1999).

It can also be helpful to examine clients' sense of spiritual identity. A spiritual identity refers to an individual's feelings of identity and worth in relation to God as well as their sense of their place and importance in the world in which they live (Richards & Bergin, 2005). People who have a healthy spiritual identity tend to enjoy greater emotional well-being and relate better to others. They are also able to connect to God and experience his love and influence in their lives more fully than those who lack a strong spiritual identity (Bergin et al., 1994; MacKenna, 2002; Richards & Bergin, 2005; Richards & Potts, 1995). Although preliminary efforts have been made to develop measures of spiritual identity (e.g., Morgan, 1999), we are not aware of any measures of spiritual identity that are ready for use in the clinical setting. Therapists may wish to informally discuss and assess their clients' sense of spiritual identity by asking questions such as:

1. Do you believe you are a child of God?
2. Do you believe you have divine worth and potential?
3. Do you feel that God loves you?
4. Do you feel that you are of divine spiritual worth?
5. Do you believe that there is any special purpose to your life?
6. Do you believe that God knows you as an individual?
7. Do you believe that you play a role in God's plan for humankind?
8. Do you have a personal relationship with God?
9. Do you believe that you are a valued creation of God?
10. Do you believe that your spiritual identity is eternal?

Therapists may also wish to examine their own spiritual development and God image perceptions. Therapists may want to ask themselves if they are relating to their clients from the viewpoint that there is a real God from whom to form an image, or if they view God as merely an object representation (Parker, 1999). Understanding their own level of God image development can help therapists to be mindful of how their views of God may be impacting how they evaluate and intervene with their clients.

Interventions. The primary aim of theistic psychotherapy is to help clients cope with and resolve their presenting concerns and to promote their long-term well being; as well as to explore how clients' spiritual beliefs may assist them in treatment and recovery (Richards & Bergin, 2005). Specific goals that therapists may wish to consider for God image change might include: (a) helping clients examine what impact their God image and relationship with God may be having on their presenting concerns, (b) helping clients look at ways their experiences with others may be contributing to their conceptions of God (c) encouraging clients to use their religious teachings to help them learn more about God's true character, (d) helping clients get in touch with their core spiritual identity, (d) helping them explore their overall level of spiritual development and set goals to overcome spiritual immaturities, (d) encouraging clients to consider ways they might foster and recognize experiences with God (Richards & O'Grady, 2005).

Although spiritual experiences cannot be manufactured, therapists can help clients draw upon practices upheld by the major world religions that may enhance their receptivity to such experiences (Kass & Lennox, 2005; Richards & Bergin, 2004; 2005). For instance many people have found prayer to be a powerful way to develop a relationship with God. Prayer has been defined as an inward communication or conversation with God or a Higher Power. Prayers can be offered verbally or silently. All of the Western world religions (Judaism, Christianity, Islam, Sikhism, and Zoroastrianism) advocate prayer (Richards & Bergin, 2005; Smart, 1994). There is evidence that people who pray receive both physical and psychological benefits (Benson, 1996; Dossey, 1993; Plante & Sherman, 2002).

Some clients, however, seem to have difficulty praying. They feel like their prayers go unheard or that they are so unworthy or unlovable that God would not want to communicate with them. These obstacles to prayer often represent a distorted understanding of the nature of God. Therapists may wish to challenge the view that God would not want to hear from the client. Therapist and client could explore the teachings of the client's spiritual or religious orientation regarding the nature and attributes of God, pointing out any discrepancies between the religious teachings and the client's God image. Client and therapist may also wish to discuss times when the client has felt that his/her prayers have or have not been answered and what those experiences meant to the client. Therapists may want to ask their clients to describe experiences and events in their lives, as well as messages from significant people in their lives, that have decreased or weakened their faith in God. It may also be helpful to discuss the pattern of prayer the client engages in and any alterations the client may find helpful in their communion with God (Richards et al., 2007).

In addition to prayer, the practices of contemplation and meditation have been engaged in by individuals all over the world for centuries (Miller, 2003; Smart, 1995). In conjunction with contemplation and meditation, spiritual imagery and mindfulness can be useful interventions for some clients. These spiritual practices involve slowing the body and mind down, surrendering control and creating a sense of peaceful focus or awareness. When these practices are approached theistically, these processes may also include communion with God (Miller, 2003, Tan & Dong, 2002). There is evidence suggesting that meditation and contemplation with spiritual meaning is more effective than meditation and contemplation void of religious content (Benson, 1996). Therapists may want to teach their clients how to slow down and be mindful in therapy and between sessions, and encourage meditation and contemplation outside of the therapy session.

Some therapists have also found it helpful to use spiritual imagery with their clients (Ball & Goodyear, 1991; Jones et al., 1992; Richards & Potts, 1995). Such imagery may be more effective if it is constructed collaboratively with the client. These practices may help clients learn to slow down enough to feel God's spirit and invite Him more fully into their lives. Parker (1999) suggests that as individuals learn to listen to the "still small voice" (1 Kings. 19:11-13), God's spirit "will take our particular developmental history into account and speak to us in ways we can hear, [and] in ways beyond our current ability to hear and invites us to listen" (p. 161).

Clients may wish to express their feelings about God and their spiritual development through talking with religious leaders, trusted friends, or their therapist. Some clients also find it helpful to process their relationship with God through journaling or through various forms of artistic expression. Therapists can help clients discover ways of understanding and developing their relationship God in a tailor made fashion (Richards et al., 2007). It is beyond the scope of this chapter to cover all of the theistic interventions for addressing God image concerns and promoting change and so we refer readers to other sources who have described a wider variety of spiritual interventions (e.g., Miller, 1999; Richards & Bergin, 2005; Richards et al., 2007; Sperry & Shafranske, 2005).

Perhaps the most important thing therapists can do to help clients in the process of discovering and developing a relationship with God is to create a safe spiritual space for them to come to regularly (West, 2000). The theistic world religions encourage people to "love their neighbors" and to reach out in service and fellowship to others, especially to those in need (Smart, 1995; Stone, 2005). Therapists can provide a safe space for clients as they embark on the sacred journey of connecting with God. Therapists can let clients know in consent forms and in intake sessions that they are comfortable discussing spiritual and religious concerns if the clients wish to do so (Richards & Bergin, 2005).

Therapists can also help create a spiritually safe environment for clients by seeking God's inspiration in their work with clients. One of the most commonly used interventions by theistic psychotherapists is praying for their clients prior to meeting with their clients and silently during the therapy session (Richards & Potts, 1995). Many theistic psychotherapists report that they have experienced God's inspiration guide them in their work with clients (Chamberlain, Richards, & Scharman, 1996; O'Grady & Richards, 2004; Richards & Potts, 1995; West, 2000), and there is some evidence suggesting that intercessory prayer can having a healing influence in the lives of those being prayed for (Plante & Sherman, 2002). Finally therapists can approach their therapy from the perspective that God is a real being who desires to be actively involved in the lives of their clients and in their own lives.

CASE REPORT

Treatment Setting and Therapist

The client was seen by Ms. Kari A. O'Grady at the Counseling and Career Center (CCC) at Brigham Young University (BYU), in Provo Utah. The Counseling and Career Center is a full service counseling center with an APA accredited internship site. It employs over 20 licensed PhD psychologists and approximately 10 to 15 other mental health professionals. The CCC provides academic support and advisement, career counseling and placement services, personal counseling services, career and psychological testing services, and a variety of educational outreach programs for students. At the time she worked with this client, Ms. O'Grady was a doctoral student in counseling psychology in BYU's APA accredited doctoral program in counseling psychology. Ms. O'Grady identifies herself as a theistic integrative psychotherapist (Richards, 2005). She is a devout member of the Church of Jesus Christ of Latter-day Saints.

Client Demographics

At the time of services, Lisa was a single, twenty-one year old, Caucasian female. She grew up in the Western United States. Her parents divorced when Lisa was ten years old. Her father remarried one year after the divorce. Her mother remarried about three years after the divorce. Lisa lived with her mother. She was the youngest of seven (three stepsiblings) children. Her mother and step father were members of the Church of Jesus Christ of Latter-day Saints (LDS). Lisa described herself as an active member of the LDS church.

Client History

Lisa's biological father was not an active member of the LDS church. He played a distant, but influential role in Lisa's life. His love was conditional and Lisa often felt demeaned and misunderstood by him. He assumed a controlling, authoritative role in the family. Lisa described her father as running their family like a business. If the children did not produce enough he would "demote or fire" them. Shortly after the divorce, Lisa's father moved to another state and remarried. After remarrying, Lisa's father became very financially successful. Despite his increase in wealth, he did not meet the financial needs of his ex-wife and the children he left behind. Lisa's mother struggled financially and continued to do so even after remarrying. At times, the children ate only one meal a day and were often unable to meet other basic material needs. Although Lisa's father abandoned the family, he maintained some level of influence and control. The children were hurt by his neglect, but often sought for his approval in the major decisions of their lives.

Lisa described her mother as passive and lacking in self-confidence. She married Lisa's father despite misgivings and married her second husband because he told her he had felt spiritual prompting that she should be his wife. She did not receive such prompting, but married him anyway, assuming that he knew what was best for them.

Lisa's stepfather was emotionally and physically abusive, though he faithfully attended church services, he did not practice the teachings of his religion and failed to assume a nurturing and protective role as the father. The children did not view him as a strong religious guide in the home. Lisa described feeling frightened as a child because there was no father to save her from her stepfather.

Assessment and Diagnosis

Lisa presented in therapy with concerns about differentiating from her family of origin. She also sought help for identity development. Further assessment revealed that Lisa had a distorted view of God in part due to the negative influences of the father figures in her life. Her therapist determined that Lisa was in need of interventions that would help her with differentiation, developing a healthy sense of her identity, and fostering a more mature image of God.

Treatment Processes and Outcomes

When Lisa first appeared for therapy, her predominated wish for therapy was to be healed from some of the pain of her childhood, and also to learn to trust her own inner experiences and definition of self. She often betrayed herself by deferring to other's judgments and directives including those of her father, despite the fact that she did not respect her father and the choices he made for his own life. She felt her identity was circumscribed into a particular label, or "confined to a box" defined by her father and older siblings. She felt frustrated that they could not view her more dimensionally and understand her character more truthfully. She had a desire to come to know who she really was for herself. Much of the focus of therapy was to help Lisa develop a stronger sense of her core spiritual identity and worth and the courage to trust and act on her own inner feelings and spiritual impressions.

According to a theistic perspective, mature spirituality includes an internal locus of control and a strong sense of one's spiritual identity and agency (Kass & Lennox, 2005; Richards & Bergin, 2005). It is in the inner part of humans–their eternal core, spirit, or heart–that people experience God's loves, guidance, and truth. As clients learn how to discern spiritual feelings and impressions they can affirm their spiritual identity and their ability to make choices and take responsibility for their own lives (Richards et al., 2007).

In their first session together, Lisa's therapist let Lisa know that she would be comfortable discussing spiritual issues or concerns if Lisa ever desired to do so. In subsequent sessions, Lisa's therapist used a number of interventions to help Lisa develop sensitivity to her own inner impressions. Some of this work in therapy included teaching Lisa to focus on her feelings and body sensations mindfully in order to help Lisa become aware of how she was experiencing her world internally. They also discussed evidences of Lisa's ability to make wise decisions for her life and why Lisa felt she needed to be the person to make those decisions. These interventions seemed to help Lisa become more in tuned to her internal, spiritual self.

During one particular session, Lisa and her therapist were discussing Lisa's relationship with God. Lisa felt that God loved her, but she was unsure that He trusted her. Near the end of the session and following a brief silent prayer by the therapist, the client and the therapist were quiet. Into the stillness came a warm, peaceful feeling experienced by both Lisa and her therapist. Lisa's therapist asked, "Do you feel that?" With tears in her eyes, Lisa responded, "It feels like absolute peace." Lisa identified the feeling as God's love and his Truth. Lisa and her therapist talked about how peaceful, spiritual feelings could serve as a pattern for knowing when truth has been found and honored.

During the course of therapy, Lisa became engaged to a devout LDS man from a healthy family background. He was helpful in her healing process and his family served as a pattern of a loving, well functioning family unit. Lisa had prayed about marrying this man and had felt a strong spiritual impression that God approved of her desire to marry him. Shortly after this experience, Lisa traveled out of town to visit her family and to announce to her father her engagement. She had some fear about doing so as she felt he would disapprove. Before traveling to her father's home, she stopped off at a family gathering that included some of her sisters, brothers, and their spouses. She felt a wish for comfort and support as she approached her father.

In the LDS church, worthy male members can hold the priesthood and administer blessings of comfort, inspiration, and healing (Ulrich, Richards, & Bergin, 2000). Lisa's father and stepfather had never been able to fulfill this role, but one of her sisters had married a man who held the priesthood. He served as a surrogate priesthood leader for Lisa's family of origin. Many of the women in Lisa's family went to this brother in law to receive answers from God. Lisa went to this brother in law for a blessing. Instead of offering a blessing of comfort and encouragement, he told Lisa in the blessing that the Lord did not want her to marry the man to whom she had become engaged.

This experience undermined Lisa's ability to trust her own spiritual impressions. After processing through Lisa's experience, Lisa's therapist challenged her brother-in-law's use of the priesthood by sharing some literature published by the church that illustrated the proper uses of the priesthood (e.g., to heal, comfort, and sustain others). According to the LDS teachings, women are equally capable as men to commune with God, and are encouraged to have their own, personal experiences with God, working out their salvation through this personal relationship with Him. The use of the priesthood to trump other's personal revelation and inspiration or experiences with God are contrary to LDS doctrine, but at times still occur (Ulrich et al., 2000). Despite this intervention, Lisa continued to question her own impressions and called off her engagement. She doubted her ability to have a personal relationship with God.

Lisa continued for several weeks to struggle with questions about whether she had made the right decision to call off her engagement. During a subsequent therapy session, Lisa's therapist handed Lisa a box of crayons and asked Lisa to draw her heart and her mind. Lisa drew her heart in red with an open center, and her mind in black shaded in gray. Her therapist then encouraged her to draw various things she thought belonged in her heart and her mind. She drew her heart in red. She represented her relationship with her fiancé in her heart. She drew her mind in darkness and depicted various scenes including the blessing. The illustration of the blessing included representations of male and female family members standing by as the blessing was given.

Lisa's therapist encouraged her to talk about the drawing. Lisa's therapist noticed that the male stick figures had arms and hands and that the female figures did not. She asked Lisa if she noticed a difference between the male and female stick figures. Lisa was surprised to notice the difference. She had not been aware she had drawn the females without arms. When asked why she may have drawn the picture this way she cried and replied, "The women can't do it by themselves." She realized that she had believed that women are unable to have a genuine relationship with God. She had formed the image of a God who favored men and had little interest in developing an individual relationship with women. Lisa then challenged her own beliefs about this distorted view of God. She also expressed how painful it had been to feel like God would not commune with her because she is a female.

During the following weeks, Lisa nurtured her relationship with God through prayer, spiritual meditation and reflection, moments of gratitude, and studying spiritual text. Her image of God became grounded in her experiences with him. She came to see Him as a loving being who was interested in her and who trusted her to make wise choices for her life. Her relationship with God gave her courage to confront family members and others that tried to usurp her ability to make decisions for her life. Near the end of therapy, her therapist asked her to write about her relationship with God. The client expressed her feelings in a poem. The poem represented her feelings about her core spiritual identity. The poem depicted her full, joyful, loving self and also expressed her rejection of the faulty labels assigned to her by family members. In the poem she indicated that is was God that "pulled her out of the mislabeled bin," and let her full self be expressed. She said the bin represented cereal bins from a local bulk grocery store. She felt like her family had put her in the "Cheerio" bin even though she may have really been "Fruit Loops" or a combination of many cereals. Her poem expressed her belief that the God knew her fully and gave her courage to fully express the love, joy, goodness, and courage she has always had within her. She then wrote a poem to her fiancée expressing her love for him and her wish to marry him soon.

The following is the therapist's case notes from Lisa's second to last visit:

> Lisa shared so many insights in therapy today that my main role was to listen to her insights and reflect them back to her. I was an onlooker in her journey. Her faith has served as a strong resource for her that seems to have moved her well beyond the work we do together in therapy. The insights that help her heal from her past, more accurately perceive her identity, develop assertiveness skills and courage, and her confidence in decision making have all been enhanced by the influence of her spiritual convictions in God and in revelatory means.

Authors' Commentary and Conclusions

Theistic psychotherapy assumes that clients' faith in God and personal spirituality can powerfully assist them in their efforts to cope, heal, and change (Richards & Bergin, 2005). Clients' perceptions of God and how they define themselves in relation to God are of critical importance to their sense of identity and psychosocial functioning. Spiritual experiences in which clients feel God's love and healing influence can be powerful catalysts for healing and therapeutic change (Richards & Bergin, 2005; Richards, 1999). From a theistic perspective, assessing and working with issues of God image in therapy are often an essential part of successful treatment.

The case of Lisa illustrates how a client's perceptions of God and self can be distorted by childhood experiences that create difficulties in developing a genuine helpful relationship with God. In the case of Lisa, her therapist helped her explore ways in which her views of God may have become distorted. Then together they confronted her childhood view and the view of some of her family members that God does not listen to or respect the needs and insights of women. This confrontation was facilitated by helping Lisa understand that such a view of God was not supported by the teachings of her religious tradition. Lisa's therapist also encouraged Lisa to find ways to develop a meaningful relationship with God including engaging in spiritual practices such as prayer, meditation, scripture study, and spiritual reflection. Lisa's personal spiritual experiences with God helped her revise her view that God would not communicate with her directly. After some of Lisa's distorted beliefs about the nature of God had been modified, Lisa was able to nurture a more mature, healthy God image.

Lisa's therapist's views of God as a loving, active God served as a resource in therapy as she silently prayed for and received guidance on how to best work with Lisa. The therapist also was able to create a safe environment in which God's love was able to be felt during a therapy session. This spiritual experience provided an opportunity for Lisa to appraise her current conceptions of God and replace them with a more accurate understanding of God as a loving, compassionate being. Finally, as Lisa developed a relationship with God, she felt His love for her and his definition of her expands her own sense of her personal spiritual identity. She came to view herself as multidimensional, capable, loving, loveable, and good. This empowered her to make important decisions in her life and to enjoy her life more fully. As illustrated in this case, theistic psychotherapists can help clients confront distortions in their views of God and self and form an image of God that is more truthful, helpful, and based on first hand experiences. When therapists do this they often become witnesses to a process of therapeutic healing and change that goes beyond the therapeutic dyad to include God's healing influence.

NOTE

1. See also Chapter 1.

REFERENCES

Ball, R. A., & Goodyear, R. K. (1991). Self-reported professional practices of Christian psychologists. *Journal of Psychology and Christianity, 10,* 144-153.
Bassett, J.F., & Williams, J.E. (2003). Protestants' images of self, God, and Satan as seen in adjective check list description. *The International Journal for the Psychology of Religion, 13,* 123-135.

Baumeister, R.F. (2005). Self and volition. In W.R. Miller & H.D. Delaney (Eds.), *Judeo-Christian perspectives on psychology: Human nature, motivation, and change* (pp. 57-72). Washington DC: American Psychological Association.

Benson, H. (1996). *Timeless healing: The power and biology of belief.* New York: Scribner.

Benson, P. L., & Spilka, B. (1973). God image as a function of self-esteem and locus of control. *Journal for the Scientific Study of Religion, 12,* 297-310.

Bergin, A. E. (1980). Psychotherapy and religious values. *Journal of Consulting and Clinical Psychology, 48,* 75-105.

Bergin, A. E., Stinchfield, R. D., Gaskin, T. A., Masters, K. S., & Sullivan, C. E. (1988). Religious life styles and mental health: An exploratory study. *Journal of Counseling Psychology, 35,* 91-98.

Brown, S., & W.R. Miller (2005). Transformational change. In W.R. Miller & H.D. Delaney (Eds.), *Judeo-Christian perspectives on Psychology: Human nature, motivation, and change* (pp. 167-184). Washington DC: American Psychological Association.

Chamberlain, R. B., Richards, P. S., & Scharman, J. S. (1996). Using spiritual perspectives and interventions in psychotherapy: A qualitative study of experienced AMCAP therapists. *Association of Mormon Counselors and Psychotherapists Journal, 22,* 29-74.

Dickie, J.R., Ajega, L.V., Kobylak, J.R., & Nixon, K.M. (2006). Mother, father, and self: Sources of young adult's God concepts. *Journal for the Scientific Study of Religion, 45,* 57-71.

Dickie, J.R., Eshleman, A.K., Shepard, A., Wilt, M.V., & Johnson, M. (1997). Parent-child relationships and children's images of God. *Journal for the Scientific Study of Religion, 36,* 25-43.

Dossey, L. (1993). *Healing words: The power of prayer and the practice of medicine.* San Francisco: HarperCollins.

Evans, C.S. (2005). The relational self: Psychological and theological perspectives (pp. 73-94). In W.R. Miller & H.D. Delaney (Eds.) *Judeo-Christian perspectives on psychology: Human nature, motivation, and change.* Washington DC: American Psychological Association.

Francis, L.J., Gibson, H.M., & Robbins, M. (2001). God images and self-worth among adolescents in Scotland. *Mental Health, Religion, & Culture, 4,* 103-108.

Freud, S. (1923/1989). *The Ego and the Id.* New York: Norton.

Gorsuch, R. (1968). The conceptualization of God as seen in adjective ratings. *Journal for the Scientific Study of Religion, 7,* 56-64.

Hall, T. W., & Edwards, K. J. (1996). The initial development and factor analysis of the Spiritual Assessment Inventory. *Journal of Psychology and Theology, 24,* 233-246.

Hall, T.W. & Brokaw, B.F. (1995). The relationship of spiritual maturity to level of object relation development and God image. *Pastoral Psychology, 43,* 373-391.

Hill, C. H., & Hood, R. W. (Eds.) (1999). *Measures of religiosity.* Birmingham, Alabama: Religious Education Press.

Janssen, J., DeHart, J.,& Garadt, M. (1994). Images of God in adolescence. *The International Journal for the Psychology of Religion, 4,* 105-121.

Jones, S. L., Watson, E. J., & Wolfram, T. J. (1992). Results of the Rech conference survey on religious faith and professional psychology. *Journal of Psychology and Theology, 20,* 147-158.

Kass, J.D., & Lennox, S. (2005). The effects of religious practices: A focus on mental health (pp. 205-226). In W.R. Miller & H.D. Delaney (Eds.) *Judeo-Christian perspectives on Psychology: Human nature, motivation, and change.* Washington DC: American Psychological Association.

Koenig, H. G., McCullough, M. E., & Larson, D. B. (2001). *Handbook of religion and health.* New York: Oxford University Press.

Krejci, M.J. (1998). Gender comparison of God schemas: A multidimensional scaling analysis. *The International Journal for the Psychology of Religion, 8,* 57-66.

Kunkel, M.A., Cook, S., Meshel, D.S., & Hauenstein, A. (1999). God images: A concept map. *Journal for the Scientific Study of Religion, 38,* 193-202.

Lawrence, R.T. (1997). Measuring the image of God: The God image inventory and the God image scales. *Journal of Psychology and Theology, 25,* 214-226.

Lee, C., & Early, A. (2000). Religiosity and family values: Correlates of God-image in a protestant sample. *Journal of Psychology and Theology, 28,* 229-239.

Levinas, E. (1981). *Otherwise than being: Or beyond essence.* Boston: Haque.

MacKenna, C. (2002). Self images and God images. *British Journal of Psychotherapy, 18,* 325-338.

Malony, H. N. (1985). Assessing religious maturity. In E. M. Stern (Ed.), *Psychotherapy and the religiously committed patient* (pp. 25-33). New York: Haworth Press.

Malony, H. N. (1988). The clinical assessment of optimal religious functioning. *Review of Religious Research, 30,* 3-17.

Miller, G. (2003). *Incorporating spirituality in counseling and psychotherapy: Theory and technique.* Hoboken, NJ: John Wiley & Sons.

Miller, W. R. (1999). *Integrating spirituality into treatment: Resources for practitioners.* Washington, DC: American Psychological Association.

Miller, W.R, & Delaney, H.D. (Eds.) (2005). *Judeo-Christian perspectives on Psychology: Human nature, motivation, and change.* Washington DC: American Psychological Association.

Morgan, D. T. (1999). *Initial development of the Multidimensional Spiritual Orientation Inventory.* Unpublished doctoral dissertation, Brigham Young University, Provo, Utah.

O'Grady, K. A., & Richards, P. S. (2004). *Professionals perceptions of the role of inspiration in science and psychotherapy.* Paper presented at the annual convention of the American Psychological Association, Honolulu, Hawaii, July, 2004.

Owen, S. D. (2004). *Spiritual intimacy: A qualitative investigation of relationships with God and their association with well-being.* Unpublished doctoral dissertation, Brigham Young University, Provo, Utah.

Paloutzian, R. F., & Ellison, C. W. (1982). Loneliness, spiritual well-being and quality of life. In L. A. Peplau & D. Perlman (Eds.), *Loneliness: A sourcebook of current theory, research and therapy* (pp. 224-237). New York: Wiley Interscience.

Pargament, K. I., Echemendia, R. J., Johnson, S., Cook, P., McGrath, C., Myers, J. G. et al. (1990). God help me: I. Coping efforts as predictors of the outcomes to significant negative life events. *American Journal of Community Psychology, 18,* 793-824.

Pargament, K. I., Kennell, J., Hathaway, W., Grenvengoed, N., Newman, J., & Jones, W. (1988). Religion and the problem-solving process: Three styles of coping. *Journal for the Scientific Study of Religion, 27,* 90-104.

Parker, S. (1999). Hearing God's Spirit: Impacts on developmental history on adult religious experience. *Journal of Psychology and Christianity, 18,* 153-163.

Plante, T. G. & Sherman, A. C. (Eds.), (2001). *Faith and health: Psychological perspectives.* New York: The Guilford Press.

Poll, J. B., & Smith, T. B. (2003). The spiritual self: Toward a conceptualization of spiritual identity development. *Journal of Psychology and Theology, 31,* 129-142.

Porpora, D.V. (2006). Methodological atheism; methodological agnosticism and religious experience. *Journal for the Theory of Social Behavior.36,* 57-75.

Richards, P. S. (1999). *Spiritual influences in healing and psychotherapy.* William C. Bier Award Invited Address, Division 36 (Psychology of Religion), Boston, MA, August 21, 1999.

Richards, P. S. (2005). Theistic integrative psychotherapy. In L. Sperry & E. P. Shafranske (Eds.), *Spiritually-oriented psychotherapy* (pp. 259-285). Washington, DC: American Psychological Association.

Richards, P. S., & Bergin, A. E. (1997). *A spiritual strategy for counseling and psychotherapy.* Washington, DC: American Psychological Association.

Richards, P. S., & Bergin, A. E. (2004). *Casebook for a spiritual strategy in counseling and psychotherapy.* Washington, DC: American Psychological Association.

Richards, P. S., & Bergin, A. E. (2005). *A spiritual strategy for counseling and psychotherapy* (2nd ed.). Washington, DC: American Psychological Association.

Richards, P. S., Hardman, R. K., & Berrett, M. E. (2007). *Spiritual approaches in the treatment of women with eating disorders.* Washington, DC, American Psychological Association.

Richards, P. S., & O'Grady, K. A. (2003). Out of obscurity: The faith factor in physical and mental health. *Contemporary Psychology: APA Review of Books, 48,* 612-614.

Richards, P. S., & Potts, R. W. (1995). Using spiritual interventions in psychotherapy: Practices, successes, failures, and ethical concerns of Mormon psychotherapists. *Professional Psychology: Research and Practice, 26,* 163-170.

Rizzuto, A. (1979). *The birth of the living God: A psychoanalytic study.* Chicago: The University of Chicago Press.

Rowatt, W.C. & Kirkpatrick, L.A. (2002). Two dimensions of attachment to God and their relation to affect, religiosity, and personality constructs. *Journal for the Scientific Study of Religion, 41,* 637-651.

Schaap-Jonker, H., Eurelings-Bontekoe, E., Verhagen, P. J., & Zock, H. (2002). Image of God and personality pathology: An exploratory study among psychiatric patients. *Mental Health, Religion and Culture, 5,* 55-71.

Smart, N. (1994). *Religions of the West.* Englewood Cliffs, NJ: Prentice Hall.

Sperry, L. & Shafranske, E. P. (Eds.) (2005). *Spiritually oriented psychotherapy.* Washington, DC: American Psychological Association.

Stone, C. (2005). Opening psychoanalytic space to the spiritual. *Psychoanalytic Review, 92,* 417-429.

Tisdale, T.C., Key, T.L., Edwards, K.J., Brokaw, B.F., Kemperman, S.R., Cloud, H. Townsend, J, & Okamoto, T. (1997). Impact on God image to personal adjustment and object relations development. *Journal of Psychology and Theology, 2,* 227-239.

Ulrich, W. L., Richards, P. S., & Bergin, A. E. (2000). Psychotherapy with Latter-day Saints (pp. 185-209). In P. S. Richards & A. E. Bergin (Eds.), *Handbook of psychotherapy and religious diversity*. Washington, DC: American Psychological Association.

West, W. (2000). *Psychotherapy and spirituality: Crossing the line between therapy and religion*. Thousand Oaks, CA: Sage.

doi:10.1300/J515v09n03_09

Chapter 10

A Liberal Protestant Pastoral Theological Approach and the God Image: The Role of God Images in Recovery from Sexual and Physical Abuse

Carrie Doehring, PhD

SUMMARY. This chapter explores the role of God images in recovery from sexual violence, using an interdisciplinary hermeneutical method that draws upon postmodern approaches to knowledge and assumes that knowledge–psychological and theological–is socially constructed. This interdisciplinary method has been developed by liberal Protestant practical theologians, and it consists of a collaborative dialogue between relevant theological and psychological studies. In reflecting upon the process of change that occurred in the case study presented in this chapter, I draw upon a psychodynamic understanding of God representations (Rizzuto, 1979) and a theological understanding of religious symbols (Neville, 1996) because these theoretical perspectives meet my criteria of contextual relevance, interdisciplinary meaningfulness, and pragmatic usefulness. These criteria provide a way to assess the contextual

---

[Haworth co-indexing entry note]: "A Liberal Protestant Pastoral Theological Approach and the God Image: The Role of God Images in Recovery from Sexual and Physical Abuse." Doehring, Carrie. Co-published simultaneously in *Journal of Spirituality in Mental Health* (The Haworth Pastoral Press, an imprint of The Haworth Press) Vol. 9, No. 3/4, 2007, pp. 211-226; and: *God Image Handbook for Spiritual Counseling and Psychotherapy: Research, Theory, and Practice* (ed: Glendon L. Moriarty, and Louis Hoffman) The Haworth Pastoral Press, an imprint of The Haworth Press, 2007, pp. 211-226. Single or multiple copies of this article are available for a fee from The Haworth Document Delivery Service [1-800-HAWORTH, 9:00 a.m. - 5:00 p.m. (EST). E-mail address: docdelivery@haworthpress.com].

Available online at http://jsmh.haworthpress.com
© 2007 by The Haworth Press. All rights reserved.
doi:10.1300/J515v09n03_10

truthfulness of religious and psychological knowledge within the framework of postmodern approaches to knowledge. This chapter illustrates how such approaches to knowledge can be utilized within the traditions of liberal Protestant pastoral theology, in pastoral psychotherapy with victims of violence. doi:10.1300/J515v09n03_10 *[Article copies available for a fee from The Haworth Document Delivery Service: 1-800-HAWORTH. E-mail address: <docdelivery@haworthpress.com> Website: <http://www.HaworthPress.com> © 2007 by The Haworth Press. All rights reserved.]*

In the 1960s and 70s, women and men broke mandates to remain silent imposed by family, church, and society and began speaking out about their experiences of sexual and physical violence.[1] They narrated the violation of sacred relationships of trust within their families and church families. They lamented the desecration of the sanctity of their bodies.[2]

As they gave voice to their experiences, they raised profound theological questions about God, human nature, evil, and sin. These questions took on a life-and-death quality for survivors, perpetrators, and those who cared for them, as they searched for who and where God was in the midst of violation and desecration. These searches for a living God led some survivors to experience God as the violated child or person,[3] and to reject images of God as the Father who sacrificed His Son.[4] Looking back on how concepts and images of God have changed since the silence about family and sexual violence was broken; it would be no exaggeration to say that these stories of violation have given rise to a theological reformation of sorts within many religiously-committed persons, communities of faith, and religious traditions.

One of the challenges in this reformation is to understand the bi-directional relationship between experiences of violence and God images: how violence can form or reinforce God images and, conversely, how God images can shape a person's response to violence, in both its immediate aftermath and the long-term process of recovery. In what ways does violence correlate with God images of an absent or judging God? Do images of a suffering God encourage victims to see their experiences of violence as the cross they must bear? Understanding the relationship between theological meanings, psychological processes, and recovery from violence has been an important and complicated task for pastoral practitioners and theologians.

In this chapter I will explore the role of God images in recovery from sexual violence, using an interdisciplinary method that draws upon postmodern approaches to knowledge and assumes that knowledge–psychological and theological–is socially constructed. After I describe this method and briefly compare it to other spiritually-oriented approaches to psychotherapy, I will present a case study and then engage theories from psychological and theological studies in order to understand the role of God images in this case study.

Given the premise that knowledge is culturally conditioned, I need to describe at the outset of this chapter my social location. I am a Euro-American, middle-class heterosexual woman who is ordained in the Presbyterian Church, USA. I have been a congregational minister for nine years full-time and seven years part-time, and have taught in liberal Protestant seminaries for fifteen years. I am also a Diplomat in the American Association of Pastoral Counselors, and licensed as a psychologist in Massachusetts and Colorado. The case study is drawn from my practice as a pastoral psychotherapist. I understand pastoral psychotherapy to be "a mode of *healing* intervention ('therapy') that is specifically grounded both in *psychoanalytic* theory and methods ('psycho-')– i.e., with a primary focus on *unconscious* mental and emotional processes–and held in a constructive, creation-affirming theology ('pastoral')" (Cooper-White, 2006 p. 8). These contexts inform the method and theories that I use in exploring the relationship between God images and violence, and this chapter will be most relevant to readers working in similar contexts.

A LIBERAL PROTESTANT
PRACTICAL THEOLOGICAL METHOD

In this chapter I use an interdisciplinary method developed by liberal Protestant practical theologians consisting of a collaborative dialogue between theological and psychological studies "in which each can challenge the other and contribute both descriptive and normative statements, coming to a deeper understanding through their essentially equal dialogue" (Poling & Miller, 1985, p. 31). This is a hermeneutical method in which psychological and theological theories, as well as psychotherapeutic approaches, are understood as texts to be interpreted.[5]

In my use of this method, I assume a postmodern approach to knowledge, namely social constructionism, proposing that knowledge about what people name as God or the sacred is continually being constructed and reconstructed in the midst of complex historical contexts and acutely intense personal circumstances. None of these constructions of religious knowledge can be said to be true in all times and places; instead they are contextual and provisional. Social constructionists understand knowledge as a process of ongoing communal construction of meaning that "draw[s] from the immense repository of intelligibilities that constitute a particular cultural tradition" (Gergen, 2001, p. 805). Biblical critical studies, or, in the social sciences, empirical psychologies of religion are examples of the cultural traditions that Gergen is describing. "In this sense, what one takes to be the real, what one believes to be transparently true about human functioning, is a by-product of communal construction" (Gergen, 2001, p. 806).

The view that all religious meanings are constructed from experience has a social and a personal dimension. Views of God, for example, are constructed by communities in various historical circumstances. These constructions become available to individuals who also construct personal beliefs through interaction with these cultural resources and their own particular circumstances and developmental histories. This social constructionist approach helps me appreciate the uniqueness and complexity of each client's experiences of both religion and violence. Borrowing the language of comparative studies of religion that use a phenomenological approach, I can describe each client as inhabiting her "religious world" that is uniquely shaped, from one moment to the next, by her experience of violence. This world of religiously-shaped violence and violently-shaped religion is a habitat–"a system of language and practice that organizes the world in terms of what is deemed sacred" (Paden, 1994, p. 10).[6] "Within a single tradition like Christianity, there are thousands of religious worlds" (Paden, 1994, p. viii).[7] In a phenomenological comparative approach religious traditions are "not static and monolithic phenomena, [they are] constantly changing and shifting [their] identity in contact and relationship with each other" (Capps, 1995, p. 339).[8]

While my use of this interdisciplinary method is informed by postmodern approaches to knowledge, I acknowledge that the 'residual tradition' of many Christian communities and individuals draws primarily upon a premodern approach to religious knowledge, in which people believe that God reveals Godself to them, and this revelation is in some circumstances–like mystical experiences–seemingly directly apprehended, without the need for formal interpretation. Modern approaches to knowledge are also widely endorsed by many religiously-committed persons, especially in terms of knowledge gained through scientific methods of research or biblical critical methods of interpretation.

In my own formulation of how postmodern, modern, and premodern approaches to knowledge co-exist in the care of persons, I often find that people draw upon premodern approaches to religious knowledge in the midst of crises to formulate images of God as immediately present with them in their powerlessness. They turn to modern constructions, particular medical knowledge or biblical scholarship, when they need to rely on expert help in constructing ways to make sense of what is happening. They sometimes implicitly or explicitly assume postmodern approaches in formulating intrinsically meaningful ways of understanding their lives, particularly if they have the wisdom to appreciate that such meaning systems are one of a number of possible ways to make sense of their lives (Doehring, 2004; 2006).

The distinction that I make between premodern, modern, and postmodern approaches to religions knowledge is helpful in understanding how the critical correlation method that I use differs from the integration method[9] used by many evangelical Christian psychologists. Many of these psychologists implicitly use a premodern approach to religious sources of authority, like Scripture. As Browning and Cooper (2004) note, "evangelicals tend to enter the dialogue [between religion and psychology] with the conviction that Scripture provides an epistemologically privileged starting point" (p. 252). Along with using premodern approaches to the bible, evangelical psychologists often draw implicitly on what they assume to be a common theological perspective[10] or what they assume to be a shared formulation of a theistic worldview.[11]

As a liberal Protestant pastoral theologian using a social constructivist approach, I can chose among many available psychological and theological perspectives. My choices are guided by three criteria:

1. Contextual meaningfulness: Are these theological and psychological perspectives meaningful in exploring the particular experiences of the person in my case study? Do they help me and my client stay creatively faithful to her religious tradition?
2. Inter-disciplinary meaningfulness: Can the theological and psychological perspectives which seem most relevant become lively conversation partners in exploring the experience of the case study?
3. Pragmatic usefulness: Do these theological and psychological perspectives, which seem relevant and related to each other in an interdisciplinary way, lend themselves to the formulation of strategies for seeking healing and justice?

In this chapter, I will draw upon a psychodynamic model of personality–object relations theory–that includes theories about the formation of representations of God and a theological perspective that focuses on religious symbols and specifically symbols of God. These perspectives are relevant because they can be used to elaborate a contextual understanding of the ways in which the woman in my case study draws upon her deepest religious beliefs in her efforts to cope with sexual violence. I will bring Rizzuto's psychodynamic perspective on representations of God into dialogue with Neville's theology of broken symbols,[12] which I will elaborate after presenting the case study. I will supplement these perspectives with pastoral theological perspectives on sexual violence, along with some research by psychologists on religious coping and sexual violence to describe how this client and I found ways for her to draw upon her religious tradition in making sense of and coping with her experience of violence.

CASE STUDY

Client History

Winifred was a thirty-year old minister in the United Church of Christ (UCC), married, with a one-year old daughter when she began therapy with me at a pastoral counseling center in Boston. She had just experienced a psychological and spiritual crisis occasioned by a three-day silent retreat intended as a time to reflect spiritually on her first year of parenthood. She chose a Jesuit retreat center because she met there once a month in a peer support group of clergy that included a spiritual director whom she trusted. She had been raised as a Roman Catholic and the retreat center reconnected her with the most positive aspects of her childhood faith, particularly in its contemporary ecumenical expressions of religious faith in its liturgy and religious symbols, which she experienced as beautiful. She and her spiritual director chose some biblical texts that focused both on God as parent and God as child.

As she meditated on these texts, she returned to an experience as a pre-teen of being raped by an older teenager who assaulted her on her way home from school. The assault had been followed by a police investigation that was an ordeal. At the time, there were no community resources for victims of sexual violence. Her parents did not know how to help her, and she struggled privately with fears that she would be attacked again.

Now, as a young mother, she felt the weight of being responsible to protect her daughter from violence. For the first time, she was aware of being angry that God hadn't protected her and of feeling abandoned by God and her parents in the aftermath of the assault. In the midst of this anger she experienced a new love and empathy for herself as a child, which was mediated by the love she felt for her daughter. Out of these feelings emerged a revelation of a loving God who had cherished her and been present with her during the violence and its aftermath, much in the same way she cherished her daughter and wanted intensely to be present with her as she faced the dangers of the world.

Presenting Problem and Treatment Plan

Winifred realized that she needed counseling when, in the weeks following the retreat, she often felt overwhelmed by anxiety and anger, which initially centered on the demands of balancing work and parenthood. Some of her dreams depicted the anxiety that suffused her roles as preacher and worship leader. She had recurrent dreams about being in the pulpit and not being able to read her sermon text. She was often critical of herself and then became aware of how much she experienced me during therapy sessions as a critical, distant parent. She agreed to shift to twice-weekly psychotherapy as a way of better understanding these dynamics. The treatment plan was to uncover the underlying sources of her anxiety through insight-oriented psychodynamic psychotherapy, in which the relationship with her therapist would evoke the dynamics of formative relationships in childhood. Winifred could experience theses dynamics within the container of the therapeutic alliance, allowing her to (1) experience a sense of psychological safety, (2) name and mourn the losses associated with her experience of violence–losses shaped by early formative relationships–and (3) reconnect with the goodness of life.[13]

Through the transference she re-experienced the ways as a child she had shut out her mother as a means of protecting herself from her mother's anxiety. While she outwardly feared becoming dependent on me, she dreamt about trying to telephone me for help and finding over and over again that the phone wouldn't work. She also dreamt about suddenly remembering she had a baby which she had "forgotten" about and hadn't fed or taken care of for hours or even days. These dreams expressed her ambivalence about being a mother, and also her ambivalence about becoming dependent on me as her therapist.

Though she knew I was religiously committed, she struggled with talking about her religious faith in therapy, imagining that I would have the same faith she identified with her mother, a faith that included strict rules to be obeyed, harsh judgment, and an authoritarian, unforgiving father God. Sometimes the way I dressed or sat reminded her of the religious sister who had been the principal in the Roman Catholic elementary school she attended. She wore a full habit, which included a wimple. The day after she was assaulted, she had been called to the principal's office, and had to recount what had happened to several police officers in the presence of the principal. This was deeply shaming. As these fears about being exposed and shamed became more conscious, her anxieties about leading worship intensified.

A breakthrough occurred in therapy when she began to imagine that intrapsychically she was two people when she came to therapy: she was a mother, bringing with her a younger version of herself. This image helped her identify the ways in which she was protecting this "little Winnie" from me, as I was cast in the role of her anxious and non-empathic mother. She also realized how she played the role of both the empathic mother she was trying to become, and the mother she had experienced growing up. Identifying herself as the anxious unavailable mother helped her see past her projection of this mother onto me, and to appreciate the mystery of who I was.

This realization became theological when she wondered how much she experienced God as the unavailable God, whom she could not rely on because this God was "incompetent" in ways similar to her experience of her mother. With this breakthrough came both sadness and joy. She felt sad about how isolated she had been, and how much she had experienced God, the world, and me through a vision shuttered by anxiety and distrust. She felt joy when she experienced a newly-found sense of freedom and apprehension of beauty in her spiritual life, much of which was mediated by the arts, including both music and literature.

Case Conceptualization: An Object Relations Perspective

Object relations theory is a post-Freudian psychodynamic model of personality that understands "the human mind [as] representational. It deals with reality and achieves mastery over it by representing it in the psychic realm" (Rizzuto, 2004, p. 12). This "reality" consists primarily of the network of formative relationships with parents, siblings, and anyone who plays a role in a child's development. Intrapsychic, or internal representations of these relationships are complex and multifaceted: "We are not talking about images, but about an extraordinarily complex set of neurological and dynamic processes organized around the perceptual and fantasized conceptions of certain realities, which are arranged as memory processes" (Rizzuto, 2004, p. 13). This model of personality is relevant in understanding the ways in which Winifred as a child constructed images of her mother as anxious and unavailable and her self as both helpless and self-reliant. As a client she re-experienced this childhood relationship in the context of therapy

In a seminal text, *Birth of the Living God*, Rizzuto (1979) describes her experiences of how clients in psychoanalysis brought "God" into the room, and her conjectures about how internal representations of the relationship between God and self are formed.

> A believer's representation of God is formed by the vast coordinates of multiple memory processes of bodily sensation, experienced affects, relational exchanges, fantasized interpretations of those exchanges, thoughts and beliefs about primary objects [that is, relationships] and objects in the present, all of which become organized by their affective and representational connection with the code word 'God.' (Rizzuto, 2004, p. 16)

Representations of God have a "mediatory psychic function which makes it possible to think about or relate to a being who is not perceptible" (Rizzuto, 2004, p. 12). Rizzuto's formulation of God representations can easily be brought into dialogue with a social constructionist approach to understanding how religious worlds are constructed out of a person's idiosyncratic experience of her familial, communal, religious and cultural contexts.

In the case study, when Winifred goes on retreat she is confronted with multiple images of God. There is the God who, like her parents, abandoned her and was "incompetent" to protect her. There are also glimpses of a God who mothered in the way she wanted to mother.[14] There is a sense of a transcendent presence apprehended through the beauty of the liturgy, the religious symbols, and the natural surroundings of the retreat center.

As therapy unfolded, the more negative images of God initially multiplied and intensified,[15] as she re-experienced formative relationships, and the anxiety, anger, and longings featured in these relationships. What emerged more clearly was the sense of being shamed and exposed in the assault and the investigation that followed, dynamics that were at the unconscious core of her identity as a minister, and which generated the conscious anxieties about leading worship. This was a "God" "made flesh" in the stern countenance of the religious sister who un-movingly heard her testimony.

In retrospect, Winifred could appreciate how much she had created a God whose limitations, similar to her mother's limitations, allowed her to be in charge. Winifred's less-than-all-powerful God left her ultimately in control, with her God representations "under the regulatory influence of psychic defenses" that helped her "to sustain . . . affective equilibrium" (Rizzuto, 2004, p. 13). The price paid for such a bargain was eruptions of anxiety whenever the dangers of violence or shameful exposure seemed imminent. The limitations of her power to protect her child from harm were made plain to her when she went on retreat.

When a breakthrough occurred in the transference, Winifred could see the ways in which she had constructed representations of God that allowed her to be in charge. She began to appreciate how much she organized her world so that she would not have to rely on anyone, including her therapist. With this breakthrough, Winifred began to engage me differently in therapy. She was much more able to be spontaneous in an unguarded way. We began together to co-construct narratives of what her childhood had been like. These became theological work when she talked about her religious and spiritual experiences. I turn now to theological perspectives on God images as religious symbols, in order to appreciate the theological dimensions of this clinical work.

Case Conceptualization Continued: A Theological Perspective on How God Is Symbolized

As a theologically-educated psychotherapist, I was able to draw upon theological perspectives in assessing and reflecting with Winifred on her experience of God. A perspective that was particularly relevant and meaningful was Robert Neville's elaboration of Paul Tillich's (1951) theology of the role of broken symbols in religious faith.

There can be no doubt that any concrete assertion about God must be symbolic, for a concrete assertion is one which uses a segment of finite experience in order to say something about [God]. . . . The segment of infinite reality which becomes the vehicle of a concrete assertion about God is affirmed and negated at the same time. It becomes a symbol, for symbolic expression is one whose proper meaning is negated by that to which it points. And yet it is also affirmed by it, and this affirmation gives the symbolic expression an adequate basis for pointing beyond itself (p. 239).

Religious symbols are formed on the boundary that de-marks what we identify as the known world and the unknown. "Religious symbols symbolize the infinite but themselves are finite" (Neville, 1996, p. x).

One of the problems that can occur with religious symbols is when a symbol becomes identified as sacred itself, and becomes worshiped and revered as if it were God. For example, the Gospel according to Mark (2:27) recounts the story of Jesus challenging the ways in which the religious laws governing the Sabbath had made the practices of keeping the Sabbath into a form of idolatry. A related problem occurs when religious symbols are used to justify social and organizational systems that maintain injustice and oppression, like gender oppression or racism. A symbol breaks when we can see the imitations and liabilities of our religious constructions. "A broken symbol is one that effectively engages us but whose limitations are known" (Neville, 1996, p. x). When symbols fail to engage people in this way, they may be dead or idolatrous (Neville, 1996, p. 62).

Neville's use of Tillich's notion of broken symbols helped me understand Winifred's religious experiences. As Winifred's symbols of God as distant, critical, shaming, and ultimately powerless became more conscious they became more "real" to Winifred, particularly in the religious context of worship, and in the dynamics of the transference as I became the parent from whom she had to protect her vulnerable childself. Bringing these symbols into consciousness upset the delicate intrapsychic balance by which, in the past, she could maintain ultimate "control" over her God, her mother, and her "world"–control that had become necessary when violence made the world unsafe and dangerous.

This balance was disrupted initially in the experience of being on retreat, when her religious experience of a living God mediated in the biblical texts and liturgy began to break through the symbols of God formed out of the traumatic events of her sexual assault and its aftermath. Unfortunately for her, these symbols were not "dead," but had taken on a tenacious psychic life of their own, in ways that Neville would describe as "demonic"–"engaging the divine but misrepresenting it"–in ways that can "lead to depravity with unbounded energy" (Neville, 1996, p. 237). Sin, in the sense of life-limiting relationships, was evident in the ways in which she objectified her mother and in turn her therapist. As well, she had constructed a false self who was in charge of a "God" who was too small.

Ultimately, the experience of the transference in psychotherapy caused the representation of the therapist as the distant critical parent to break. As fissures appeared in this representation, so also the symbol of a limited, distant God began to crack. However, before the constricting representations finally toppled, there was a time of intense anxiety, when the psychic and spiritual regime constructed in the aftermath of the assault was experienced as having a demonic life of its own. The psychic container formed through the trials of psychotherapy became a background of safety that held Winifred psychically and spiritually. From the shards of broken religious symbols she began piecing together transformative symbols. These mosaics contained many remnants from her early childhood faith, along with her love of the arts that had kept her spiritually alive throughout her childhood and adult spiritual life.

Interventions: The Work Generated by the Transference

Another way to describe this transformative process is to say that the dynamics of the transference triggered an intrapsychic earthquake, uncovering an embedded theology that had been latent in her childhood and constructed in her experience of trauma. This theology was the best she could construct on her own, at that stage in her faith development. In her experience of becoming a mother, this theology became inadequate, because it basically was built upon a distrust of the world and God. Giving up this embedded theology was risky because it meant that she would have to trust others, and at moments this felt too dangerous. Her relationship with her therapist, along with the God she had glimpsed on retreat became the fragile connections that began to form a web of life in which she could feel held and to which she could entrust her child.

Duration of Treatment, Termination, and Therapeutic Outcomes

Winifred was in treatment for three years, and therapy ended when she relocated to begin a graduate degree program in counseling. From a social constructivist perspective, one of the outcomes of therapy was that Winifred now had narrative ways of understanding the sources of her anxiety. When she experienced anxiety, she could empathically connect with the childhood experiences that generated anxiety, and she could understand this anxiety from the perspective of her adult alliance with me as her therapist. She also could name the ways in which her religious faith and vocation had been shaped by both her formative relationships and her experience of violence. She now had a narrative framework for naming the embedded images of God that surfaced under stress, and she could draw more readily upon her adult experiences of religious faith and theological education to deliberate over these embedded theologies, in terms of their relevance to her adult life. Having co-constructed narrative ways of understanding the stress associated with her ministerial roles, she experienced much less stress, becoming more relaxed and spontaneous, particularly in leading worship, preaching, and in her practice of pastoral care. The lessening of anxiety and the deepening of self empathy enabled her to enjoy her work and to imagine a new future for herself, one that included further studies and training in pastoral theology.

CONCLUSION

This chapter illustrates an interdisciplinary approach to psychotherapy with victims of violence, an approach that draws upon postmodern approaches to both psychological and religious knowledge. This approach allows me to appreciate the unique ways in which people construct images of themselves, God, and the world that help them cope with violence. The modality of pastoral psychotherapy provides a form of care that allows these images to be experienced in the therapeutic relationship, and then understood as therapist and client co-construct meanings that can be psychological and theological. In reflecting upon the process of change that occurred in this particular case study, I drew upon a psychodynamic understanding of God representations and a theological understanding of religious symbols because these theoretical perspectives met my criteria of contextual relevance, interdisciplinary meaningfulness, and pragmatic usefulness. These criteria provide a way to assess the contextual truthfulness of religious and psychological knowledge within the framework of postmodern approaches to knowledge. This chapter illustrates how such approaches to knowledge can be utilized within the traditions of liberal Protestant pastoral theology, in pastoral psychotherapy with victims of violence.

NOTES

1. "We are hearing a lot about sexual violence because many women are beginning to break the silence and tell about their experiences. The taboos about speaking the truth are being set aside, and shocking stories are being heard" (Poling, 1991, p. 11).
2. "When our very beings are violated through physical and sexual violence, this is a desecration of the inner sanctuary" (Doehring, 1993, p. xv).
3. "Some victims of rape and abuse have found hope in the crucifixion in the sense that, through his suffering, Jesus stands in solidarity with their suffering and there is no suffering that is unknown to God" (Cooper-White, 1995, p. 94)
4. "*Abuse of power is a theological problem.* Sexual violence is not just a function of a pathological self or oppressive institutions and ideologies of society. It is also hid-

den in the images of God in the Bible... The theme of the violence of God in the Bible and in church beliefs under some conditions provides latent sanctions for certain forms of human violence" (Poling, 1991, p. 155).

"The problem with the theory of substitutionary atonement [Jesus as the substitute sacrifice for sinners] in relation to the issue of sexual violence is the image of an abusive God against which the children of creation have no power or moral claim. The omnipotence and perfection of God create a unilateral relationship in which humans are in constant danger from an enraged God. The only protection is for the children to be submissive and obedient to God by praising the father and the son and living sanctified lives" (Poling, 1991, p. 170).

"Sometimes Jesus's crucifixion is misinterpreted as being the model for suffering. Since Jesus went to the cross, according to this interpretation, persons should bear their own crosses of irrational violence (for example, rape) without complaint. Rather than the *sanctification of suffering*, Jesus's crucifixion remains a witness to the horror of violence. It is not a model of how *suffering should be borne*, but a witness to God's desire that no one should have to suffer such violence again" (Fortune, 2005, p. 140).

5. Among Protestant practical theologians, Browning and Cooper (2004) have most fully elaborated the use of hermeneutic philosophy for "uncovering the religious or visional levels of the various modern psychologies" (p. ix).

6. "The concept of world provides a tool for understanding and analyzing the plurality, contextuality and self-positing nature of religious cultures" (Paden, 2000, p. 334).

7. "Religious language and behavior are not just beliefs and acts *about* the world, but actual ways through which a world comes into being" (Paden, 1994, p. 54). "The notion of world calls attention to the radical cultural and geographical diversity among and within religious systems" (Paden, 1994, p. 55).

8. "If the comparative approach acknowledges many worlds, it does so not to 'agree' with them on the one hand or to reduce them to 'merely' human projections on the other, but rather to approach the subject matter in a manner appropriate to the goals of understanding and description. The comparativist's polycentric universe is not in itself a person or metaphysical position . . . but a phenomenological premise required by the field of study" (Paden, 1994, p. 168).

9. In surveying this broad and varied literature, Eck (1996), Worthington (1994), and Collins (2000) all note that no agreement on a theoretical-conceptual method of "integration" has emerged.

10. See, for example, Johnson's (1997) theologically-oriented article, in the 25th anniversary issue of the *Journal of Psychology and Theology*. Johnson develops the theological concept of the kingdom of God and the components of what he calls kingdom psychology.

11. While not explicitly privileging the Bible as a unique source of religious authority, Richards and Bergin have proposed a theistic approach to psychotherapy in which a one-sentence proposition about God-stated as a premodern faith claim-is presented as the core belief common to all five world religions.

12. Pastoral theologian Deborah Hunsinger (1995) also engages Rizzuto's psychodynamic perspectives on God representations with a theological perspective. In her work, she uses Rizzuto to assess whether God representations are functional or dysfunctional; she uses theologian Karl Barth to assess whether a God representation is theologically adequate or inadequate.

13. These goals have been identified by Herman (1992). Elsewhere I have described these goals using the metaphor of reconsecration of the inner sanctum of the psyche: "Recovery involves, first, creating safety and trust, enough to empower one to return to the scene of desecration. Next, one must sift through the rubble and reconstruct the experience of desecration, while mourning the loss of the inner sanctum and all that was associated with it. The final stage of recovery will be to build new inner sanctums and reconsecrate them. Reconsecration may happen in the ordinary moments of reconnecting with everyday life, when one experiences the sanctity of life, the blessedness of creation, and the goodness of one's body (Doehring, 1993, p. 137)."

14. "Theologian Jane Grovijahn [1997], in her study of sexual abuse survivors' narratives, has idenitifed ways in which the inner God imago may also be split by the traumatic experience into one or more versions of "Good God," "God gone wrong," and "no-God" (Cooper-White, 2006).

15. "When the child's development has taken place in an emotionally an religiously meaningful environment, the representation of the divinity may be multifaceted and complex. On the other hand, disturbed relationships during development . . . may present a divine being dominated by few and stark traits" (Rizzuto, 2004, p. 20).

REFERENCES

Browning, D. S., & Cooper, T. D. (2004). *Religious thought and the modern psychologies* (2nd ed.). Minneapolis: Fortress.

Capps, W. (1995). *Religious studies: The making of a discipline.* Minneapolis: Fortress.

Collins, G. R. (2000). An integrative view. In E. L. Johnson & S. L. Jones (Eds.), *Psychology and Christianity: Four views* (pp. 101-129). Downers Grove, IL: InterVarsity Press.

Cooper-White, P. (1995). *Tamar's cry: Violence against women and the church's response.* Minneapolis: Fortress.

Cooper-White, P. (2006). *Many voices: Pastoral psychotherapy in relational and theological perspective.* Minneapolis: Augsburg.

Doehring, C. (1993). *Internal desecration: Traumatization and representations of God.* Lanham, MD: University Press of America.

Doehring, C. (2004). The challenges of bridging pastoral care experiences and postmodern approaches to knowledge. *Journal of Pastoral Theology* 14 (1), 1-14.

Doehring, C. (2006). *The practice of pastoral care: A postmodern approach.* Louisville: Westminster John Knox.

Eck, B. E. (1996). Integrating the integrators: An organizing framework for a process of integration. *Journal of Psychology and Christianity, 15,* 101-115.

Fortune, M. M. (2005). *Sexual violence: The sin revisited.* Cleveland: Pilgrim.

Gergen, K. J. (2001). Psychological science in a post-modern context. *American Psychologist, 56 (10),* 803-813.

Grovijahn, J. (1997). *A theology of survival.* Unpublished PhD dissertation. Graduate Theological Union, Berkeley, CA.

Herman, J. (1992). *Trauma and recovery: The aftermath of violence–From domestic abuse to political terror.* New York: BasicBooks.

Hunsinger, D.V.D. (1995). *Theology and pastoral counseling: A new interdisciplinary approach.* Grand Rapids: Eerdmans.

Johnson, E. L. (1997). Christ, the Lord of psychology. *Journal of Psychology and Theology, 25,* 11-27.

Neville, R. (1996). *The truth of broken symbols.* New York: SUNY.

Paden, W. E. (1994). *Religious worlds: The comparative study of religion* (2nd ed.). Boston: Beacon.

Paden, W. E. (2000). World. In Willi Braun & Russell T. McCutcheon (Eds.), *Guide to the Study of Religion* (pp. 334-347). London: Cassell.

Poling, J. N., & Miller, D. E. (1985). *Foundations for a practical theology of ministry.* Nashville: Abingdon.

Poling, J. N. (1991). *The abuse of power: A theological problem.* Nashville: Abingdon.

Richards, P. S., & Bergin, A. E.. (2005). *A spiritual strategy for counseling and psychotherapy* (2nd ed). Washington, DC: American Psychological Association.

Tillich, P. (1959). *Theology of culture.* New York: Oxford University Press.

Rizzuto, A. M. (1979). *Birth of the living God: A psychoanalytic study.* Chicago: University of Chicago.

Rizzuto, A. M. (2004). Psychodynamic processes in religious and spiritual life. *Pastoral Sciences, 23(2),* 9 - 28.

doi:10.1300/J515v09n03_10

PART III
FUTURE DIRECTIONS

Chapter 11

Measurement Issues
in God Image Research and Practice

Nicholas J.S. Gibson, PhD

SUMMARY. People think and feel about God in a far more complex way than is acknowledged by current measurement approaches. A review of the social cognition literature as it applies to the representation of God in mind provides a helpful corrective and allows a more sophisticated perspective on what can be measured and how

Correspondence concerning this chapter should be addressed to Nicholas Gibson, Psychology and Religion Research Group, Faculty of Divinity, West Road, Cambridge, CB3 9BS, UK (E-mail: njsjg2@hermes.cam.ac.uk).

This work was supported by John Templeton Foundation grant 10701 to Fraser Watts and John Polkinghorne.

[Haworth co-indexing entry note]: "Measurement Issues in God Image Research and Practice." Gibson, Nicholas J.S. Co-published simultaneously in *Journal of Spirituality in Mental Health* (The Haworth Pastoral Press, an imprint of The Haworth Press) Vol. 9, No. 3/4, 2007, pp. 227-246; and: *God Image Handbook for Spiritual Counseling and Psychotherapy: Research, Theory, and Practice* (ed: Glendon L. Moriarty, and Louis Hoffman) The Haworth Pastoral Press, an imprint of The Haworth Press, 2007, pp. 227-246. Single or multiple copies of this article are available for a fee from The Haworth Document Delivery Service [1-800-HAWORTH, 9:00 a.m. - 5:00 p.m. (EST). E-mail address: docdelivery@haworthpress.com].

doi:10.1300/J515v09n03_11

to measure it. Such a review reveals multiple limitations with current measurement approaches and indicates the benefits that the introduction of cognitive techniques may bring. The review also suggests specific improvements that could be made in the use of existing quantitative methods in research and clinical practice. doi:

10.1300/J515v09n03_11 *[Article copies available for a fee from The Haworth Document Delivery Service: 1-800-HAWORTH. E-mail address: <docdelivery@ haworthpress.com> Website: <http://www.HaworthPress.com> © 2007 by The Haworth Press. All rights reserved.]*

A moderate familiarity with the psychology of religion literature might lead one to the conclusion that measuring mental representations of God is a straightforward and exact task. After all, so many measures exist that an entire chapter of Hill and Hood's (1999b) *Measures of Religiosity* is devoted to reviewing them. Moreover, a multiplicity of papers have been published in which researchers have explored correlative relationships between these measures and other variables of interest. It is unfortunate, then, that the measurement of representations of God is neither straightforward nor exact. At best, current approaches to measurement give only a partial picture of how believers and unbelievers represent God in mind; at worst, current approaches may provide meaningless or even misleading data.

My purpose in this chapter is not to duplicate the work of Hill and Hood (1999b) in reviewing specific measures. Rather I wish to reflect at a more fundamental level on the endeavor of measurement as it pertains to mental representations of God. First, I will consider what we are trying to measure in more detail by drawing on the social cognition literature to give a clearer picture of how God is represented in mind. Second, I will critique existing measurement approaches in the light of this framework. Finally, I will consider how we may circumvent the problems inherent in current approaches and make some recommendations for the assessment of representations of God in clinical and pastoral work and future research.

WHAT ARE WE MEASURING?

With few exceptions, measurement of mental representations of God has been concerned with isolating individual differences in content, and that particularly with regard to the character of God. This content is variously termed the *God concept*, *God image*, or *God representation*. The lack of consensus regarding what these terms signify well illustrates the inadequate conceptual basis in extant work for what we are trying to measure (Spilka, 2000). Some psychologists of religion use all three terms interchangeably (e.g., Hill & Hall, 2002), while others make explicit distinctions between them, as in this volume. Rizzuto (1979) argued for a propositional level God concept and multiple emotional-related God images, all composing the God representation. Other workers, however, have simplified Rizzuto's structure and refer instead to a God concept and a God image as though each were a single construct (e.g., Hoffman, 2005; Lawrence, 1997). In such cases, the God concept is defined similarly to Rizzuto, as an intellectualized, theological, or cognitive understanding of God. The God image, however, receives an inconsistent treatment. Despite drawing directly on Rizzuto's distinctions, Lawrence (1997) uses *God image* and *God representation* interchangeably, though with a preference for the former. Hoffman (2004) meanwhile does not refer to a God representation at all, and defines the God image as "a person's emotional experience of God" (p. 2), the content of which may be undifferentiated and at an unconscious level.

What are we to make of all this inconsistency? Though use of specific terms has been haphazard, a common theme is that of researchers trying to find ways to refer to two types of content regarding God, one that is propositional or doctrinal in nature ("head knowledge") and one that is emotional and experiential in nature ("heart knowledge"). In terms of the language used to describe these two contrasting mental representations, *God concept* is usefully retained to refer to propositional level knowledge. Inconsistent use of the terms *image* and *representation* together with the potential confusion created through lack of awareness of their technical senses within particular psychological subdisciplines suggests that these terms could helpfully be abandoned altogether except in their general sense; talk of *images* in particular is open to misinterpretation, suggesting literal pictorial images. Given the schematic nature of experiential mental representations, it would seem most sensible to follow the majority of social and cognitive psychologists working within the dominant information processing paradigm in using the alternative term *schema* (Fiske & Linville, 1980; see also Fiske & Taylor, 1991), and I will do so in the remainder of this chapter.

Nomenclature aside, being able to distinguish between these two quite different ways of holding knowledge about God is vital. Unfortunately, psychologists of religion have neglected affect and emotion in their theories, choosing instead to focus on propositional beliefs (cf. Hill, 1994, 1995; Watts, 1996). Yet as Rizzuto (1979) and Watts and Williams (1988) have acknowledged, information about God at these two levels can be in conflict, and empirical researchers need to investigate this possibility. There is a gradual recognition of the need to address this neglect within the study of religion, and several workers have made efforts to account for emotional beliefs in recent models of religious belief (Hall, 2003; 2004; Hill & Hood, 1999a; Watts, in press; see also Pyysiäinen, 2004). Indeed, this volume is an attempt to redress the balance specifically within the study of how people think about God.

Simply distinguishing between propositional God concepts and experiential God schemas is not sufficient, however. Accurate measurement requires a still more sophisticated description of how God is represented in mind. We need to understand something about what a mental representation of God actually is–how it is structured, when it is used, and how it relates to other mental representations. Help is at hand from the social cognition literature, a subdiscipline of social psychology that has applied the theory and findings of cognitive psychology to the representation of social phenomena. In particular, much of what we can expect to be true about how God is represented can be inferred from what we already know about how people represent information about themselves, about other people, and about relationships with other people. The following brief review of the functioning of social-cognitive schemas will provide a richer framework from which to consider issues of measurement.

COGNITIVE SCHEMAS FOR GOD

Fiske and Taylor (1991) define a schema as "a cognitive structure that represents knowledge about a concept or type of stimulus, including its attributes and the relations among those attributes" (p. 98). People unconsciously use schemas as conceptual frameworks to organize their experience and knowledge: schemas influence what people pay attention to, how they store new information, what they can remember, and how they make decisions. As such, once laid down, schemas are relatively stable, and people try to make new experiences or information fit the existing content of a schema rather than altering the schema to fit new data (Neisser, 1976). The precise cognitive structure of a social schema is not yet clear, but it has aspects both of a collection of specific examples of encounters of whatever the schema represents and of generalizations abstracted across multiple experiences (Fiske & Taylor, 1991; Park, 1986; Sherman & Klein, 1994).

It should be clear then, that a person's schema for God will consist of far more than a simple list of attributes. Rather, as McIntosh (1995) has suggested, "a God schema might include, for example, assumptions about the physical nature of God, God's will or purposes, God's means of influence, and the interrelations among these beliefs" (p. 2). It is important to note that people's God schemas will differ not just in content but also in structure, degree of organization, and personal relevance. Since social schemas share similar functional properties regardless of content (Fiske & Taylor, 1991), we can draw on what social psychologists have discovered about self-schemas, person schemas, and relational schemas to help us understand several important aspects of how God schemas work.

People Hold Multiple Schemas for God

A simplistic assumption made by the majority of researchers is that people hold a single concept or image of God. This is unlikely to be the case. Just as people have been shown to have schemas for possible future selves such as *ideal self* and *ought self* in addition to *actual self* (Higgins, 1987, 1989; Markus & Nurius, 1986), people are likely to have multiple schemas for God. These may include *the God I believe in* (or *the God I don't believe in*), *the God I'm supposed to believe in, the God I wish existed, the God my friend believes in, the Christian God, the Muslim God, the Bearded Old Man Who Lives in the Clouds*, and so on. Any attempt to measure how a person represents God in mind may therefore need to measure several different schemas for God, or at least specify a particular schema of interest. While instructional variations may be able to distinguish among different concepts (e.g., Gibson, 2006; Schaap-Jonker, Eurelings-Bontekoe, Zock, & Jonker, in press) few studies have acknowledged that any distinctions are even necessary.

People Differ in the Complexity of Their God Schemas

A related concept is that of *self complexity* (Linville, 1985; 1987). Some individuals view themselves in terms of multiple roles (e.g., professor, wife, daughter, violinist) while others in terms of only one or two principal roles. Multiple roles have been shown to act as a protective buffer against negative life events (Niedenthal, Setterlund, & Wherry, 1992) and suggest that those with a high degree of self complexity may have a more compartmentalized organization of self-knowledge than a unitary self construct would allow. Just as people differ in self complexity, so too do people differ in the complexity of their God schemas. Such differences are easily observed by comparing faith traditions; for example, a Jewish individual may conceive simply of YHWH, a Christian may view God in terms of the multiple persons within the Trinity of Father, Son, and Holy Spirit. However, individuals are likely to differ in the complexity of their God schemas even within a given tradition: one Christian, for example, may view Jesus in terms of multiple roles (e.g., savior, friend, king, judge, lover, creator, Son of God), whereas another Christian may view Jesus in terms of just one or two principal roles (cf. Roof & Roof, 1984). Sound assessment of a Christian's God schemas must therefore consider the possibility of differences in content both between different persons of the Trinity and also within the different roles each person plays.

God Schemas Are Dynamic

If a believer does have multiple God schemas, each with its own complexity, it seems unlikely that he or she will be able to maintain all of these ideas in mind at the same time. This leads us to the concept of a *working God schema*. Markus and Kunda (1986) note that only a portion of one's self-knowledge is accessible or salient at any given moment, and changes in mood or situation can trigger shifts in this working self-concept. Similarly, it seems likely that the way in which people think about God will change dynamically according to the constraints of mood and situation (Hill & Hall, 2002; Thurston, 1994). A charismatic worship service, a Bible study, and sitting in a foxhole while under fire are each likely to activate different God schemas.

Occasionally more than one God schema may become salient simultaneously. Just as salient discrepancies between, for example, *ideal self* and *actual self* lead to feelings of loss, sadness, and dejection (Higgins, Bond, Klein, & Strauman, 1986; Higgins, Shah, & Friedman, 1997), we can predict that making salient a disparity between two God schemas also leads to specific emotions. Precisely which emotions obtain will depend in a complex way on motivational goals: for example, a salient discrepancy between *the God I'm supposed to believe in* and *the God I actually believe in* may lead to feelings of doubt, skepticism, or challenge, depending on whether the individual noticing the discrepancy is a struggling believer, an apostate, or a seeker, respectively. It may even be the role of the therapist to bring two or more schemas into dialogue.

God Schemas Are Hierarchical

Schemas are organized in relation to each other in loose hierarchies such that, for example, schemas for individual traits are superordinate to schemas for self (Rogers, Kuiper, & Kirker, 1977). Trait-level schemas are powerful ways of organizing social information (Markus, 1977; Markus, Smith, & Moreland, 1985) and it is important to note that where the schema for a given trait is poorly elaborated it is unlikely to be used at the level of person schemas. This suggests that if an individual does not possess a schema for a given trait then it will not contribute toward that individual's overall God schema. A person may understand what a given trait word means, such as *forgiving*, but unless that definition has been fleshed out with ideas of what forgiveness looks like, what it feels like to forgive and to be forgiven, how forgiveness can be distinguished from excusing, pardoning, explaining away, and so on, the idea of a forgiving God may not mean very much. Another important aspect in measurement, then, is to consider how people understand God's various attributes in the first place.

God Schemas Are Relational

A considerable body of research indicates that the representation of social information is not necessarily discrete. Rather, information about other persons is held in a rich overlapping schematic network centered on the self and significant others. Relational schemas consist of representations of self and of others together with an interpersonal script for typical patterns of interaction generalized from past experience (for reviews see Andersen & Chen, 2002; Andersen, Chen, & Miranda, 2002; Aron, Aron, Tudor, & Nelson, 1991; Baldwin, 1992, 1999, 2001; Markus et al., 1985). Preliminary evidence from questionnaire measures suggests an overlap between representations of self and Jesus and of self and God (Piedmont, Williams, & Ciarrocchi, 1997; Ciarrocchi, Piedmont, & Williams, 2002). Hill and Hood (2002) have also suggested this possibility, noting that one example of an internal script is an individual's attachment style (cf. Kirkpatrick, 1999). This has implications for measurement of representations of God because the strength of connection between God schemas and self schemas will affect the influence God schemas have on a person (McIntosh, 1995).

REVIEW OF EXISTING MEASUREMENT TOOLS

With a clearer idea of the complexity of what we are trying to measure, we can now assess examples of existing tools for the measurement of representations of God.

Quantitative Tasks

Psychologists of religion have used a wide variety of survey-based quantitative techniques to investigate mental representations of God (Hill & Hood, 1999b). Scales designed specifically include adjective check lists (e.g., Gorsuch, 1968), semantic differentials (e.g., Benson & Spilka, 1973; Francis, Robbins, & Gibson, 2006), Likert-scale responses to a series of items (e.g., Lawrence, 1991, 1997) or short statements (e.g., Lindeman, Pyysiäinen, & Saariluoma, 2002), and the ranking of attributes (e.g., Lalljee, Brown, & Hilton, 1990). Another approach is to adapt a measurement technique from personality psychology; for example, Piedmont and colleagues have used Gough and Heilbrum's (1983) Adjective Check List to measure perceptions of God within the five-factor personality framework (Piedmont, Ciarrocchi, & Williams, 2002). While survey-based measures, when reliable and valid, have proved their worth in the measurement of many religious dimensions (Hill, 2005), it is difficult to say how much studies employing these methods can tell us about how God is represented–either in general, or in a given person.

Survey measures of God share flaws common to self-report measures in general. One issue with any survey-based measure of representations of God is that self-report measures suffer multiple problems with validity: failure to discriminate within certain samples; bias toward specific populations, limitations with what can be measured with closed-ended questions, the requirement of adult-level reading abilities, and the effects of a social desirability response set. Critical reviews of measurement issues in psychology of religion have mentioned all of these problems (Batson, Schoenrade, & Ventis, 1993; Gorsuch, 1990; Hill & Pargament, 2003; Slater, Hall, & Edwards, 2001) yet too many workers seem to shrug them off as if they somehow do not apply to them!

Survey measures may ignore important aspects of God representations. Survey measures can only provide data in response to the questions asked, and here lies another problem: the selection of items. Most researchers have used attributes of their own selection, terms of biblical origin, or terms from previous lists to attain some sort of comparison value between studies. For example, Lawrence (1991, 1997) constructed a 156-item inventory with eight subscales designed to measure different aspects of a respondent's God image. Unfortunately, such an approach can ignore important aspects of people's representations of God. Indeed, a factor analysis of Lawrence's inventory yielded ten factors, of which seven contained items from at least two of his theoretical eight scales, making it quite uncertain what scores on these scales actually represent. A related problem is that the meaning of specific items may change from individual to individual. For example, Hutsebaut and Verhoeven (1995) found that the factor some items loaded onto changed according to whether the group was believers, doubters, or unbelievers. This is certainly an issue for anyone trying to use instruments standardized on a Christian population to measure representations of God among populations who may be questioning their belief in God.

Survey measures may be limited to propositional beliefs. Information about God held at a schematic level cannot easily be verbalized and must be first translated into propositional (conceptual) form (Watts, in press). When responding to direct measurement techniques such as surveys people are therefore actually providing answers from their conceptual knowledge. It is clear, then, that no survey method can provide a pure read-off of a person's God schemas. For this reason, attempts such as that of Hall, Tisdale, and Brokaw (1994) to divide questionnaires up into those that measure what they call *God concept* (e.g., Loving and Controlling God Scales, Benson & Spilka, 1973; e.g., Religious Concept Survey, Gorsuch, 1968) and those that measure what they call *personal experience of God* (e.g., God Image Inventory, Lawrence, 1991; e.g., God Questionnaire, Rizzuto, 1979) are probably not helpful. Indeed, Hoffman, Jones, Williams, and Dillard (2004) failed to find a hypothesized empirical distinction between the God concept (as measured by the Religious Concept Survey, Gorsuch, 1968) and the God image (as measured by the God Image Scales, Lawrence, 1997). The best that can be hoped for is that a survey, when used appropriately, will pick up conceptual knowledge that has been colored by schematic knowledge.

Survey measures provide poor indicators of underlying cognitive structures. The vast majority of studies attempting to measure representations of God do so to explore correlations between these representations and other variables of interest (Gibson, 2006; Spilka, 2000). The problem is that correlative use of survey methods provides little indication of the organization of representations of God in relation to the rest of a person's cognitive functioning. Even where we can demonstrate a correlation between representations of God and some other variable, we are no wiser with regard to the causal links between the two. Suggesting a causal link is often too tempting to avoid, however. A typical conclusion from one of these studies is that of Benson and Spilka (1973): on finding that self-esteem is positively related to loving, accepting God images, and negatively related to rejecting images, they concluded that self-esteem may be a major determinant of God images. But alternative causal stories are equally conceivable: high self-esteem could be the product of a positive God image; alternatively some third intercorrelated variable such as attachment style might mediate both self-esteem and God image. Even when using sophisticated statistical techniques such as factor analysis (Gorsuch, 1968) or concept mapping (e.g., Kunkel, Cook, Meshel, Daughtry, & Hauenstein, 1999) to elucidate the structure of representations of God, it is unclear whether the conceptual structures indicated are replicated at the schematic level.

Qualitative Tasks

Qualitative methodologies provide a way of avoiding many of these limitations, and several psychologists of religion have explored such techniques, particularly when working with children. These have included asking open-ended questions (Hutsebaut & Verhoeven, 1995; W. C. Nye & Carlson, 1984), extended interviews (Rizzuto, 1979; Hay & Nye, 1998; R. Nye, 1999), writing a letter to God (Heller, 1986), or interpreting images and drawings (Bassett et al., 1990; Bassett, Perry, Repass, Silver, & Welch, 1994). There are of course drawbacks with qualitative measures, including the lack of standardization, time-consuming data collection and analysis, and difficulty in developing metrics for comparing individuals or groups. Nevertheless, qualitative techniques have the particular advantage of allowing respondents to use their own vocabulary to describe their beliefs about and experiences of God, and judicious use of analytical tools such as grounded theory can provide a powerful method for hypothesis generation and potentially even model testing (Denzin & Lincoln, 2005).

Cognitive Tasks

A new approach to measuring religious belief that avoids many of the problems associated with self-report measures is to adapt indirect measurement techniques from the cognition and emotion and social cognition literatures (Gibson, 2006). These techniques typically involve measuring participants' speed or accuracy in performing tasks in such a way that reveals the underlying cognitive structures and processes. Although no general review of these techniques exists to my knowledge, there are several helpful reviews of their use within cognitive, social, and clinical psychology (Eysenck & Keane, 2005; Musch & Klauer, 2003; Williams, Watts, MacLeod, & Mathews, 1997).

Measuring God's powers. Most of the techniques mentioned so far have been employed to measure beliefs about God's character. Indeed, psychologists of religion have given little consideration to how people think about God's supernatural properties, such as being everywhere at once, knowing everything, and being able to do anything. Powers like these stretch our understanding, and although Christians will readily affirm in a questionnaire that God possesses these powers, some psychologists have questioned the ability of people to use these beliefs in their everyday thinking about God.

Barrett and colleagues used a technique that involved experimental participants listening to a story and subsequently being asked to recall whether information was featured in the story (Barrett, 1998; Barrett & Keil, 1996; Barrett & VanOrman, 1996). In comprehending a narrative the reader's conceptual knowledge is used to draw inferences that are not made explicit in the text (Bransford & McCarrell, 1974), and Barrett used this principle to demonstrate that in understanding stories about God Christian adults often used an anthropomorphic concept of God that was inconsistent with their stated beliefs about God's supernatural attributes. So, for example, a participant might state in a questionnaire that God is everywhere simultaneously, but subsequently mistakenly recall a narrative featuring God as though God could not simultaneously be in two places. It is still an open question, however, as to whether the effects observed here are limitations in people's cognitive capacities or rather that people are capable of using theologically correct information about God's powers, albeit only under certain circumstances or motivational conditions. A blocked goal might be just one such circumstance, and indeed, it seems likely that a person who gets angry at God for not acting to avert some disaster is at some level conceiving of God as omnipotent–there is after all no point in getting angry at someone who is powerless to act. Considerable further work is needed here to understand how cognitive representations of God's powers interact representations of God's character.

Measuring God's character. Cognitive techniques can also be used to investigate how people represent God's character, and cognitive schemas for persons have several properties making them amenable to investigation measuring biases in memory for material. For example, when people make a series of decisions about whether a given adjective describes a given target person, their subsequent recall for the adjectives in a surprise memory test varies according to the intimacy of the target that the adjective was paired with (Symons & Johnson, 1997). Words rated for familiar but non-intimate targets, such as Tony Blair, are recalled less frequently than words rated for self or for familiar and intimate targets, such as mother; indeed the more intimate the target the closer the recall to that for self. God is familiar to everyone, but intimate only to some, and an investigation using this technique found that an advantage of self-referent recall over God-referent recall for was observed for atheists and non-evangelical Christians but not for evangelical Christians (Gibson, 2006). Even though both Christian groups described God similarly on a self-report test, use of this indirect test suggested that God was intimate for the evangelical group in a way that was not true for the non-evangelical Christian group. Numerous other recall paradigms exist that could be adapted to the study of how people think about God (e.g., see Puff, 1982)

Another indirect measurement holding considerable promise is the use of judgment speed as a measure of attitude accessibility (Fazio, Sanbonmatsu, Powell, & Kardes, 1986). Psychologists of religion have suggested using timing techniques to measure religious beliefs for more than four decades (Hill, 2005; Slater et al., 2001; Strunk, 1966) but only now are researchers beginning to apply them to the measurement of representations of God. Gibson (2006), for example, reports the results of several experiments suggesting that timing measures are sensitive both to how accessible people's God schemas are but also their affective valence. Other timing techniques that could prove promising but have yet to be applied to God schemas include the Implicit Association Test (IAT); Greenwald, McGhee, & Schwartz, 1998), the Go/No-go Association Task (Nosek & Banaji, 2001), the Affective Simon Task (de Houwer & Eelen, 1998), and the Extrinsic Affective Simon Task (de Houwer, 2003a), along with further variations of each of these (for reviews see de Houwer, 2003b; Fazio & Olson, 2003; Spence, 2005).

RECOMMENDATIONS FOR THE MEASUREMENT OF REPRESENTATIONS OF GOD

While I am optimistic about the development of cognitive techniques for the measurement of representations of God, I also recognize that for many researchers and mental health professionals, quantitative questionnaire-based measures and qualitative interviews are the only viable techniques for current work. Given this, I offer several suggestions of how to use self-report measures in a more sophisticated fashion that takes into account what we know about cognitive schemas for God.

Manipulate Survey Instructions to Make Any Disparity Between God Concepts and God Schemas Salient

Given that people hold multiple God schemas that themselves vary in complexity, survey instructions should specify exactly how respondents should think about God while completing any survey. For example, the survey could specify "Please answer the questions about Jesus as you have directly experienced him." Since social desirability and theologically correctness can still influence the answers, however, a more powerful approach would be to make the disparity between different concepts and/or schemas salient to the respondent. Initial research has indicated that asking participants to access more than one God concept simultaneously can reveal differences (Gibson, 2006; Schaap Jonker et al., in press), but further research is needed to determine which pairs of instructions would best generate dissonance for respondents. Potential pairs of instructions might include "What I believe in my head" versus "What I believe in my heart"; "What I know in my head" versus "What I know emotionally"; "What I should believe" versus "What I experience"; "How I wish I experienced God" versus "How I do experience God"; and so on. It is not yet clear whether any disparity is more salient when all of the items for one instruction are answered before moving to the second or whether answering each pair of instructions for each item in turn is a better approach.

Use Questionnaires That Measure in More Than One Dimension for Each Item

Another strategy that would provide a richer data set is to ask respondents to make more than one judgment about each item. Instead of having a single Likert scale in response to a given item, we could also ask respondents to make a further judgment for the same item to clarify their first. If, for example, the first judgment is about how well a trait word describes the Holy Spirit as the respondent has experienced him, the second judgment might ask "How central to your view of the Holy Spirit is this attribute?", "How certain are you that the Holy Spirit is as you have described him?", or "How much emotion do you feel about your rating?"

Manipulate Which Schemas Are Active
When the Questionnaire Is Given

As discussed above, God schemas are dynamic in nature. If the particular God schema of interest is not salient or active at the time at which the participant completes the survey, its influence on the answers given is unlikely to be observed. This suggests the need to consider the social context in which the questionnaire is being delivered and whether particular situations or interventions would be more likely to activate the schema or schemas of interest. For example, surveys could be given shortly after a church service or Bible study, in a location rich with religious sensory cues and associations, or following a period in which the participant prayed, wrote a letter to God, described a religious experience, or interacted with religious artifacts or images. Researchers may even consider going beyond correlational studies and create experimental situations in which different schemas are activated for different groups or are primed under different conditions.

Consider How Belief in God and His Supernatural Powers Interacts
with Belief in God's Character

What it means to believe in God is an issue deserving of more attention, especially with regard to how it is measured. Belief in God is normally measured by a forced-choice self-report task, though sometimes the belief status of research participants is not even reported (e.g., Kunkel et al., 1999). Quite what answers on such a scale mean, however, is likely to vary considerably depending on the centrality and elaboration of God schemas in a person's thinking. For example, one person might report not believing in God but have a well-developed and highly affective schema of the God she does not believe in (cf. Exline, 2004; Novotni & Petersen, 2001) whereas another person might similarly report not believing in God but not have given the character of God much thought. Similarly, it is not always clear what a person who says he believes in God actually means, for example, regarding their expectation of God's ability to act upon the world. Considerably more could be said about God's supernatural powers but suffice it here to say that much work needs to be done to integrate psychology of religion with the growing literature on this topic within the cognitive science of religion (for reviews see Barrett, 2000, 2004).

Use a Mixture of Quantitative and Qualitative Methodology

Objective research into the way people represent God cannot be bounded either by theological prescriptions of what God is like or by the investigator's presuppositions of what God is supposed to be like. Qualitative methodologies allow researchers' assumptions to be questioned and can provide richer data than quantitative methods, suggesting that quantitative and qualitative approaches could helpfully be used side by side. Hammersley (1996) affirms the importance of methodological eclecticism, noting the possibility of triangulation from more than one method to counteract different threats to validity, and of using qualitative methods to generate hypotheses, research strategies, or questionnaire items for quantitative measures, or to debrief participants after quantitative work.

Measure Relational Schemas

Given that information about God is also held in relational schemas, a fruitful way into God schemas not discussed thus far would be to measure different aspects of people's relationship with God. Several approaches are possible here. The first is to measure people's feelings toward God. Rather than asking participants what God is like, this approach involves asking how people feel about God's character and actions. Although Christians can be reluctant to report anger toward God because of fear that it is morally wrong (Exline, 2004), they may still be more willing to do this than to report that their view of God himself is negative. Several preliminary scales have been developed to assess this dimension and this represents a promising line of future work (Exline, Fisher, Rose, & Kampani, 2005; Murken, 1998; Schaap Jonker, Eurelings-Bontekoe, Zock, & Jonker, 2006). A second approach is to measure the quality of relationship that exists in attachment terms; inferences can easily be made about the God schemas present in an avoidant relationship relative to a secure relationship. Two measures are helpful here: Sim and Loh's (2003) measure of the presence of an attachment relationship and Beck and McDonald's (2004) measure of style of attachment to God. A third approach is one that I have not seen taken elsewhere but that nonetheless merits exploration, and that is to consider people's perceptions of what God thinks or feels about them. Theologians make a number of claims from the Bible for God's attitudes toward humans and it would be interesting to systematically investigate how people engage with these ideas in their everyday thinking.

REFERENCES

Andersen, S. M., & Chen, S. (2002). The relational self: An interpersonal social-cognitive theory. *Psychological Review, 109*(4), 619-645.

Andersen, S. M., Chen, S., & Miranda, R. (2002). Significant others and the self. *Self and Identity, 1*(2), 159-168.

Aron, A., Aron, E. N., Tudor, M., & Nelson, G. (1991). Close relationships as including other in the self. *Journal of Personality and Social Psychology, 60*(2), 241-253.

Baldwin, M. W. (1992). Relational schemas and the processing of social information. *Psychological Bulletin, 112*(3), 461-484.

Baldwin, M. W. (1999). Relational schemas: Research into social-cognitive aspect of interpersonal experience. In Y. Shoda & D. Cervone (Eds.), *The coherence of personality: Social cognitive bases of consistency, variability, and organization* (pp. 127-154). New York: Guilford Press.

Baldwin, M. W. (2001). Relational schema activation: Does Bob Zajonc ever scowl at you from the back of your mind? In D. K. Apsley & J. A. Bargh (Eds.), *Unraveling the complexities of social life: A festschrift in honor of Robert B. Zajonc* (pp. 55-67). Washington, DC: American Psychological Association.

Barrett, J. L. (1998). Cognitive constraints on Hindu concepts of the divine. *Journal for the Scientific Study of Religion, 37*(4), 608-619.

Barrett, J. L. (2000). Exploring the natural foundations of religion. *Trends in Cognitive Sciences, 4*(1), 29-34.

Barrett, J. L. (2004). *Why would anyone believe in God?* Oxford, England: AltaMira.

Barrett, J. L., & Keil, F. C. (1996). Conceptualizing a nonnatural entity: Anthropomorphism in God concepts. *Cognitive Psychology, 31*(3), 219-247.

Barrett, J. L., & VanOrman, B. (1996). The effects of image-use in worship on God concepts. *Journal of Psychology and Christianity, 15*(1), 38-45.

Bassett, R. L., Miller, S., Anstey, K., Crafts, K., Harmon, J., Lee, Y., et al. (1990). Picturing God: A nonverbal measure of God concept for conservative Protestants. *Journal of Psychology and Christianity, 9*(2), 73-81.

Bassett, R. L., Perry, K., Repass, R., Silver, E., & Welch, T. (1994). Perceptions of God among persons with mental retardation: A research note. *Journal of Psychology and Theology, 22*(1), 45-49.

Batson, C. D., Schoenrade, P., & Ventis, W. L. (1993). *Religion and the individual.* Oxford, England: Oxford University Press.

Beck, R., & McDonald, A. (2004). Attachment to God: The Attachment to God Inventory, tests of working model correspondence, and an exploration of faith group differences. *Journal for Psychology and Theology, 32*(2), 92-103.

Benson, P., & Spilka, B. (1973). God image as a function of self-esteem and locus of control. *Journal for the Scientific Study of Religion, 12,* 297-310.

Bransford, J. D., & McCarrell, N. S. (1974). A sketch of a cognitive approach to comprehension: Some thoughts about understanding what it means to comprehend. In D. S. Palermo & W. B. Weimer (Eds.), *Cognition and the symbolic processes* (pp. 189-229). Hillsdale, NJ: Erlbaum.

Ciarrocchi, J. W., Piedmont, R. L., & Williams, J. E. G. (2002). Image of God and personality as predictors of spirituality in men and women. *Research in the Social Scientific Study of Religion, 13,* 55-73.

de Houwer, J. (2003a). The extrinsic affective Simon task. *Experimental Psychology, 50*(2), 77-85.

de Houwer, J. (2003b). A structural analysis of indirect measures of attitudes. In J. Musch & K. C. Klauer (Eds.), *The psychology of evaluation: Affective processes in cognition and emotion* (pp. 219-244). Mahwah, NJ: Erlbaum.

de Houwer, J., & Eelen, P. (1998). An affective variant of the Simon paradigm. *Cognition and Emotion, 12*(1), 45-61.

Denzin, N. K., & Lincoln, Y. S. (Eds.). (2005). *The SAGE handbook of qualitative research* (3rd ed.). London: Sage.

Exline, J. J. (2004). Anger toward God: A brief overview of existing research. *Psychology of Religion Newsletter, 29*(1), 1-8.

Exline, J. J., Fisher, M. L., Rose, E., & Kampani, S. (2005). *Emotional atheism: Anger toward God predicts decreased belief.* Unpublished manuscript, Case Western Reserve University.

Eysenck, M. W., & Keane, M. T. (2005). *Cognitive psychology: A student's handbook* (5th ed.). Hove, England: Psychology Press.

Fazio, R. H., & Olson, M. A. (2003). Implicit measures in social cognition research: Their meaning and uses. *Annual Review of Psychology, 54*, 297-327.

Fazio, R. H., Sanbonmatsu, D. M., Powell, M. C., & Kardes, F. R. (1986). On the automatic activation of attitudes. *Journal of Personality and Social Psychology, 50*(2), 229-238.

Fiske, S. T., & Linville, R. S. (1980). What does the schema concept buy us? *Personality and Social Psychology Bulletin, 6*, 543-557.

Fiske, S. T., & Taylor, S. E. (1991). *Social cognition* (2nd ed.). New York: McGraw-Hill.

Francis, L. J., Robbins, M., & Gibson, H. M. (2006). A revised semantic differential scale distinguishing between negative and positive God images. *Journal of Beliefs and Values, 27*(2), 237-240.

Gibson, N. J. S. (2006). *The experimental investigation of religious cognition.* Unpublished doctoral dissertation [available from http://www.divinity.cam.ac.uk/pcp/personnel/nicholas.html#PhD], University of Cambridge, Cambridge, England.

Gorsuch, R. L. (1968). The conceptualization of God as seen in adjective ratings. *Journal for the Scientific Study of Religion, 7*, 56-64.

Gorsuch, R. L. (1990). Measurement in psychology of religion revisited. *Journal of Psychology and Christianity, 9*(2), 82-92.

Gough, H. G., & Heilbrum, A. B. (1983). *The adjective check list manual.* Palo Alto, CA: Consulting Psychologists Press.

Greenwald, A. G., McGhee, D. E., & Schwartz, J. L. K. (1998). Measuring individual differences in implicit cognition: The implicit association test. *Journal of Personality and Social Psychology, 74*(6), 1464-1480.

Hall, T. W. (2003). Relational spirituality: Implications of the convergence of attachment theory, interpersonal neurobiology, and emotional information processing. *Psychology of Religion Newsletter, 28*(2), 1-12.

Hall, T. W. (2004). Christian spirituality and mental health: A relational spirituality paradigm for empirical research. *Journal of Psychology and Christianity, 23*, 66-81.

Hall, T. W., Tisdale, T. C., & Brokaw, B. F. (1994). Assessment of religious dimensions in Christian clients: A review of selected instruments for research and clinical use. *Journal of Psychology and Theology, 22*(4), 395-421.

Hammersley, M. (1996). The relationship between qualitative and quantitative research: Paradigm loyalty versus methodological eclecticism. In J. T. E. Richardson (Ed.), *The handbook of qualitative research methods for psychologists and the social sciences* (pp. 159-174). Oxford, England: The British Psychological Society.

Hay, D., & Nye, R. (1998). *The spirit of the child.* London: Fount.

Heller, D. (1986). *The children's God.* Chicago: University of Chicago Press.

Higgins, E. T. (1987). Self-discrepancy: A theory relating self and affect. *Psychological Review, 94*(3), 319-340.

Higgins, E. T. (1989). Self-discrepancy theory: What patterns of self-beliefs cause people to suffer? In L. Berkowitz (Ed.), *Advances in experimental social psychology* (Vol. 22, pp. 93-136). San Diego, CA: Academic Press.

Higgins, E. T., Bond, R. N., Klein, R., & Strauman, T. (1986). Self-discrepancies and emotional vulnerability: How magnitude, accessibility, and type of discrepancy influence affect. *Journal of Personality and Social Psychology, 51*(1), 5-15.

Higgins, E. T., Shah, J., & Friedman, R. (1997). Emotional responses to goal attainment: Strength of regulatory focus as moderator. *Journal of Personality and Social Psychology, 72*(3), 515-525.

Hill, P. C. (1994). Toward an attitude process model of religious experience. *Journal for the Scientific Study of Religion, 33*(4), 303-314.

Hill, P. C. (1995). Affective theory and religious experience. In R. W. Hood, Jr. (Ed.), *Handbook of Religious Experience* (pp. 353-377). Birmingham, AL: Religious Education Press.

Hill, P. C. (2005). Measurement assessment and issues in the psychology of religion and spirituality. In R. F. Paloutzian & C. L. Park (Eds.), *Handbook of the psychology of religion* (pp. 43-79). New York: Guilford Press.

Hill, P. C., & Hall, T. W. (2002). Relational schemas in processing one's image of God and self. *Journal of Psychology and Christianity, 21*(4), 365-373.

Hill, P. C., & Hood, R. W., Jr. (1999a). Affect, religion and unconscious processes. *Journal of Personality, 67*(6), 1015-1046.

Hill, P. C., & Hood, R. W., Jr. (Eds.). (1999b). *Measures of religiosity.* Birmingham, AL: Religious Education Press.

Hill, P. C., & Pargament, K. I. (2003). Advances in the conceptualization and measurement of religion and spirituality: Implications for physical and mental health research. *American Psychologist, 58*(1), 64-74.

Hoffman, L. (2004, October). *Cultural constructions of the God image and God concept: Implications for culture, psychology, and religion.* Paper presented at the annual meeting of the Society for the Scientific Study of Religion, Kansas City, MO.

Hoffman, L. (2005). A developmental perspective on the God image. In R. H. Cox, B. Ervin-Cox & L. Hoffman (Eds.), *Spirituality and psychological health* (pp. 129-147). Colorado Springs: Colorado School of Professional Psychology Press.

Hoffman, L., Jones, T. T., Williams, F., & Dillard, K. S. (2004, March). *The God image, the God concept, and attachment.* Paper presented at the annual meeting of the Christian Association for Psychological Studies, St Petersburg, FL.

Hutsebaut, D., & Verhoeven, D. (1995). Studying dimensions of God representation: Choosing closed or open-ended research questions. *International Journal for the Psychology of Religion, 5*(1), 49-60.

Kirkpatrick, L. A. (1999). Attachment and religious representations and behavior. In J. Cassidy & P. R. Shaver (Eds.), *Handbook of attachment: Theory, research, and clinical applications* (pp. 803-822). New York: Guilford Press.

Kunkel, M. A., Cook, S., Meshel, D. S., Daughtry, D., & Hauenstein, A. (1999). God images: A concept map. *Journal for the Scientific Study of Religion, 38*(2), 193-202.

Lalljee, M., Brown, L. B., & Hilton, D. (1990). The relationships between images of God, explanations for failure to do one's duty to God, and invoking God's agency. *Journal of Psychology and Theology, 18*(2), 166-173.

Lawrence, R. T. (1991). *The God Image Inventory: The development, validation, and standardization of a psychometric instrument for research, pastoral and clinical use in measuring the image of God.* Unpublished doctoral dissertation, The Catholic University of America, Washington, DC.

Lawrence, R. T. (1997). Measuring the image of God: The God Image Inventory and the God Image Scales. *Journal of Psychology and Theology, 25*(2), 214-226.

Lindeman, M., Pyysiäinen, I., & Saariluoma, P. (2002). Representing God. *Papers on Social Representations, 11*(1), 1-13.

Linville, P. W. (1985). Self-complexity and affective extremity: Don't put all of your eggs in one cognitive basket. *Social Cognition, 3*(1), 94-120.

Linville, P. W. (1987). Self-complexity as a cognitive buffer against stress-related illness and depression. *Journal of Personality and Social Psychology, 52*(4), 663-676.

Markus, H. R. (1977). Self-schemata and processing information about the self. *Journal of Personality and Social Psychology, 35*(2), 63-78.

Markus, H. R., & Kunda, Z. (1986). Stability and malleability of the self-concept. *Journal of Personality and Social Psychology, 51*(4), 858-866.

Markus, H. R., & Nurius, P. (1986). Possible selves. *American Psychologist, 41*(9), 954-969.

Markus, H. R., Smith, J., & Moreland, R. L. (1985). Role of the self-concept in the perception of others. *Journal of Personality and Social Psychology, 49*(6), 1494-1512.

McIntosh, D. N. (1995). Religion-as-schema, with implications for the relation between religion and coping. *International Journal for the Psychology of Religion, 5*(1), 1-16.

Murken, S. (1998). *Gottesbeziehung und psychische Gesundheit: Die Entwicklung eines Modells und seine empirische Überprüfung [God relationship and* mental health: The development of a model and its empirical testing]. Münster, Germany: Waxmann.

Musch, J., & Klauer, K. C. (Eds.). (2003). *The psychology of evaluation: Affective processes in cognition and emotion.* Mahwah, NJ: Erlbaum.

Neisser, U. (1976). *Cognition and reality: Principles and implications of cognitive psychology.* San Francisco: W. H. Freeman.

Niedenthal, P. M., Setterlund, M. B., & Wherry, M. B. (1992). Possible self-complexity and affective reactions to goal-relevant evaluation. *Journal of Personality and Social Psychology, 63*(1), 5-16.

Nosek, B. A., & Banaji, M. R. (2001). The Go/No-go Association Task. *Social Cognition, 19*(6), 625-666.

Novotni, M., & Petersen, R. (2001). *Angry with God.* Colorado Springs, CO: Piñon Press.

Nye, R. (1999). Relational consciousness and the spiritual lives of children: Convergence with children's theory of mind. In K. H. Reich, F. K. Oser & W. G. Scarlett (Eds.), *Being human: The case of religion* (Vol. 2, pp. 57-82). Lengerich, Germany: Pabst.

Nye, W. C., & Carlson, J. S. (1984). The development of the concept of God in children. *Journal of Genetic Psychology, 145*(1), 137-142.

Piedmont, R. L., Ciarrocchi, J. W., & Williams, J. E. G. (2002). A components analysis of one's image of God. *Research in the Social Scientific Study of Religion, 13*, 109-123.

Piedmont, R. L., Williams, J. E. G., & Ciarrocchi, J. W. (1997). Personality correlates of one's image of Jesus: Historiographic analysis using the Five-Factor Model of personality. *Journal for Psychology and Theology, 25*, 364-373.

Puff, C. R. (Ed.). (1982). *Handbook of research methods in human memory and cognition.* New York: Academic Press.

Pyysiäinen, I. (2004). Intuitive and explicit in religious thought. *Journal of Cognition and Culture, 4*(1), 123-150.

Rizzuto, A. M. (1979). *The birth of the living God: A psychoanalytic study.* London: University of Chicago Press.

Rogers, T. B., Kuiper, N. A., & Kirker, W. S. (1977). Self-reference and the encoding of personal information. *Journal of Personality and Social Psychology, 35*(9), 677-688.

Schaap Jonker, H., Eurelings-Bontekoe, E. H. M., Zock, H., & Jonker, E. R. (2006). *Development and validation of the Dutch Questionnaire God Image.* Manuscript submitted for publication, Kampen Theological University, The Netherlands.

Schaap Jonker, H., Eurelings-Bontekoe, E. H. M., Zock, H., & Jonker, E. R. (in press). The personal and normative image of God: The role of culture and mental health. *Archive for the Psychology of Religion.*

Sim, T. N., & Loh, B. S. M. (2003). Attachment to God: Measurement and dynamics. *Journal of Social and Personal Relationships, 20*(3), 373-389.

Slater, W., Hall, T. W., & Edwards, K. J. (2001). Measuring religion and spirituality: Where are we and where are we going? *Journal of Psychology and Theology, 29*, 4-21.

Spence, A. (2005). Using implicit tasks in attitude research: A review and a guide. *Social Psychological Review, 7*(1), 2-17.

Spilka, B. (2000, October). *God images: Broadening psychological perspectives and research.* Paper presented at the annual meeting of the Society for the Scientific Study of Religion, Houston, TX.

Strunk, O., Jr. (1966). Timed-cross examination: A methodological innovation in the study of religious beliefs and attitudes. *Review of Religious Research, 7*, 121-123.

Symons, C. S., & Johnson, B. T. (1997). The self-reference effect in memory: A meta-analysis. *Psychological Bulletin, 121*(3), 371-394.

Thurston, N. S. (1994). Exemplary approach to operationalizing psychoanalytic theory and religion: Commentary on "The relationship of God image to level of object relations development." *Journal of Psychology and Theology, 22*(4), 372-373.

Watts, F. N. (1996). Psychological and religious perspectives on emotion. *International Journal for the Psychology of Religion, 6*(2), 71-87.

Watts, F. N. (in press). Implicational and propositional religious meanings. *International Journal for the Psychology of Religion.*

Watts, F. N., & Williams, J. M. G. (1988). *The psychology of religious knowing.* Cambridge, England: Cambridge University Press.

Williams, J. M. G., Watts, F. N., MacLeod, C., & Mathews, A. (1997). *Cognitive psychology and emotional disorders* (2nd ed.). Chichester, England: John Wiley.

doi:10.1300/J515v09n03_11

Chapter 12

God Image Psychotherapy:
Comparing Approaches

Glendon L. Moriarty, PsyD
Michael Thomas, MA
John Allmond, MA

SUMMARY. This chapter compares the seven different God image therapy approaches outlined in Part II of this book. These approaches include: attachment therapy, existential-integrative psychotherapy, neuroscientific therapy, rational emotive behavior therapy, time-limited dynamic psychotherapy, liberal protestant pastoral psychotherapy and theistic psychotherapy. First, similarities and differences are explored. Next, God image psychotherapy integration is discussed. General psychotherapy integration models are reviewed and applied to the different God image approaches. Finally, the chapter closes with a table that compares each orientation across the following categories: background and assumptions, God image development, God image difficulties, God image change, strengths and weaknesses. doi:10.1300/J515v09n03_12 *[Article copies available for a fee from The Haworth Document Delivery Service: 1-800-HAWORTH. E-mail address: <docdelivery@*

[Haworth co-indexing entry note]: "God Image Psychotherapy: Comparing Approaches." Moriarty, Glendon L., Michael Thomas, and John Allmond. Co-published simultaneously in *Journal of Spirituality in Mental Health* (The Haworth Pastoral Press, an imprint of The Haworth Press) Vol. 9, No. 3/4, 2007, pp. 247-255; and: *God Image Handbook for Spiritual Counseling and Psychotherapy: Research, Theory, and Practice* (ed: Glendon L. Moriarty, and Louis Hoffman) The Haworth Pastoral Press, an imprint of The Haworth Press, 2007, pp. 247-255. Single or multiple copies of this article are available for a fee from The Haworth Document Delivery Service [1-800-HAWORTH, 9:00 a.m. - 5:00 p.m. (EST). E-mail address: docdelivery@haworthpress.com].

Available online at http://jsmh.haworthpress.com
doi:10.1300/J515v09n03_12

GOD IMAGE PSYCHOTHERAPY: COMPARING APPROACHES

There are seven approaches, or theoretical orientations, that are laid out in Part II of this volume. The goal of this chapter is to catalog this material so key information can be quickly identified. Another goal is to provide an efficient way for the different approaches to be compared. These goals are met through narratives on the similarities and differences of the God image approaches, and through an overview of God image psychotherapy integration. The chapter closes with a table that draws the material together for comparative analysis.

Similarities

The seven approaches outlined in this chapter have much in common. Each orientation values the therapeutic alliance and recognizes the importance of aligning with the client in order to collaboratively identity and resolve God image difficulties. As is the case with many religious/spiritual approaches, each orientation, in one way or anther, is highly sensitized to ethical issues. Authors were careful to warn about the need for informed consent, the importance of client autonomy, and the mindfulness needed to not explicitly or implicitly impose one's beliefs on the client.

The approaches also share agreement on how the God image develops. The authors suggest that relationships are the key ingredient in God image development; in particular, early childhood relationships with primary caregivers seem to be of fundamental importance. In addition, many of the approaches tie God image development to the development of the self: as the self changes, the God image changes.

Many other nuanced similarities exist that were not captured in this narrative or the below table. One has to wonder if we were to observe each of these contributors in the therapy room if there might not be far more similarities of style that are difficult to capture with words. Would the observing eye be able to distinguish between time-limited dynamic psychotherapy and a liberal protestant pastoral approach? How about theistic psychotherapy and neuroscientific therapy? There is a lot of common ground shared amongst these different approaches, but there are also important differences.

Differences

There are several differences that characterize these varied approaches. One primary difference is that some approaches seem more comfortable giving room to other factors, besides parenting and self-esteem, to influence God image development. These perspectives provide more space for cultural and religious variables, suggesting that factors like denominational background and racial identity are important factors in shaping the God image. Other contributors would likely agree with these inclusions, but they did not proactively frame them in their discussions.

Another difference lies in the deliberate inclusion of God in the therapy room. These authors suggest that God is an active and potent force that can transform the God image. Spiritual disciplines like prayer and mediation are easily employed. Other authors likely see these as valuable assets, but they might not be as comfortable using them in the therapeutic relationship.

A third difference is the explanation of how God image difficulties develop. There is much agreement on how the God image develops in general, but less so as to how God image *difficulties* develop. These descriptions and their corresponding explanations for God image change are much more closely tied to their theoretical roots. For example, Time-Limited Dynamic Psychotherapy describes God image difficulties as arising through maladaptive relational experiences and suggests that change occurs through corrective relational experiences. Rational Emotive Behavioral Therapy, on the other hand, explains God image difficulties through negative schemas, or deeply held beliefs, and states that God image transformation occurs through challenging God image beliefs.

When exploring differences between orientations, one has to wonder if these distinctions actually exist. Is there true variation or are we just using different words to describe the same phenomenon? Are we capturing distinct constructs or getting lost in semantics? We are reminded of the metaphor of the three blind men describing different parts of the same elephant. It does not seem we will ever truly know how distinct these approaches are; however, it appears safe to assume that the different perspectives give us language to better understand different parts of the emotional experience of God. Another way of looking at these approaches, instead of comparing similarities and differences, occurs through the lens of psychotherapy integration.

God Image Psychotherapy Integration

Psychotherapy integration refers to the way that different theoretical orientations (e.g., psychodynamic, cognitive-behavioral, humanistic) are synthesized or integrated (Norcross & Goldfried, 2005). There are a variety of ways that psychotherapy integration occurs. The common factors approach is an early and popular model of integration. This model looks at the shared features, or universal factors, that are common to all approaches (e.g., sense of hope, therapeutic alliance) and highlights the variables that seem to be the most effective. Another approach is known as theoretical integration. This approach synthesizes theories; an example of this is Young's Schema Theory in which relational dynamics are integrated with cognitive-behavioral principles.

It seems likely that as the God image field develops, there will be opportunities for these models to be applied to the different God image approaches. There were several similarities outlined above, but there are likely more robust common factors that are shared across the different approaches to God image therapy. If these factors could be successfully distilled, then they would help clinicians, regardless of their orientation, better aid clients struggling with religious issues. Similarly, there may be benefit in integrating different theoretical approaches to the God image. Integrating REBT with a depth approach like attachment therapy or existential therapy might yield insight into understanding how deep thought patterns affect the emotional experience of God.

A third approach to psychotherapy integration, and one that is gaining increasing support from clinicians and researchers, is technical eclecticism, which is characterized by Larry Beutler's (2002) prescriptive psychology (Norcross & Goldfried, 2005). The main idea is that a client's problems should be deliberately matched with an empirically supported treatment that has been shown to effectively address that problem. Contrast this perspective with the normal approach in which the clinician identifies with a particular orientation (e.g., "I'm psychodynamic") and treats a variety of disorders from that same perspective. For example, a psychodynamic clinician who treats personality issues, phobias, and generalized anxiety solely through psychodynamic psychotherapy. David Barlow (2001) has persuasively argued that a more appropriate approach would be for that clinician to use empirically supported approach with each of the disorders. In keeping with the above example, the clinician would use psychodynamic therapy to address the personality issues, behavioral therapy to treat the phobia, and cognitive therapy to address the generalized anxiety.

Technical eclecticism seems to be where the field of clinical psychology is increasingly moving. It is likely that the clinical psychology of religion will shift in this direction as well. There will probably be an increased need to match a particular orientation with a specific God image issue. What might this look like? Maybe more deeply ingrained God image difficulties would respond better to spiritually oriented approaches rooted in TLDP, attachment, or liberal protestant pastoral approaches. Similarly, perhaps a person who has generalized anxiety symptoms and corresponding God image worries would be more effectively helped with an REBT approach. Likewise, maybe a seeker who is struggling with a lack of genuineness in their faith would be best served with an existential-integrative therapy. The future challenge for clinicians who work with God images issues may be to move out of a theoretical orientation 'ghetto' and into a more spiritually-oriented prescriptive psychotherapy approach. The goal is to match the client's specific religious or spiritual problem with a tailored therapy solution.

We have to first define the distinct approaches before we begin to establish deliberate and integrated God image interventions. Developing a solid understanding of the different approaches is fundamental to any future progress. Table 1, although far from complete, is a good stating point to gain a thorough understanding of different perspectives on God image therapy.

TABLE 1

APPROACH	BACKGROUND AND PHILOSOPHICAL ASSUMPTIONS	GOD IMAGE DEVELOPMENT	GOD IMAGE DIFFICULTIES	GOD IMAGE CHANGE	STRENGTHS AND WEAKNESSES
Attachment (Jacqueline Noffke & Todd Hall; Chapter 4)	*Background:* Stems from attachment theory, affective neurobiology, and emotional information processing. *Philosophical Assumptions:* Implicit representations of God are brought about through emotional attachment to one's caregivers developed during infancy. God is a legitimate external object with which believers can relate.	The God image develops through the early experiences an individual has with his/her caregivers. The way in which a person's emotional needs are met may generalize this early experience to his relationship and attachment style to God. Repeated relational experiences with primary caregivers (attachment figures) are encoded in implicit memory as implicit relational representations—a gut level sense of "how to be with" significant others. These implicit relational representations then function as an "attachment filter" with God as one becomes attached to God, biasing an individual's experiences of God toward that of human attachment relationships.	God image difficulties arise from problems in an individual's attachment to his/her primary caregiver(s). For example, many insecurely attached individuals experience God as controlling, less nurturing and caring, and/or distant. These negative messages received by the individual cause neural networks to be formed that cause an individual to view their other relationships through the same lens with which they experienced their early caregiver(s).	Transformation of the God image involves both nonverbal relational information from the therapist and an integration of this code with the symbolic, verbal code. New relational experiences recruit new neural networks that lay down the neural basis for a different way of experiencing, representing, and being with God. Imagery-based inner healing exercises or intense spiritual experiences elicited through worship can connect with believers' maladaptive implicit representations of God and provide reparative experiences that then transform general models of relating.	*Strengths:* This theory brings together several strands of research on God image development and maintenance including: attachment theory, neurobiology, and emotional information processing. This theory also holds that God exists and is able to be actively involved in the therapy process. *Weaknesses:* This theory of treatment may be rather time consuming as it requires an "attachment" bond to be formed between the therapist and client. More research needs to be conducted to determine the efficacy of this mode of therapy.
Time Limited Dynamic Therapy (TLDP), (Glendon Moriarty; Chapter 5)	*Background:* TLDP has its roots in psychoanalytic thought, the brief therapy paradigm, and in empirical research. It was created and empirically tested by Hans Strupp and colleagues at Vanderbilt University in the 1980's. *Philosophical Assumptions:* TLDP assumes that interpersonal problems are learned in the past, maintained in the present, and acted out in the therapeutic relationship.	The God image develops along with the changing self through life stages, such as the developmental stages defined by Erik Erikson. For example, if a child experiences his caregiver as loving and trustworthy in the infancy stage, he will later find that others, including God, can be trusted. Likewise, if the child can trust and separate from his caregiver in a healthy manner, he will experience God as mature and encouraging of his autonomy.	God image difficulties occur when there is unsuccessful resolution of a life stage or the formation of a cyclical maladaptive pattern. For example, if the child's caregiver neglects or abuses him, the child will conclude that others, the universe, and God cannot be trusted. The child may not grow and emotionally separate from the caregiver in this case. Though he may lack insight into this problem later in life, his behavior will be characterized by a fear that if he grows too much or becomes too independent, then God will be unhappy and abandon him.	As the self changes, the God image changes. God image change occurs through internalization, which is the gradual process by which people learn to treat themselves as others treat them. Improvement in relational patterns learned in therapy results in the resolution of God image problems.	*Strengths:* TLDP is heavily influenced by empirical research, includes techniques that both directly and indirectly change the God image, and is a focused, short term therapy. *Weaknesses:* It can be challenging for experienced therapists to unlearn other therapeutic strategies in becoming a participant-observer in therapy and maximize the efficacy of TLDP techniques. Similarly, it can be challenging for less experienced therapists to avoid getting "hooked" into dysfunctional relational patterns. Additionally, the patient needs to have one main, identifiable relational pattern that is maladaptive for TLDP to be most effective.
Existential-Integrative (Louis	*Background:* Existential psychotherapy originated	God image development in this approach is very	Difficulties occur when the patient fails, for	Primary means of change is self-	*Strengths:* This approach values the

| Hoffman, Chapter 6) | from the writings of Rollo May in the 1950's and 60's and is considered a branch of the third force of psychology or humanistic/ phenomenological therapies. It shares a focus on subjectivity, experience, personal freedom, human potential, and dignity with humanistic psychology, but differs in that it places more emphasis on darker realities such as suffering, evil, and human limitation. Existential therapy can be integrated with other approaches that are consistent with its foundation to address God image difficulties. *Philosophical Assumptions:* Assumes that people can become freer by becoming conscious of influences that control them, of which they were previously unaware. By becoming free, they can then become more responsible and moral in life. Assumes that a genuine, satisfying therapeutic relationship is more important than interventions or techniques. | complex and not over-simplified. It can include a variety of relational experiences outside of those with traditional caregivers. Such relational experiences may occur with the church, religious leaders, and the world in general. God image development cannot necessarily be fully understood through scientific research alone and usually involves God or other conceptions of the transcendent. The following themes, and the related challenges that may be faced regarding them, are also involved in God image development: 1) freedom and responsibility, 2) the human tendencies toward expansion and constriction, and 3) genuineness of relationship. | whatever reason, to individuate his faith. A lack of individuation may occur due to an establishment of false security. Difficulties may also occur when the patient views himself or herself as either inherently too "bad" or too "good," both of which can be psychologically destructive. Finally, the patient may experience difficulties as a result of a lack of genuine relationships with others, including God. This lack may be the result of an impaired ability to trust or an insufficient knowledge of how to attain genuine relationship. | awareness and experience. As the patient becomes increasingly self-aware, he or she becomes more able to respond responsibly to his freedom, genuinely engage with others as well as his or her faith, and experience genuine intimacy to the depths of his or her desire. Through a mutually disclosing and genuine therapeutic relationship, the patient gains understanding. He or she learns more about personal freedom, will, and the potential to trust God enough to share pain, anger, and hurt, even when it is directed at God. Tension within the therapeutic relationship is not avoided, but embraced and utilized for discussion and growth. | human potential for *genuine, vulnerable* relationship that involves trust and unmatched engagement. The approach challenges accepted thoughts and creates opportunity for meta-cognitions as well as critical reflection on reality. Existential therapists are optimistic about the therapist's ability to overcome transference and promote a genuine relationship that will facilitate meaningful growth. *Weaknesses:* Patients would ideally possess capacity for deeper insight and an ability to explore topics that may cause discomfort and present difficult challenges. Some patients may be resistant to such an approach. Due to the time required for therapist and patient to establish an authentic, genuine relationship, therapy tends to be long-term. |
| Neuroscience and God Image (Fernando Garzon, Chapter 7) | *Background:* The field of neuroscience has grown significantly in recent decades and has led to the development of the subfield, neurotheology. This subfield is defined as an exploration of how the mind/brain operates in regards to one's relationship to God. *Philosophical Assumptions:* Neuroscientific findings can inform strategies in the areas of interpersonal problems and God image. Such findings provide information on understanding unconscious processes. Differences between the God concept and God image may be linked to differences in the implicit versus explicit memory coding systems, differences between left and right brain functions, and/or the effects of trauma on neural development. | Neural network development begins in the early stages of life and is influenced by environmental interactions including relationships with caregivers. Neural networks involved in these early stages of life set the groundwork for interpersonal attachment and, therefore, influence the God image. The God image (the emotional, subjective experience of God) is linked to right brain function; therefore, it is conceivable through the lens of neuroscience that one could have a negative God image, but a positive God concept (the intellectual experience of God) which is linked with left brain function. | Negative experiences with early life relationships and interactions, including traumatic experiences, can impact how the wiring of the amygdala and other structures involved in the memory systems progress. Trauma can lead to 1) the secretion of increased levels of stress hormones, 2) the strong activation of the amygdala (which is involved in implicit memory), and 3) temporary impairment of the hippocampus (which is involved in explicit memory and the memory consolidation process). | God image change can occur via a variety of ways according to this approach. A positive therapeutic experience may facilitate change in the composition of neural networks associated with authority figures and, hence, influence the God image even if God is not directly addressed in therapy. Since neural networks can be activated through human imagination, Scripture meditation, and contemplative prayer may also produce change in neural networks and pathways. This approach sheds light on the fact that treatments which involve strategies to | *Strengths:* This approach integrates respected findings of various disciplines including neurology, psychology, and theology. It promotes synthesis and understanding of a variety of other-discipline findings including the influence of early relationships on later life attachment style, the importance of an empowering therapeutic relationship, and recognition of the impact that trauma can have on interpersonal development. *Weaknesses:* More research, empirical support, and understanding is needed regarding the relationship between neural development and the God image. Additionally, this approach can be |

TABLE 1 (continued)

				activate right hemispheric and implicit memory processes warrants at least increased consideration and research.	controversial due to the variety of beliefs and worldviews that many professionals possess regarding neuroscientific findings (i.e. reductionistic versus non-reductionistic).
Rational Emotive Behavior Therapy (REBT); (Brad Johnson, Chapter 8)	*Background:* REBT has its roots in Cognitive Behavioral Therapy and Cognitive theory. It was formed by Albert Ellis and focuses primarly on the irrational beliefs that dictate a client's negative emotional/psychological consequences. *Philosophical Assumptions.* REBT assumes that it is not an activating event which causes an emotional disturbance, but rather an irrational belief which causes the disturbance.	Research has found that a person's God image most likely develops parallel to 1) an individual's relationship with his/her early caregivers, and 2) an individual's level of self-esteem.	God image difficulties develop due to negative self perception schemas. The way in which an individual perceives him/her self correlates highly with the way in which this individual believes God thinks and feels towards him/her. Consequently, negative schemas both develop and maintain negative God images.	God image change is made through the therapist and client working to make sense of the "B" (beliefs) in the ABC model. Through the therapist combating irrational beliefs about self and God through a "Cognitive disputation," this is a debate or challenge to the client's irrational belief system. This should be done with care and it is recommended that the therapist consult with a relevant religious leader.	*Strengths:* REBT has been found to be effective in the treatment of many psychological disorders. *Weaknesses:* Ethical considerations should be thoroughly thought through whenever working with a client's God image or religious beliefs. Appropriate training and knowledge of the client's religious system should be a prerequisite for ethical practice. God image modification should always be done collaboratively with a client, and never against their will or desire.
Theistic Psychotherapy; (Kari A. O'Grady & P. Scott Richards; Chapter 9)	*Background:* Grounded in the worldview of the major theistic world religions, including Judaism, Christianity, and Islam. Theistic psychotherapy is an integrative approach in which therapists use spiritual interventions combined with a variety of standard mainstream techniques, including psychodynamic, behavioral, humanistic, cognitive, and systemic. *Philosophical Assumptions:* Assumes that God exists, that humankind is the creation of God, and there are spiritual processes at work in the relationship between God and humankind.	The development of God image is a complex process that may include influences from religious theology and tradition, popular culture, family and peer influences, gender, and age. Actual experiences with God can have a powerful influence on individuals' representations of God. Getting to know God better can affect an individual's God image. God is not merely a representation to be perceived but also a reality to be experienced first hand.	Some individuals have trouble developing a relationship with God because they have not been able to overcome their childhood associations with his image. Difficulties can also occur when people sin and do not repent or do not believe they can be forgiven for their failures. Sin makes it difficult for people to connect to God because it fosters a distorted view of self.	Many interventions are used to guide clients toward a more healthy experience of God. These interventions may include the following: prayer in or out of session, meeting with a religious leader, spiritual imagery, contemplation and meditation, challenging distorted views of the nature of God, and finding the real God or a safe person to meet with regularly.	*Strengths:* Assumes that a loving God is real and active in the therapy process. *Weaknesses:* May not be indicated with clients who do not describe themselves as religious/spiritual or with certain approaches to approaching religious/spiritual belief.
Liberal Protestant Pastoral Theological Approach (Carrie Doehring, Chapter 10) (Specifically in the role of God images in the recovery from sexual and physical abuse)	*Background:* An interdisciplinary method that draws upon postmodern approaches to knowledge; psychodynamic theory; object relations theory *Philosophical Assumptions:* Knowledge-psychological and theological-is socially constructed	There is a complex, bi-directional relationship between experiences of violence and God images: how violence can form or reinforce God images and, conversely, how God images can shape a person's response to violence, in both its immediate aftermath and the long-term process of recovery.	God image difficulties can arise due to problems and/or hurts an individual experiences (violence, abuse, etc.). God image difficulties can also arise due to the way an individual responds to a problem or wounding experience.	God image change is found when an individual's unconscious beliefs about God, caregivers, and/or past relationships, which have remained hidden within the person as anxieties or depression, become conscious to the individual in a safe environment where new, more accurate thinking about God can be experienced.	*Strengths:* Often goes to the root of problems and changes deep, ingrained patters of relating with self, others, and God. *Weaknesses:* Often this style of therapy may take several years; may not be as effective with individuals who have lower levels of insight

REFERENCES

Barlow, D.H., (2001). Clinical handbook of psychological disorders. New York: Guilford Press.

Beutler, L. (2002). The Dodo bird is extinct. *Clinical Psychology: Science and Practice,* 9, 30-34.

Norcross, J. (2005). A primer on psychotherapy integration. In Norcross, J., & Goldfried, M.R. (Eds.), Handbook of psychotherapy integration. Oxford: Oxford University Press.

doi:10.1300/J515v09n03_12

Chapter 13

Diversity Issues
and the God Image

Louis Hoffman, PhD
Sandra Knight, PhD
Scott Boscoe-Huffman, MA
Sharon Stewart, MA

SUMMARY. The research and theory on the God image has neglected considering important diversity issues. Despite this, it is evident that culture, gender, and sexual orientation significantly impact the way people experience God. The paper begins by building a basis for understanding the how various forms of diversity, including cultural diversity and religious diversity, impact the God image. Specific applications of women, LGBT, and black God images are explored. It is purported that while white males are able to base religious experience and a God image off of similarities to God, women, LGBT individuals, and people of color are placed in a position of relating to God based upon dissimilarity. Implications for future research and therapy developments are discussed. doi:10.1300/J515v09n03_13 *[Article copies available for a fee from The Haworth Document Delivery Service: 1-800-HAWORTH. E-mail address:*

[Haworth co-indexing entry note]: "Diversity Issues and the God Image." Hoffman, Louis et al. Co-published simultaneously in *Journal of Spirituality in Mental Health* (The Haworth Pastoral Press, an imprint of The Haworth Press) Vol. 9, No. 3/4, 2007, pp. 255-279; and: *God Image Handbook for Spiritual Counseling and Psychotherapy: Research, Theory, and Practice* (ed: Glendon L. Moriarty, and Louis Hoffman) The Haworth Pastoral Press, an imprint of The Haworth Press, 2007, pp. 255-279. Single or multiple copies of this article are available for a fee from The Haworth Document Delivery Service [1-800-HAWORTH, 9:00 a.m. - 5:00 p.m. (EST). E-mail address: docdelivery@haworthpress.com].

Available online at http://jsmh.haworthpress.com
doi:10.1300/J515v09n03_13

DIVERSITY ISSUES AND THE GOD IMAGE

Postmodernism jolted contemporary culture into increased awareness of diversity issues. Pluralism is a reality. Religious diversity,
cultural diversity, gender issues, and sexual orientation issues are commonplace in today's psychotherapy offices. However, many therapists
do not feel confident in dealing with the majority of diversity issues.
This becomes even more complicated when interfacing different forms
of diversity such as religious diversity, cultural diversity, and sexual
orientation. Although therapists may feel competent in one of these
realms, it is much less frequent to find therapists who feel competent to
deal with multiple forms of diversity in the same individual.

The current volume, along with the preponderance of papers on the
topic at professional conferences, suggests that the importance of the
God image construct is now being accepted. Despite this, few papers
address the psychological importance of diversity issues in understanding the way people experience God (Hoffman, 2004; Hoffman, Hoffman
et al., 2005; Hoffman, Knight, Boscoe-Huffman, & Stewart, 2006). The
other chapters of this book represent a multiplicity of different theoretical approaches to understanding the God image; however, this is only a
starting point. Future research and theoretical development needs to
show increased attention to gender, race, culture, religious differences,
socioeconomics, and sexual orientation. The purpose of this chapter is
to (1) review and critique the relevant literature, (2) highlight important
content domains, (3) address applications of diversity issues, and (4)
suggest important considerations for future development.

CRITIQUE OF CURRENT GOD IMAGE LITERATURE

Some of the earliest writings on the God image were by Feuerbach
(1841/1989), Freud (1913/1950, 19271961), and Nietzsche (1892/1954)
although they did not use the language of "God image." Both Freud and
Feuerbach maintained that the idea of God was a social *creation* based
upon an illusion. Rizzuto (1979) and Lawrence (1997) developed a clearer
articulation of the broader experience of God in differentiating between the
God image and the God concept. The contributions of Rizzuto and Law-

rence brought the God image theory into greater relevance and prominence while moving toward understanding the God image as a *social and personal construct.*

This distinction between a social *creation* and social *construction* is significant. According to Freud (1913/1950, 1927/1961), the experience of God is an illusion based on wish fulfillment. Most contemporary theorists do not deny these influence how God is experienced; however, they also maintain there is a reality of God which is distorted by these processes. Although the social creationÿ does not!exist and is merely a projection, the social construction approach allows for the possibility that God does exist, although individuals are unable to purely know or experience God. A social constructionist approach advocates that the human understanding of God is still a social construction intended to approximate or reflect God as clerly as possible; however, the transference process limits the success of this endeavor.

Theoretical developments of God as a social construction remained closely tied to the experience of God being based primarily upon early caregiver relationships and has been supported in the research literature (Brokaw & Edwards, 1994; Hoffman, Jones, Williams, & Dillard, 2004; Tisdale et al., 1997). Research supporting caregiver influences does not deny, but often neglect, other important factors influencing the development of the God image. For example, they do not take into account developmental factors (Hoffman, 2005), gender issues (Foster & Babcock, 2001; Krejci, 1989; Nelson, Cheek, & Au, 1985; Roberts, 1989), and various other forms of diversity (Hoffman, 2004; Hoffman, Hoffman et al., 2005; Hoffman et al., 2006).

Two primary errors exist in the contemporary understanding of the God image in interaction with the neglect of diversity issues. First, if God does exist and interacts with the world, then consideration needs to be given to the various forms of diversity. The majority of theistic religions believe that God influences the world and, at least occasionally, interacts with human beings. This remains true whether God is understood as a theistic being separate from the world, the Ground of all Being (i.e., God as being itself; see Tillich, 1951), the world and everything in it (i.e., pantheism), or as all things are in God (i.e., panentheism). If there is a God factor in the experience of God, most psychologists and researchers remain skeptical of the ability to quantify this experience. Although agreeing that any God factor cannot be quantified, this does not mean that it should be neglected. However, with notable exceptions such as William James (1902/1997), American psychology continues to be highly pragmatic and functional, often neglecting unseen or unquantifiable factors, such as God.

This first issue has important influences in reference to particular diversity issues, including religious diversity. Most Pentecostal and charismatic Christian traditions profess a high pneumatology emphasizing the role of the Holy Spirit. Similarly, many African American and Latin American theologies emphasize God's divine intervention. Native American spirituality often views the relationship with the Great Spirit as highly related to events in the world. For many of these individuals, neglecting the reality of God in psychological conceptualizations or treatment is offensive if not dangerous.

Many therapists assume these beliefs are superstitious or false attributions to God. Although it is not necessary to agree with the client's worldview, it is important to recognize the tension between the therapist's and client's belief systems to avoid imposing values on the client. Typically, therapists are most likely to impose their values on clients when they do not show respect for the client's beliefs or assume agreement (Hoffman, Grimes, & Mitchell, 2004).

The second error in contemporary theory related to diversity is the assumption that the God image is primarily or exclusively determined by parental influences. As cited above, research supports the influence of the parental relationship on the experience of God. Few theoretical approaches would deny this. However, as reflected in the various theoretical chapters in this book, the degree to which parental relationships are believed to influence the experience of God varies greatly.

Many researchers and theorists assume that the degree to which the parental factor influences how a person experiences God is consistent over time. Research and theory, however, suggests that the degree to which the God image is dependent upon parents may change due to the influence of therapy (Sorenson, 2004; Tisdale et al., 1997) and development (Hall & Brokaw, 1995; Hoffman, 2005; Hoffman, Hoffman et al., 2005). This critique could be applied to other factors. The assumption of stability fits with classic psychoanalytic, object relations, and self psychology perspectives that the personality is established at a young age and primarily stable thereafter. However, contemporary psychoanalysis and the other depth psychotherapies along with many solution-focused approaches view the personality as more malleable and fluid. Furthermore, problems may arise when treating the experience of God as merely an aspect of personality.

The position of this chapter proposes that factors influencing the God image vary between individuals. For example, the God image of someone who grows up privileged may be less culturally influenced than that of someone who grew up struggling with discrimination. Similarly, a person diagnosed with a chronic illness at an early age may have a God image influenced more by health issues than someone who grows up with good physical health.

What Are the Factors?

This section proposes some of the factors which influence an individual's experience of God. This list is not exhaustive and will need refinement following new theoretical and research developments. The intent of this exploration is to provide a starting point to facilitate the expansion of theory and research. The factors include: (1) caregiver relationships, (2) other significant relationships, (3) church experience, (4) world experiences (e.g., general experience of the world as a safe or unsafe place), (5) gender, (6) sexual orientation, (7) cultural experience, (8) God concept/beliefs, (9) wish fulfillment/compensation, (10) personality factors, (11) psychological health, (12) ability/disability, (13) self-image/self-esteem, and (14) developmental factors (including religious/spiritual/faith development and psychological development). Additional factors which may need further consideration include biological factors and direct relational factors with God.

Many of these factors are interrelated and influence each other. For example, the world experience and cultural experience may be highly related for some individuals. A person who grows up consistently having people stare at them or treat them differently because of their skin color or sexual preference often experience the world differently from someone who does not have this experience.

The degree to which these factors influence the God image varies. For some, parental influences may be the primary factor. For others, culture may be more important. Clinicians who assume that God image is solely determined by parental influences may encounter difficulties by searching for problems in parental relationships with individuals who have a negative experience of God when it does not exist. Conversely, clinicians may assume that individuals have a negative God image if they had conflicted relationships with their parents. If the client does not present in a manner consistent with this premise, clinicians may assume that the client is denying, repressing, or suppressing their *true* experience of God. Clinicians would better serve their clients by remaining open to discovering how the God image develops and changes in these individuals over time.

TYPES OF DIVERSITY

Two categories of diversity will be discussed. First, religious and spiritual diversity need to be addressed. Various theoretical and research perspectives suggest that the experience of God may be partially independent of religious belief (Hall & Brokaw, 1995; Hoffman, 2005; Hoffman, Hoffman et al., 2005; Sorenson, 2004; Tisdale et al., 1997). In other words, some factors influence the experience of God regardless of religious affiliation. Freud (1913/1950, 1927/1961) agreed with this perspective purporting that the experience of God is created through projection and wish fulfillment.

The majority of God image theory and research assumes the Judeo-Christian worldview. Although there are similarities across the theistic traditions, there are also important differences. Even if the differences in beliefs are small, they are important and may impact the broader experience of God.

Examining differences within the broad religious traditions also warrants consideration. As stated, Christianity has received the most of the attention so far. Some research studies have considered how denominational affiliation impacts psychological health; however, no significant differences have been found in the current research (Koenig, McCullough, & Larson, 2001). The reason for this is likely multifaceted. First, in contemporary Christian culture, there is often more variance in theological beliefs within a particular denomination while there is increasing similarity between denominations. Additionally, many people are not familiar with the specific beliefs of their church and may not join a church or denomination based upon similarity of belief. If different beliefs do influence how a person experiences God, denominational differences may not be a good test of this hypothesis. Furthermore, if these differences are small, as hypothesized herein, it would require a very large sample for these variations to emerge at significant levels.

The second category includes various other factors identified as diversity issues including race, culture, ethnicity, gender, socioeconomic status, ability/disability, and sexual orientation. Thus far, the only factors examined empirically at any depth are gender, race, and ethnicity (Foster & Babcock, 2001; Hoffman, Hoffman et al., 2005; Krejci, 1989; Nelson, Cheek, & Au, 1985; Roberts, 1989). In the initial study conducted by Hoffman, Hoffman et al., (2005) significant differences emerged between people of color and people who identified themselves as Caucasian. Although this study was limited by the sample size, the preliminary results suggest that additional differences are likely to surface in a larger, more diverse sample.

Consideration of diversity's impact on the experience of God commonly finds expression in contemporary theology, but rarely receives mention in the God image literature. Slave theology (Hopkins, 1996, 2001), black theology (Noel, 1996), feminist perspectives (Daly, 1993; Grey, 2001), womanist viewpoints (Baker-Fletcher, 1996) and sexual orientation (Graham, 1997) have been explored in the theological literature. Most of this writing emerged from liberal or progressive approaches to Christian theology. From a psychological viewpoint, this investigation should be expanded into other Judeo-Christian traditions as well as other religious and spiritual traditions.

Pathways from Diversity to the God Image

Additional issues are important to address in order to promote a better understanding of how diversity impacts the experience of God. Factors which influence the God image, such as diversity and development, emerge through both direct and indirect means. The dynamic nature of these interrelationships is highly complex. A simple linear model will not suffice.

Whether the experience of God develops through a correspondence (correlation model) or compensational process is a fundamental debate. This issue has received much attention in the attachment and spirituality literature (Hall et al., 2005; Kirkpatrick, 1997, 1998, 2004; Kirkpatrick & Shaver, 1990).[1] Unfortunately, few of these findings have been applied to the God image specifically. Contributions of Hall and colleagues (Halcrow, Hall, Hill, & Delaney, 2004; Hall & Porter, 2004; Hall et al., 2005) addresses this issue. In general, the correlation model assumes that the God image develops parallel to the child's experience of their primary caregiver or caregivers. Conversely, the compensation model purports that the individual uses God as an *ideal attachment figure* to compensate for what was lacking in their early caregiver relationships. The former model is based on a transference process while the latter is based upon a projection and wish fulfillment process.

The current literature reflects the implicit belief that one or the other model is correct. The God image literature generally endorses the correspondence model while much of the attachment research supports the compensation model. Both models contain partial truths. The compensation model may be a better fit with some individuals while the correlation model may apply with others. This indicates that confounding factors may have influenced previous research findings. A multi-causal conceptualization would shift the focus of research by requiring researchers to first identify which model better fits a particular individual. Quantitative research, particularly when based on objective measures with implicit theoretical assumptions, is limited in its ability to discover these differences. Future research may need to give more attention to qualitative approaches.

For most individuals, parents are the primary attachment figure forming the basis of the child's relational experience during the formative years. However, some individuals are exposed to other competing emotional or relational processes which impact their God image. For example, individuals exposed to traumatic events may have their God image more determined by the trauma than their relationship with their parents. Similar effects occur when growing up experiencing discrimination, racism, sexism, or consistently feeling different than others, such as Lesbian, Gay, Bisexual, and Transgender (LGBT) individuals. In other words, diverse populations who are exposed to prejudice and discrimination are more likely to have other formative experiences impacting their God image.

In addition to the more direct influences discussed above, there are also indirect cultural influences to be considered. Cultural differences in child rearing practices, family relationships, and spiritual experience also influence the God image. Particular cultural groups, women, and LGBT individuals are more likely to be discriminated against which changes their experience of the world. Due to the many interrelated factors which influence individual's experience of God, it will be difficult for research, particularly quantitative research, to sort out the complexities involved in this formative process.

APPLICATION WITH SPECIFIC GROUPS[2]

LGBT God Images[3]

Before addressing the development of the God Concept and God Image with LGBT clients, a brief discussion on the relationship between homosexuality and religion is necessary. The majority of the theistic world religions maintain that homosexuality is sinful. Hendershot (2001) indicates that many religious organizations, especially those which are fundamentalist, have become actively involved in presenting to parishioners and to the public that homosexuality is sinful. In addition, some religious organizations have gone as far as lobbying the government to ban same-sex relationships. Melton (1991) found that 72% of religious organizations and churches surveyed condemned homosexuals and homosexuality as being an abomination in the eyes of God; however, this is beginning to change. Studies by Ellison and another by Mafferty (cited in Rodriguez & Ouellette, 2000) found that a few Christian denominations and denominational groups, such as the United Church of Christ, Integrity in the Episcopal Church, Dignity in the Roman Catholic Church, and Lutheran's Concerned were affirming of LGBT individuals.

Religious perspectives on homosexuality can be placed into three broad categories (Hoffman et al., 2006). The first group maintains that being homosexual is sinful. Generally, this group purports that homosexuality is a choice and reflects a sinful pattern in one's life. Within this group, there are varying opinions about whether this is a conscious choice, when the choice occurred, and how easy it is to make a different choice. Typically, this group, which is intolerant of homosexuality in any form, believes that homosexuality can be changed.

A second group, which represents the middle position, believes homosexual behaviors are sinful, but that LGBT individuals are not bad people (Hoffman et al., 2006). People in this group are likely to align themselves with the statement "love this sinner, hate the sin." Although they express a more tolerant attitude toward LGBT individuals, they believe engaging in sexual intimacy with individuals of the same sex is sinful. It is believed to be a viable option to remain a homosexual and lead a life of celibacy. Individuals in this second group may or may not see homosexuality as a choice and may or may not believe it can be changed.

The third group maintains that homosexuality, including engaging in same-sex intimacy, is not sinful (Hoffman et al., 2006). In general, sexual acts are viewed as not sinful if expressed in the confines of a committed relationship with a partner. This group tends to believe that homosexuality is not a choice and cannot be changed. This is often referred to as an affirming or welcoming perspective.

The idea of God in itself is very troubling for many LGBT individuals. They experience rejection and judgment from many in the church while being told about God's love and grace. This paradoxical message provides an important experiential basis for their God image, which becomes more powerful than their early experiences with parents. Perhaps more than any other example, the experience of LGBT individuals reveals the oversimplification of previous theories which have not taken into account other relational influences in additional to parental relationships. Although it is common for many people in the LGBT community to leave organized religion, many continue to wrestle with profoundly painful spiritual issues (Bouldrey, 1995; Graham, 1997). Rejection by one of the primary support systems in their spiritual lives creates ambivalent feelings which may result in years of emotional turbulence for many LGBT individuals. Many others leave behind any belief in a transcendent other (i.e., God) altogether.

Early parental relationships provide a rudimentary basis for an experience of God with LGBT individuals; however, this basis often becomes overpowered by painful experiences with the church. Graham (1997) points out that there are generally two alternatives provided by the church for LGBT individuals. First, they can attempt to convert to a heterosexual orientation. Second, they can lead a life of celibacy. Neither of these solutions provides comfort or an answer as to why LGBT individuals must maintain a war with their natural longings. Although Christianity frequently maintains a position stating that all humans are at war with their nature, heterosexual individuals have acceptable outlets for their sexual longings. This is not offered to LGBT individuals.

Psychology has long criticized religion, in particular Christianity, for its approach to sexuality. Freud's critique of the Victorian era was that repression of sexuality was unsuccessful. Psychoanalysis purports that when a basic desire or aspect of our existential nature is repressed it will find an outlet through other means (i.e., the desire or drive will find an expression elsewhere). Generally, this is through more destructive means of which the person is often unaware or which they feel they cannot control. Existence cannot be contained through repression or denial (Becker, 1973).

The sexual revolution freed people to experience their sexuality more completely, even within the confines of a marriage relationship. This has greatly diminished many problems of sexuality.[4] This freedom is only granted to heterosexuals in Christian communities. LGBT individuals are expected to repress and deny this basic aspect of their personhood. Psychoanalytic theory helps to explain the various potential implications of this repression. Although some may be able to successfully live a life of celibacy without complications, this is not the norm. LGBT individuals have no more success containing their sexuality through celibacy than heterosexual persons. This suggests that individuals' sexual impulses will find expression through other means, which may lead to anxiety, guilt, depression, sexual promiscuity, and sexual dysfunction.

The meaning and purpose of sex has been constructed and reconstructed throughout history. In an evolutionary perspective, sex originally was for the purpose of reproduction and survival of the species. However, somewhere along the way sex became intimately connected with other aspects of relationships and intimacy. This process has been paralleled in the church's understanding. At times during the history of Christianity, sex was considered to be solely for reproductive purposes, and some churches, such as the Catholic Church, still maintain this position to a degree. Gradually, the church has placed sex in the context of a broader relational understanding. For married couples, sex is often understood to be, and maybe even expected to be, part of a healthy intimate relationship. A healthy sex life increases the depth of intimacy and the overall health of the relationship. Furthermore, research suggests involvement in long-term committed relationships enhances mental health (Kurdek, 1986).

As the cultural understanding of sexual nature has changed, so has the meaning and purpose of sex. Although many competing views of sexuality emerged in today's society, some consistencies surfaced in Christianity's view of sexuality. Within this context, there is a difference between how sex is talked about amongst the typical Christians and amongst the Christian leadership or purveyors of values.[5] The meaning of sex has evolved to be a natural part of a healthy, intimate relationship beyond procreation. Furthermore, there remains a cultural value that being in a committed, monogamous, sexual relationship is normal, healthy, and beneficial. Yet many in the LGBT community are not given the same access to these benefits. Even within many churches which purport to be affirming, many LGBT individuals do not feel that they have the same privileges as heterosexual congregants. They often experience that their sexual orientation is tolerated, not embraced. They may be told their behavior is okay as long as they don't "flaunt it." Their experience remains that there is something wrong with them or that they have to hide aspects of themselves. In other words, heterosexual individuals can embrace their wholeness, while this is not supported for LGBT individuals.

An additional consideration in the treatment of LGBT individuals is the importance placed upon their sexual being. The heterosexual community often defines the homosexual person in terms of their sexual orientation. In other words, sex is seen to be more central to their identity than it is for most heterosexuals. For many LGBT individuals, this then becomes internalized and they experience themselves primarily as sexual beings. When their sexual identity is also internalized as something fundamentally flawed, they may experience an alienation from their relationships and God.

Recent trends in psychoanalysis have de-emphasized, though not discounted, early life influences while accentuating later life influences (Mitchell, 1988; Stark, 2000). This can be extended to God image theory. Although parents may form the initial God image, later in life authority figures provide the basis for ongoing God image development. Cultural analysis suggests that culture, politics, and power issues also need to be included in these later life influences. Other factors include churches, popular religion, government, and other political organizations. In considering these factors, it now becomes likely that influences on the God image would become more diffuse. Although these other external factors may not significantly influence the God image of individuals who are not subjected to prejudice and discrimination, they are more likely to impact the God image of LGBT individuals.

As God image influences become more diffuse for LGBT individuals, they become more problematic. Despite strides in the realm of political rights, there still remain disproportionate privileges. Despite increasing openness within the general public and the church, there remains a common lack of acceptance of homosexuality. It remains a common message to LGBT individuals that there is something fundamentally wrong with them. Similarly, the common phrase, "Love the sinner, hate the sin," reinforces the message that something which is natural in others is wrong in them.

It can be maintained that throughout history the message of original sin stated there is something fundamentally wrong with all human beings. This claim, however, is a universal. When LGBT individuals are told there is something wrong with them they are told this in the context of saying that what is wrong with them is acceptable for non-homosexuals.

The process of accepting one's sexual identity is a challenging and painful process, especially for individuals coming from a religious background. Many LGBT individuals fear losing both their family and religious support systems through the coming out process. This apprehension often creates barriers to achieving a healthy sexual identity.

Spiritual and sexual identity development frequently intersects creating intense fear and anxiety. Hoffman et al. (2006) maintain that the early stages of spiritual development in which beliefs are often rigid and based upon external authority can lead to identity foreclosure as a heterosexual. This causes the individual to repress their sexual identity which prevents the development of an authentic self. Similarly, acceptance of oneself as LGBT may cause religious individuals to reject or question their faith which states that their sexual identity is sinful or wrong. Stated differently, these two developmental lines can not be fully understood apart from each other.

In summary, the God Image for the LGBT community will frequently be based primarily upon broader experiences, as opposed to primarily parental influences. This does not discount the influence of parents, but places them secondary to other life experiences. There continues to be a strong need for the development of resources to assist LGBT individuals in reconciling and integrating their spirituality with their authentic self.

Female God Images

Three fundamental influences on the God Image in women are addressed in this section. First, historically God has been talked about in primarily masculine terms. Although some argue that both males and females are created in God's image, most descriptors tend to suggest that men are made more so in God's image than women. Second, many religious texts, including the Christian scriptures, often rely on masculine terminology and have been interpreted as placing women as second class citizens within the religious community. Third, returning to the topic of sexuality, women have often been taught that this very natural part of the female experience is not natural to them, but is to men. In this regard, some comparisons can be drawn between the experience of women and the experience of LGBT individuals. There are many other aspects of the female experience which influence the God image; however, this section will focus on these three realms.

God has not always been perceived in masculine terms as has often been assumed within many traditional religious groups. Stone (1978) offers historical and archeological evidence that God has also be conceived of as female. However, this has often been discounted or written out of history through the development of the patriarchal religions dominating Western culture. This has been extended into language which often exclusively, or nearly exclusively, relies of masculine terminology.

In recognizing the impact of male descriptors of God on women's God images, language should be recognized as having an experiential component. Although it appears rational to state that the masculine descriptors such as "he," "him," and "man" refer to both men and women, it is not experienced as inclusive by many women. Most academic writing now requires the uses of gender inclusive language; however, religion continues to rely on language referring to God as solely being male.

Enns (1997), in her introduction to feminist theory and psychotherapy, discusses this in the context of psychological diagnosis. The Diagnostic and Statistical Manual of Mental Disorder, Fourth Edition (DSM-IV; American Psychiatric Association, 2002) is argued to have a gender bias. A noteworthy example is the bias toward seeing independence as healthy and dependence or interdependence as pathological. The bias in psychology toward a more masculine, logical, and independent approach as healthy and moral also has been addressed in Gilligan's (1993) classic text *In a Different Voice*. In stating the male cognitive approach is logical, it appears to suggest the more common feminine approach of relational knowledge is illogical or irrational. This gender bias also can be illustrated in writing style. As feminist writers have maintained, an embodied, subjective writing style reflects a more authentic expression of the feminine way of being. The objective, third-person approach is more demonstrative of the masculine approach to knowing and communicating. The maintenance of this objective, third-person style of writing as the only appropriate scholarly writing reflects an inherent gender bias.

Understanding the feminine as that which is not masculine has been a common approach to understanding gender differences in Western culture. Within this context, that which is masculine is generally perceived as what is good. This is even supported by psychological research. In examining masculine and feminine self-concepts in regards to the ideal self, both men and women desired to be more masculine than they perceived themselves to be (Best & Williams, 2001).

If the feminine is implicitly determined, in part, by what is not masculine, and God is identified as masculine, then the feminine is separated from God. This is a common experience of God for women. The difficulties in this line of thinking have often been overshadowed by parallels in the broader female experience. It has been implied in Western culture that women derive their value through men as the more powerful other. If this is true, then it would not seem so unnatural for women to also receive value through the Other that is God; however, the psychological consequences remain damaging to women. Although men are able to derive their value through being made in God's image and through how they are similar to God, women are placed in the position of deriving their value through being different, the other, and dependent.

Theologically, this does not sound so troubling from many traditional Judeo-Christian approaches which assume a patriarchal hierarchy. Psychologically, however, problems emerge. The difference in relationships between husband and wife can be rationalized as complementary. However, when God is the other, what does the woman have to offer to complement God? This creates a relational bond based upon a person's lack of inherent value. The experiential component of this process can lead to a God image which is built upon fear, distance, and insecurity.

A second factor is the place of women in religion and the church within the context of history and culture. Horney (1967), in the first book of psychology devoted to the feminine perspective, typifies the process in which women, through various means, are viewed to be less significant than men. She argues that women are often placed in the role of something to be feared by men. Examples of this fear can be seen throughout religious history. Eve was the temptress who led Adam astray into a life of sin. Mary Magdalene was portrayed as a prostitute. This cycle was repeated by the casting of women in the role of sexual temptresses who led men astray into a life of sin. Christianity frequently constructed views of women in which they were associated with sin, evil, and temptation. The masculine was constructed as the good and moral leadership that needed to stay pure in spite of the influences of the female. Although these statements typify a mode of thinking rarely explicitly expressed today, the remnants of this viewpoint remain in many of the cultural practices of Judeo-Christian religion.

Many more examples, including the prohibition against female priests, women being excluded from religious readings during many religious services, and females being seated separately in some Synagogues, Mosques, and Churches, exemplify the differences in treatment, freedoms, and characterizations of men and women in the church. The changes in religious practice that have brought greater liberty for women do not abolish the historical or current impact of these issues on women who often continue to experience the church as a place for men first and women second.

Experientially, these occurrences reinforce a God image in which females perceive God as loving and caring, but also experience the self as negative or inferior. Although this may emphasize grace, it does so at the cost of self-worth. As discussed earlier, theologically this is consistent with many approaches to theology which emphasize God's grace and humanity's sin or fallen state. What remains problematic is that women remain aware that the same is not true for men who are able to value most or all aspects of themselves. The God image then is based on a discriminatory process similar to their experience of being discriminated against in the world.

Sexuality, our final point of discussion, has been doubly abusive for women. As discussed previously, historically, women's sexuality was associated with being a temptress leading men into sin. In this sense, women were sexual beings, but their sexuality was associated with sin. Furthering this process, men frequently projected their sexual desires, which were unacceptable from a religious viewpoint, onto women. In this way, men were able to disown their anxiety about their sexuality while women were vilified in a male defense.

In contemporary times, women's sexuality has been disembodied. This can be seen as either a continuation of the process discussed above or as a new direction in female sexuality. A pure woman is expected to be nonsexual. A commonplace example of this is differing standards on male and female promiscuity. Men's sexuality is seen as natural, healthy, and acceptable, even if it at times leading them astray. Conversely, women's sexuality is seen as unnatural, pathological, and unacceptable. Although men are encouraged to embrace their sexuality, at least in heterosexual society, women are encouraged to hide or suppress it.

A religious symbol of this can be seen in the Virgin Mary (Daly, 1973). For some Christians, the insistence of Mary's virginity throughout her life, even after the birth of Jesus, is seen as necessary in order to maintain her purity and sinlessness. This is illustrated in the ongoing reference to Jesus's mother as "the Virgin Mary" even in reference to her after Jesus's birth. For some women, this insistence on the virginity of Mary represents a need to deny the one's sexual nature.

Sexuality is part of the normal, healthy identity of both men and women; however, in many religious circles, only men have been allowed to embrace this. Although the blatant expressions of this double standard are not as common explicitly today, it still remains in the implicit and unconscious realms in much of the Judeo-Christian religions.

Women have been deprived of many of the privileges of men in religious culture. This social reality has psychological consequences for women's experience of God. Although religious groups have made many positive changes and recognized many of the detrimental consequences of the historical treatment of women, they have not done an adequate job of dealing with the psychological consequences of this history.

Black God Images[6]

A proliferation of writing on African American religious experience from theological, social, and anthropological perspectives provides fertile ground for integration of God image theory. Many analyses of slave theology and its importance for African American spirituality have been included. What has not been addressed as thoroughly is the psychological impact of slave theology in the lives of African Americans in contemporary times.

The unique aspects of slave theology and black religious tradition emphasized the role of God's divinity and issues of liberation (Hopkins, 1996, 2001; Noel, 1996). This theme in Black culture would appear to have positive implications for the God image. These must be balanced, however, with other cultural influences which are more suggestive of God as being that which is different.

The positive influences of portraying God as liberator expands the awareness of the role of religion and conceptions of God in the lives of the Black community (Hopkins, 1996, 2001; Noel, 1996). Pinn's (2001) discussion of the influences on Black theology brings an awareness of its complexity. In emphasizing the limitations of historical knowledge he asserts, "A clear and uncontaminated link between the past and present does not exists" (Pinn, 2001, p. 110). Yet we must not neglect the importance of history in the development of religious concepts and approaches. Pinn recognizes this: "Theology, at its best, is dependent upon cultural production as a means to understand the expression and substance of religious experience" (p. 106). An important addition to these recognitions for Black theology is the influence of White and Euro-American theologies. Pinn notes that much of Black theology, as with other liberation theologies, is reactive against external influences. In this development, God and religion is experienced as liberating. This is seen in many Black cultural expressions of religion that emphasize themes of liberation in the midst of suffering. Furthermore, the form or structure of religion tends to be display more freedom than most American or European expressions of religion which tend to be more stoic.

This historic role of God and religion in the liberation process for Blacks may explain why *religion* remains central for Black Christianity while many others in the United States tend to prefer *spirituality*. For example, Hoffman, Hoffman et al. (2005) found that individuals identifying as religious but not spiritual had a positive relationship to the individual's God image for White individuals, but not for people of color.

Although this study did not have a large enough sample to look specifically at African Americans distinct from people of color, it is likely that this finding would hold true with a larger sample allowing for a more discrete analysis. Stated succinctly, religion tends to be experienced differently within Black Christianity.

It would, however, be an oversimplification to describe the God image for Blacks as being solely based on this experience of God as liberator. Belton (1995), in his reflection on growing up as a black, gay man reveals another important aspect of the Black experience of God. His depictions describe how he was drawn to early images of Jesus which he saw as being erotic. As he was enticed by these images, he was also struck by how this Jesus of Middle Eastern decent was portrayed as white. This was true even in the Black homes and churches where he grew up. Belton discussed his struggle with this depiction of Jesus who was so different than he was. To him, it appeared that Jesus was a white man sent to a nonwhite culture to save them. God, here, is experienced even from within his own culture as being different from himself. Otherness, again, is the basis for salvation. This was even more stringently reinforced by the predominantly white culture which surrounded him. It is interesting to note that for Belton, growing up Black appears to have been more challenging to his experience of God than growing up as a gay man.

This situation taps into a common experience among all of the groups discussed in this chapter. As pointed out by Guthrie (2004) in his book *Even the Rat Was White*, there has been a white male standard that has emerged in Western psychology. This is also true in much of Western religion. The white, heterosexual male has been the standard by which all other groups are compared. Whatever is typical of a white male is seen as better. One disturbing example that Guthrie mentions pertains to the early finger tapping tests. Individuals from different cultures were tested for finger tapping quickness. It was demonstrated that other groups were often quicker than white males. The interpretation of this was that these other groups had quicker finger tapping ability because they were designed for manual labor. It seems that, regardless of the issue, Western society has been able to find a way to state the white male way is better no matter how perverse of an interpretation was necessary to accomplish this.

In applying this to the God image, white males are often afforded ways to relate directly to God that other groups are not. White males are able to relate to God more through their similarities to God, while other groups are placed in a position of relating to God based upon difference.

Although most theistic traditions base relationships with God on difference or being separate from God, white males are in the privileged position of being assumed closer or less different from God than other groups. This is not only an offensive process, but it also reduces God and creates a psychological consequence for many individuals from diverse backgrounds. The God image is one of many problems with this social reality.

The God image as discussed throughout this paper reflects the complexity of this psychological construct. Within the example of the Black experience of God, it can be seen that culture has brought competing emotional influences. Although the experience is often of God as liberator, this liberator is more like a white male than a Black male or female. These competing influences on the God image for the Black community creates a diversity of experiences of God, most of which are complex integrations of positive and negative experiences.

Similar to the experience of women and LGBT individuals, God's goodness or grace is based in that which is different from the self. Again, although many theologies highlight that this is true for all humanity, within the white male experience God is still portrayed as being more similar. Additionally, this is only one aspect of the God image. The portrayal and experience of God as liberator, and the power of Black spirituality, also contribute to a very rich, satisfying, and complex experience of God within Black culture.

FACTORS FOR FUTURE RESEARCH

The field of psychology is only beginning to examine the way people experience God. It is critical that future research take diversity issues into consideration. One primary limitation is methodological. Lawrence's (1997) God Image Scales provided a useful starting point, but the limitations of this measure are becoming increasingly clear (Hoffman, Grimes, Acoba, & Leung, 2005).[6] Additionally, future research must include both quantitative and qualitative methods. If, as is purported in this chapter, the factors influencing the God image vary in individuals, qualitative research will be needed to ascertain how these differences emerge. In general, more qualitative and mixed methodology research is needed to better direct future theory and quantitative research.

Future research must be intentionally inclusive of various ethnicities, cultures, ages, physical abilities, religious affiliations, and sexual orientations. International studies should also be included. As God image studies become more inclusive of diversity factors, new questions are likely to emerge about the interaction between factors. Researchers and theorists need to remain open to exploring new hypotheses and perspectives on multifactorial relationships to avoid the limitations and errors of previous research.

The methodological innovations by Gibson demonstrated in chapter 12 along with the growing acceptance of qualitative studies provide important new opportunities in understanding how people experience God. Yet, all of this is just a beginning. If the psychological and religious communities are to grow in their understanding of how people experience God, it will be essential to remain open to new perspectives and interpretations.

NOTES

1. See also chapter 3

2. This portion of the paper was adapted from a portion of two earlier paper, "The God Concept and God Image as Cultural Constructs" presented at the 2004 Society for of the Scientific Study of Religion and "Religious Experience, Gender, and Sexual Orientation." Complete reference information is available in the reference section.

3. In this chapter, we consider Lesbian, Gay, Bisexual, and Transgender (LGBT) experience together; however, it is important to note that there are significant differences for each of these experiences. This is another form of diversity which should be considered in future theory and research.

4. This is not to state that we now live in a society which is primarily healthy in regards to our sexuality. There continue to be many problems in regards to sexual repression, as is arguably evidenced by the recent scandals in the Catholic and Protestant Churches. Additionally, the sexual revolution has brought with it new realms of sexual problems. However, as a cultural phenomenon, sexual repression has become much less of a problem than in the Victorian era.

5. Tanner (1997) provides a discussion of changing views of culture across time. She contrasts "high culture" perspectives, from which culture is manufactured by the elites, to a "low culture," where culture is understood as coming from the people. It could be maintained that in church, at least in regards to some issues, there remains a "high culture" production of norms and values. However, even if the values are established by the church hierarchy and leadership, these values are interpreted and played out differently by members of the church. Thus, the meaning of the values is changed.

6. In this chapter, we are focusing on black God images in the United States primarily.

7. See also Chapter 12.

REFERENCES

American Psychological Association. (2002). *Diagnosis and statistical manual of mental disorders* (Text Revision.). Washington, D.C.: Author. Baker-Fletcher, K. (1996). *Sisters of dust, sisters of spirit: Womanist wordings on God and creation.* Minneapolis, MN: Fortress Press.

Becker, E. (1973). *The denial of death.* New York: The Free Press.

Belton, D. (1995). My father's house. In B. Bouldrey (Ed.), *Wrestling with the angel: Faith and religion in the lives of gay men* (pp. 11-20). New York: Riverhead Books.

Best, D. L. & Williams, J. E. (2001). Gender and culture. In D. Matsumoto (Ed.), *The handbook of culture and psychology* (pp. 195-219). New York: Oxford University Press.

Bouldrey, B. (1995). Editors introduction. In B. Bouldrey (Ed.), *Wrestling with the angel: Faith and religion in the lives of gay men* (pp. ix-xiii). New York: Riverhead Books.

Brokaw, B. F. & Edwards, K. J. (1994). The relationship of God image to the level of object relations development. *Journal of Psychology and Theology, 22,* 352-371.

Daly, M. (1993). *Beyond God the father.* Boston, MA: Beacon.

Enns, C. Z. (1997). *Feminist theories and feminist psychotherapies: Origins, themes, and variations.* New York: Harrington Park Press.

Feuerbach, L. (1989). *The essence of Christianity* (G. Eliot, Trans.). Amherst, NY: Prometheus. (Original work published in 1841)

Foster, R. A. & Babcock, R. L. (2001). God as man versus God as woman: Perceiving God as a function of the gender of God and the gender of the participant. *The International Journal for the Psychology of Religion, 11(2),* 93-104.

Freud, S. (1950). *Totem and taboo* (J. Stratchey, Trans.). New York: Norton & Company. (Original work published in 1913)

Freud, S. (1961). The future of an illusion (J. Stratchey, Trans.). New York: Norton & Company. (Original work published in 1927)

Gibson, N. J. S. (2004, October). *Overcoming methodological boundaries the experimental investigation of religious cognition.* Paper presented at the joint meeting of the Society for the Scientific Study of Religion and Religious Research Association, Kansas City, MO.

Gilligan, C. (1993). *In a different voice: Psychological theory and women's development.* Cambridge, MA: Harvard University Press.

Graham, L. K. (1997) *Discovering images of God: Narratives of care among lesbians and gays.* Louisville, KY: John Knox Press.

Grey, M. (2001). *Introducing feminist images of God.* Cleveland, OH: Pilgrim Press.

Guthrie, R. B. (2004). *Even the rat was white: A historical view of psychology* (2nd ed.). Boston, MA: Pearson.

Halcrow, S., Hall, T. W., Hill, P. C., & Delaney, H. (2004, July) *A multidimensional approach to the correspondent and compensatory attachment to God.* Paper presented at the annual convention of the American Psychological Association, Honolulu, HI.

Hall, T. W. & Brokaw, B. F. (1995). The relationship of spiritual maturity to level of object relations development and God image. *Pastoral Psychology, 43,* 373-391.

Hall, T. W., Halcrow, S., Hill, P., Delaney, H., & Teal, J. (2005, April). *Attachment and spirituality.* Paper presented at the Christian Association for Psychological Studies International Conference, Dallas, TX.

Hall, T. W. & Porter, S. L. (2004). Referential Integration: An emotional informaiton processing perspective on the Process of Integration. *Journal of Psychology and Theology, 32,* 167-180.

Hendershot, H. (2001). Holiness codes and holy homosexuals: Interpreting gay and lesbian Christian subculture. *Camera Obscurra, 45,* 15-18.

Hoffman, L. (2004, October). *Cultural constructs of the God image and God concept: Implications for culture, psychotherapy, and religion.* Paper presented at the Joint Annual Meeting of the Society for the Scientific Study of Religion and the Religious Research Association, Kansas City, MO.

Hoffman, L. (2005). A development perspective on the God image. In R. H. Cox, B. Ervin-Cox, & L. Hoffman (Eds.). *Spirituality and psychological health* (pp. 129-147). Colorado Springs, CO: Colorado School of Professional Psychology Press.

Hoffman, L., Grimes, C. S. M., & Acoba, R. (2005, November). *Research on the experience of God: Rethinking epistemological assumptions.* Paper presented at the Society for the Scientific Study of Religion Annual Meeting, Rochester, NY.

Hoffman, L, Grimes, C. S. M., & Mitchell, M. (2004, July). *Transcendence, suffering, and psychotherapy.* Paper presented at the Bi-annual Conference of the International Network for Personal Meaning, Vancouver, British Columbia, Canada.

Hoffman, L., Hoffman, J. L., Dillard, K., Clark, J., Acoba, R., Williams, F., & Jones, T. T. (2005, April). *Cultural diversity and the God image: Examining cultural differences in the image of God.* Paper presented at the Christian Associationfor Psychological Studies International Conference, Dallas, TX.

Hoffman, L., Jones, T. T., Williams, F., & Dillard, K. (2004, March). *The God image, the God concept, and attachment.* Paper presented at the Christian Association for Psychological Studies International Conference, St. Petersburg, FL.

Hoffman, L., Knight, S. K., Boscoe-Huffman, S. & Stewart, S. (2006, August). *Religious experience, gender, and sexual orientation.* Paper presented at the American Psychological Association Annual Convention, New Orleans, LA.

Hopkins, D. N. (1996). Theological method and cultural studies: Slave religious culture as a heuristic. In D. N. Hopkins & S. G. Davaney (Eds.), *Changing conversations: Religious reflection and cultural analysis* (pp.161-180). New York: Routledge.

Hopkins, D. N. (2001). Self (co)constitution: Slave theology from everyday cultural elements. In D. Brown, S. G. Davaney, & K. Tanner (Eds.), *Converging on culture: Theologians in dialogue with cultural analysis and criticism* (pp. 89-105. New York: Oxford University Press.

Horney, K. (1967). *Feminine psychology.* New York: W. W. Norton & Company.

James, W. (1997). Varieties of religious experience. New York: Touchstone. (Original work published 1902)

Kirkpatrick, L. A. (1997). A longitudinal study of changes in religious beliefs and behavior as a function of individual differences in adult attachment style. *Journal for the Scientific Study of Religion, 36,* 207-217.

Kirkpatrick, L. A. (1998). God as a substitute attachment figure: A longitudinal study of adult attachment style and religious change in college students. *Personality and Social Psychology Bulletin, 24,* 961-973.

Kirkpatrick, L. A. (2004). *Attachment, evolution, and the psychology of religion*. New York: Guilford Press.

Kirkpatrick, L. A. & Shaver, P. R. (1990). Attachment theory and religion: Childhood attachments, religious beliefs, and conversion. *Journal for the Scientific Study of Religion, 29*, 315-334.

Koenig, H. G., McCullough, & Larson, D. B. (2001). *Handbook of religion and health*. New York: Oxford University Press.

Krejci, M. J. (1998). Gender comparison of God schemas: A multidimensional scaling analysis. *The International Journal for the Psychology of Religion, 8(1)*, 57-66.

Kurdek, L.A. & Schmitt, J.P. (1986). Relationship quality of partners in heterosexual married, heterosexual cohabiting, and gay and lesbian relationships. *Journal of Personality and Social Psychology, 51(4)*, 711-720.

Lawrence, R. T. (1997). Measuring the image of God: The God image inventory and the God image scales. *Journal of Psychology and Theology, 25*, 214-226.

Melton, J. G. (1991). *The churches speak on homosexuality*. Detroit, MI: Gale Research.

Moriarty, G., Hoffman, L., Grimes, C. S. M., & Gattis, J. (2005, April). *God and attachment: Using integration techniques to working models*. Paper presented at the Christian Association for Psychological Studies International Conference, Dallas, TX.

Nelsen, H. M., Cheek, N. H., Jr., & Au, P. (1985). Gender differences in images of God. *Journal for the Scientific Study of Religion, 24(4)*, 396-402.

Nietzsche, F. (1954). *Thus spoke Zarathustra: A book for none and all* (W. Kaufmann, Trans.). New York: Penguin. (Original work published in 1892)

Noel, J. A. (1996). The post-modern location of black religion: Texts and temporalities in tension. In D. N. Hopkins & S. G. Davaney (Eds.), *Changing conversations: Religious reflection and cultural analysis* (pp.79-99). New York: Routledge.

Pinn, A. B. (2001). In the raw: African American cultural memory and theological reflection. In D. Brow, S. G. Davaney, & K. Tanner (Eds.), *Converging on culture: Theologians in dialogue with cultural analysis and criticism*. New York: Oxford University Press.

Rizzuto, A. M. (1979). *The birth of the living God: A psychoanalytic study*. Chicago: University of Chicago Press.

Roberts, C. W. (1989). Imagining god: Who is created in whose image? *Review of Religious Research, 30(4)*, 375-387.

Rodriguez, E., & Ouellette, S. (2000). Gay and lesbian Christians: Homosexual and religious identity integration in the members and participants of a gay-positive church. *Journal for the Scientific Study of Religion, 39(3)*, 333-347.

Sorenson, R. L. (2004). *Minding spirituality*. Hillsdale, NJ: Analytic Press.

Stone, M. (1978). *When God was a woman*. New York: Barnes and Noble.

Tanner, K. (1997). *Theories of culture*. Minneapolis, MN: Fortress Press.

Tillich, P. (1951). *Systematic theology* (Vol. 1). Chicago: University of Chicago Press.

Tisdale, T. C., Key, T. L., Edwards, K. J., Brokaw, B. F., Kemperman, S. R., & Cloud, H (1997). Impact of God image and personal adjustment, and correlations of the God image to personal adjustment and object relations development. *Journal of Psychology and Theology, 5*, 227-239.

doi:10.1300/J515v09n03_13

EPILOGUE

Postscript

This volume marks the appearance of an exciting contribution to the field of Psychology of Religion, specifically God image research, and its implications for psychotherapy. Psychology of Religion is truly a 20th Century product with William James' *Varieties of Religious Experience* (1902) the seminal and founding work, which was followed by periods of rich and fertile contributions, but also extended periods of stagnation. This complex history is captured well in David M. Wulff, *Psychology of Religion: Classic and Contemporary*, 1997, a must for any serious student of the field.

In 1979, however, the publication of Ana-Maria Rizzuto, *The Birth of the Living God*, gave fresh new impetus to the field which is even now inspiring further reflection and inquiry. This volume stands in that tradition, even if the methodologies have shifted away from Psychoanalytic and Object-Relational frameworks toward a much wider range of Psychological methodologies and therapies. This broadening is valuable and necessary, since Psychology as a broad field is seeking to engage Spirituality very directly, as well as the deeper layers of human subjectivity. The Psychoanalytic tradition does, however, need to be revisited in this regard, especially since contemporary models of Psychoanalytic thought through constructs such as Intersubjectivity Theory and Relational Psychoanalysis, for example, have taken significant steps beyond Rizzuto's work. This Psychoanalytic contribution is miss-

[Haworth co-indexing entry note]: "Postscript." Schmidt, Willilam S. Co-published simultaneously in *Journal of Spirituality in Mental Health* (The Haworth Pastoral Press, an imprint of The Haworth Press) Vol. 9, No. 3/4, 2007, pp. 281-284; and: *God Image Handbook for Spiritual Counseling and Psychotherapy: Research, Theory, and Practice* (ed: Glendon L. Moriarty, and Louis Hoffman) The Haworth Pastoral Press, an imprint of The Haworth Press, 2007, pp. 281-284. Single or multiple copies of this article are available for a fee from The Haworth Document Delivery Service [1-800-HAWORTH, 9:00 a.m. - 5:00 p.m. (EST). E-mail address: docdelivery@haworthpress.com].

Available online at http://jsmh.haworthpress.com
doi:10.1300/J515v09n03_14

ing from this volume as Dr. Rizzuto notes in her Foreword, but it will hopefully be included in subsequent articles.

The value of this volume is clear, however, first of all in its helpful historical overview of current research, but also as it moves in clinical directions. The heart of the book is this application section which covers seven specific clinical and therapeutic approaches to working with God image material in therapy. Any practitioner can relate to one or more of these modalities, and to have pathways for engaging God image material from within these approaches is invaluable. The volume ends with methodological reflections, along with issues of diversity as places of further stretching of our conceptual boundaries.

The volume raises numerous theoretical and not just clinical questions. Among these is perhaps the classic question for the field of Psychology of Religious Experience, namely, the nature of representability of imaginal life itself. More directly, is the God-experience always mediated (via standard structures of consciousness or experience), or is it ever unmediated, i.e., direct and "unfiltered" so to speak? In other words, is the God image a representation only, and can it ever bypass standard emotional or relational pathways? If our mind/brain filters and processes here and now experience through prior established perceptual/conceptual pathways, how "pure" or uncontaminated can any so-called "new" experience really be?

This question becomes vital as one contemplates the evolution of God image representations over the course of a spiritual life-time, and as one considers accompanying others in searching out the meaning of their God images. As several of our authors note, a parentally-determined God image often forms the predominant characteristics of one's God representations, and spiritual maturation requires that these inherited and internalized images be sorted out from all subsequent sources.

All mental and emotional processes including religious and spiritual, utilize images and operate in channels that allow for recognizeability and familiarity even as they may reveal something new. Hence, religious and spiritual discourse generally relies on modes such as symbol, metaphor, analogy, ritual, and narrative, etc., to communicate its "truth." These of necessity reach back into experiences that approximate the current manifestation or experience. So, when we say God is experienced as Love, we must of necessity draw upon all prior patterns of loving known to us. But for many these modes of having known love do not form a sufficient explanation for the loving pattern they come to know as God.

For some spiritual sojourners, the experience of God-love is not simply akin to loving another love-object, but is more like becoming one with love-itself. This seems to move us beyond representational object patterns toward "being" patterns, in this instance a oneness with Being known as love. If God is not simply one object alongside other objects then at some point image-ness recedes into being-ness. At some point analytic discourse reaches the limits of language and logic, and yet experiential realness is nevertheless claimed by practitioners of states of oneness, for example. Perhaps Psychology is no longer the lens which can penetrate into these mysteries, yet Psychology is certainly an indispensable resource for describing the interwovenness of all psychic life, including encompassing and value-laden states of consciousness.

A reader of this volume will have noticed an awkwardness for some authors about claims regarding the so-called "realness" of God. It is a limitation of much research in this field that no claims about God are intended or even allowed. At first glance this attempt to retain scientific purity seems noble and necessary. And yet, its limitation is that few researchers or practitioners then own their theological or spiritual assumptions. I am most pleased that this volume has been greatly strengthened by contributions from persons across a wide theological range from conservative to liberal, but what is at stake here within the field is the wider question of which experiential pathways are allowed for study and examination. While several authors noted the important difference between "God image" research and "God content," with the latter an inappropriate focus for a study such as this, it might move the field along more effectively if these assumptions were in fact articulated as part of the assumptive base that any researcher brings into encompassing questions of this sort.

The very question about the "realness" of God largely presumes the "otherness" of God as theistic or "God-as-object" which can be studied along the psychological pathways depicted in this volume. This is vital for sorting the archeological layers of the God image that persons utilize in their spiritual self-understandings. However, tracking the shifts this image undergoes over the course of a spiritual life-time requires an awareness of a broader sense of "Sacred" reality which one could perhaps call God-as-subject, i.e., more immanently available and operating at a deep subjective and interior levels, and hence intimately interwoven with the full dimensions of subjective life. This is where Psychology must engage the conversation partners of Philosophy, Theology, and Spirituality, so that these explorations can be framed within the grand panorama of spiritual experience across the wide sweep of Spiritual traditions across the ages.

A rich foundation has been laid by the contributors of this volume, and it is exciting to see Psychology re-engaging its deepest historical roots, but also being willing to venture into the wide sea of meaning-making, and comprehensive spiritual experience.

William S. Schmidt, PhD
Editor
Journal of Spirituality in Mental Health
Associate Professor
Institute of Pastoral Studies
Loyola University Chicago

Index